SAUNDERS MONOGRAPHS IN PHYSIOLOGY

Other Monographs in Physiology

Cohn: *Clinical Cardiovascular Physiology*

Granger, Barrowman, Kvietys: *Clinical Gastrointestinal Physiology*

CLINICAL ENDOCRINE PHYSIOLOGY

GEORGE A. HEDGE, Ph.D.
E.J. Van Liere Professor and Chairman, Department of Physiology,
West Virginia University Medical Center,
Morgantown, West Virginia

HOWARD D. COLBY, Ph.D.
Professor and Chairman, Department of Biomedical Sciences,
University of Illinois College of Medicine at Rockford,
Rockford, Illinois

ROBERT L. GOODMAN, Ph.D.
Associate Professor, Department of Physiology,
West Virginia University Medical Center,
Morgantown, West Virginia

A SAUNDERS MONOGRAPH IN PHYSIOLOGY

W. B. SAUNDERS COMPANY
Philadelphia/London/Toronto/ Sydney/Tokyo/Hong Kong

W.B. SAUNDERS COMPANY
A Division of
Harcourt Brace & Company

The Curtis Center
Independence Square West
Philadelphia, PA 19106

Library of Congress Cataloging-in-Publication Data

Hedge, George A.
    Clinical endocrine physiology.

    (A Saunders monograph in physiology)
    1. Endocrine glands.   I. Colby, Howard D.
II. Goodman, Robert L. (Robert Leonard)   III. Title.
IV. Series.   [DNLM: 1. Endocrine Glands—physiology.
2. Hormones—physiology.   WK 102 H453c]
QP187.H44   1987   612'.04   86-20317
ISBN 0-7216-1414-0

Listed here is the latest translated edition of this book together with the language of the translation and the publisher.

Portuguese—First Edition—Interlivros Edicoes Ltda. Rio de Janeiro, Brazil

Acquisition Editor: Marty Wonsiewicz

Production Manager: Frank Polizzano

Manuscript Editor: Edna Dick

Illustration Coordinator: Kenneth Green

Indexer: Sarah Wilkerson

Clinical Endocrine Physiology   ISBN   0-7216-1414-0

Last digit is the print number: 9   8   7   6

PREFACE

This textbook has been written to be used primarily by first-year medical students, but we believe that it will be of value to students in other biological and health related sciences as well. Part of the impetus for writing the book was the recognition that fewer and fewer departments of physiology are able to agree on a single comprehensive text to be used in their survey courses, many of which are taught by groups of instructors. Because of this team teaching, there is now a trend toward the use of individual monographs for the various sections of physiology courses. Moreover, curricula are being compressed such that students have less and less time to devote to each area. Thus, if a monograph is to be useful, it must be "digestible" over a period of only a few weeks. These factors have been prominent in our minds as we organized and wrote this text. While we have attempted to make the book both current and complete, we have also worked very diligently to make it "reader friendly." We have resisted the temptation to simply collect the individual efforts of three authors and bind them into a single cover. Instead, all three of us have read, discussed, and revised the entire text, including figures and tables. As a result, the book has the benefit of multiple author input combined with a homogeneity of style that we believe our readers will appreciate. This joint authorship developed very naturally from our combined efforts in teaching endocrinology to a variety of health science students over nearly a decade at the West Virginia University Health Science Center.

We have arranged the chapters of this book in a sequence that we have found to be optimal in our courses. To the extent possible, we have also presented the material within each chapter in a standardized sequence. There are some topics that are discussed to varying degrees in more than one chapter. This was done in an attempt to make each chapter reasonably self-contained and understandable independent of other chapters. As a result, the chapters beyond the first two need not be used in the order we have chosen to present them. Nearly all of the figures have been prepared specifically for this textbook; we have attempted to keep them simple, well-focused, and closely correlated with the text. There are several generic figures that are repeated throughout the text, and each time these appear, the new version contains an additional element or some shading to emphasize its specific message. The sections on clinical application do not represent an attempt to teach clinical endocrinology. Instead, they are used to provide examples of diagnostic or clinical principles that reinforce the basic principles of endocrine physiology. Each chapter ends with a list of references to further reading. This reading is not required for the understanding of the material presented, but it will provide a starting point for the student who is interested in information beyond the scope of this text.

The combined effort required for the production of this book is not restricted to the three authors. First, our families have contributed by tolerating considerable encroachment on the time that they so richly deserve from us. Also, we are very appreciative of the superb efforts of Miss Diane Kinney in preparing the manuscript and Ms. Marianne Peterson of the WVU Medical Center Photo/Illustration unit, who drew the figures. In spite of our best efforts, there will undoubtedly be errors in this book, and unfortunately, these will have to be discovered by our readers. We sincerely hope that no one will hesitate to inform us of these errors as they are recognized.

G. A. HEDGE

H. D. COLBY

R. L. GOODMAN

CONTENTS

4

5

PART III: ENDOCRINE SYSTEMS

6

7

8

REPRODUCTIVE FUNCTION IN THE MALE

9

FEMALE REPRODUCTION 189

10

PREGNANCY AND LACTATION 223

11

FETAL ENDOCRINOLOGY 245

16

PART I

INTRODUCTION

GENERAL PRINCIPLES OF ENDOCRINOLOGY

INTRODUCTION

Definitions

Endocrinology can be defined quite simply as the study of endocrine systems. The primary function of endocrine systems is to regulate physiological processes by means of a group of chemical messengers called hormones. Although the strict definition of a hormone is often debated, it is still quite useful to **define a hormone** as a chemical substance that is released by an endocrine organ into the blood in which it travels to another site in the body where it exerts its effect. In contrast, **exocrine** organs release their products into specialized ducts rather than blood vessels.

Organization and Functions of Endocrine Systems

The simplest endocrine system consists of (1) an endocrine gland that secretes a hormone, (2) the hormone itself, and (3) a target tissue that responds to the hormone. However, most endocrine systems are considerably more complex than this. For example, a given hormone may be secreted by more than one endocrine gland, a hormone may affect many different tissues, several endocrine glands may be functionally connected (by hormones) within a system, and the result of the action of a hormone on its target tissue may influence the secretion of that hormone. Regardless of the degree of organizational complexity, the basic function of any endocrine system is still that of **regulation.**

The nature of such regulation may vary depending upon what the system is designed to accomplish. In many instances, endocrine systems maintain a constant internal environment in spite of perturbations; such systems are responsible for holding the concentrations of many constituents of plasma within their normal ranges. In other cases the mission will be to induce, rather than resist, change. For example, certain endocrine organs are activated in response to stressful events in either the internal or the external environment, and the hormones secreted are important in adapting to the stress. Another function of endocrine systems is that of coordination of the activities of various tissues toward a common goal. Tissues such as muscle, liver, and fat all respond to hormones in a fashion that ensures that their contributions to overall intermediary metabolism are acting in concert. Finally, endocrine systems also provide coordination of function in a temporal sense. This type of regulation is particularly apparent in reproductive endocrinology, in which normal function requires extremely specific patterns of change in the secretion of various hormones.

Types of Hormones

Hormones are generally categorized according to their biochemical structure or to their function. Structurally, all established hormones are (1) **peptides or proteins,** (2) **steroids,** or (3) **amino acid derivatives.** The structural relationships among the various steroid hormones derived from the common precursor cholesterol have been recognized for many years. Only more recently, however, has it become apparent that many peptide hormones also are members of structural families derived from common precursors. The structural classification of hormones is of more than biochemical interest in that it allows one to predict important functional information about a given hormone. For example, the solubility properties of a hormone (i.e., hydrophilic or lipophilic) are determined by its structure, and this factor determines the way in which a hormone is transported in blood and the general mechanism by which it exerts its effects. In addition to this structural classification, hormones are also classified functionally as **tropic** or **nontropic hormones.** A tropic (or trophic) hormone is secreted by one endocrine gland and has as its primary function the regulation of another endocrine gland. The secretion of the tropic hormone is in turn under the regulation of the hormone from the gland it regulates.

Receptors and Endocrine Specificity

The sites at which a hormone exerts its effects are often referred to as the "target" tissues or organs for that hormone. Some hormones have a single target tissue, while others have many. Regardless of the number, all target tissues for a hormone contain **receptors** for that hormone. Receptors are sites either on or in cells of the target tissues that bind the hormone as it is delivered by the blood, and as a consequence of this binding, a reaction (or a series of reactions) is initiated that culminates in the final effect of the hormone. Interaction with the receptor is the essential first step in the hormone's action.

An important characteristic of hormone receptors is that they are highly specific in their binding function. They will recognize and bind only a certain hormone even though they are simultaneously exposed to many other hormones, some of which may be structurally similar to the one bound. This illustrates that endocrine communication has its specificity built into the receiving end, not into the transmission of the information. That is, hormones are distributed indiscriminately by the blood, but they exert their effects where they encounter specific receptors. This is quite different from the way in which specificity of communication is built into the other major regulatory system of the body, the nervous system. In this case, the sites between which the communication occurs are structurally connected by a nerve fiber. At the receiving end, a mediator is released for quite restricted distribution, but it has little chemical specificity in that it could activate receptors in many other locations if delivered there.

Techniques of Endocrine Study

Many of the classical endocrine research techniques have been designed to mimic the disease states caused by hyposecretion or hypersecretion of hormones. A reduction in circulating hormone levels can be accomplished by surgically removing the organ that secretes the hormone, destroying the organ with radiation, or blocking its secretion pharmacologically. Such procedures often mimic the disease states closely, and the resulting symptoms can be reversed by administration of the appropriate hormone. The diseases caused by hypersecretion can be studied by treatment with high doses of exogenous hormones or, in some cases, by electrical or chemical stimulation of endocrine tissues.

The traditional approaches of ablation and hormone treatment provide rather crude but basic information about a hormone's origin and its actions. These approaches are still widely used during early stages of modern endocrine investigation, but subsequent stages now involve increasingly sophisticated questions, and answers are provided by the application of modern technology. For example, hormone receptors can now be isolated and characterized, and passive immunization techniques can be used to neutralize endogenous hormone pools. Also, recombinant DNA technology has allowed the cloning of hormone genes, one result of which is that bacteria can now be induced to produce certain human hormones in large supply.

An integral part of all endocrine investigation (laboratory and clinical) is the measurement of hormone levels in body fluids. This technology has also advanced rapidly over the past few decades. The techniques currently available for hormone measurement will be presented in Chapter 2.

HORMONE BIOSYNTHESIS, STORAGE, AND SECRETION

Peptide Hormones

The synthesis of peptide hormones is similar to that of most cellular proteins, in that they are made on ribosomes, using a messenger RNA (mRNA) blueprint for the amino acid sequence. However, because hormones are destined to be released by the cell, they must be segregated from intracellular proteins. This segregation is achieved by packaging hormones into secretory vesicles, a process that begins at the site of their biosynthesis. Cytosolic proteins are synthesized on free ribosomes, but hormones (and other exported proteins) are synthesized on ribosomes attached to rough endoplasmic reticulum (RER) and the completed polypeptide is released into the RER cisternae. Once inside the RER, these proteins remain sequestered in a membrane-bounded compartment until released from the cell.

Biosynthesis. Since protein hormones are synthesized on membrane-bound ribosomes, there must be some mechanism for attachment of either the mRNA or nascent polypeptide chain to the RER membrane. The key to understanding this mechanism was the discovery that hormones are synthesized as larger precursor proteins, known as **preprohormones**. These precursors are converted first to prohormones and then to hormones by sequential proteolytic cleavages as they move from the RER to secretory vesicles (Fig. 1–1).

The "pre" segment (or signal peptide) of the preprohormone appears to provide the mechanism for attachment to RER. This segment is the first portion of the molecule synthesized and it contains lipophilic amino acids. Synthesis of preprohormones is thought to begin on free ribosomes, but as the pre-segment emerges it attaches to RER membrane, pulling the ribosome with it. Whether this initial attachment is to a specific receptor or occurs because of the lipophilic nature of the pre-segment is not known. Once the ribosome contacts the RER membrane, it remains attached until hormone synthesis is completed. This attachment ensures that the growing polypeptide chain is extruded into the RER lumen so that the completed protein is released inside the RER. The final step in hormone biosynthesis is cleavage of the pre-segment by a peptidase on the inner side of the RER membrane. This reaction is rapid. (It may occur before complete synthesis of the preprohormone.) It is so efficient that the only structure normally found within the RER is prohormone.

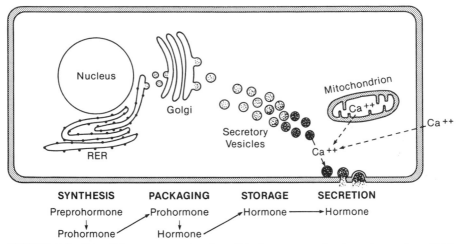

FIGURE 1–1. Subcellular components of peptide hormone synthesis and secretion. RER, rough endoplasmic reticulum.

Packaging and Storage. After their release into the RER, the prohormones are transported to the Golgi apparatus (Fig. 1–1). The Golgi consists of a series of parallel, elongated cisternae; it functions to concentrate hormones and package them into secretory vesicles. Prohormones are transported to the Golgi in membrane-bounded vesicles that pinch off from the endoplasmic reticulum nearest the Golgi and coalesce with the proximal Golgi membrane, dumping their contents into its cisterna. Prohormones then travel through the Golgi until they reach the cisterna nearest the plasma membrane. Here they are packaged into secretory vesicles, which pinch off from the outer membrane and migrate toward the plasma membrane.

The Golgi also appears to be the site of conversion of prohormones to hormones. For some hormones (e.g., insulin) this cleavage occurs at the same time as, or shortly after, vesicle formation so that the secretory vesicles contain equal concentrations of hormone and "pro" segment. For others (e.g., parathyroid hormone), cleavage occurs earlier so that secretory vesicles contain primarily hormone. In addition, this reaction is not as efficient as removal of the pre-segment; consequently small amounts of prohormone are sometimes found in secretory vesicles. The functional significance of the pro-segment is not clearly understood. In some instances, it may be important for formation of disulfide bonds within the hormone. Whatever its function, a prohormone is not absolutely essential for hormone biosynthesis or packaging because some hormones bypass this stage completely.

Once packaged, hormones are stored in secretory vesicles, released outside the cell, or degraded by lysosomal enzymes after fusion of the vesicles with lysosomes. Under normal conditions, most of the hormone is stored so that a multitude of secretory vesicles are stacked up in the cytoplasm. This storage of hormone in a readily releasable form allows the gland to respond rapidly to any demands for increased secretion without the necessity of first increasing hormone biosynthesis.

Secretion. Protein hormones are released from the cell by the process of **exocytosis.** The secretory vesicle approaches the cell surface, its membrane fuses with the plasma membrane, and the vesicle then opens, releasing its contents into the extracellular fluid (Fig. 1–1). As a result of this process, the vesicle membrane is incorporated into the plasma membrane and the entire contents of the vesicle are released. Thus, in addition to hormone, pro-segments and prohormone may also be secreted by endocrine glands. However, these substances usually have little or no biological activity.

The molecular mechanism of exocytosis is not well understood. The process requires energy (ATP), Ca^{++}, and an intact cellular cytoskeleton (microtubules and microfilaments). Further, it appears to be regulated by cytoplasmic Ca^{++} concentrations. Thus, the key link in stimulus-secretion coupling is an increase in cytosolic Ca^{++}. This increase can result from either an influx of extracellular Ca^{++} or the release of Ca^{++} sequestered in the mitochondria or endoplasmic reticulum (see Fig. 1–1). Elevated Ca^{++} levels then initiate exocytosis by binding to a protein mediator. The identity of this protein remains a mystery. However, there are currently three popular candidates: (1) actin in the microfilaments, which could provide a force for pulling the secretory vesicle up to the plasma membrane; (2) calmodulin, a Ca^{++} receptor known to mediate many of the intracellular actions of this cation; and (3) synexin, a protein capable of producing fusion of secretory vesicles. The process of Ca^{++}-activated exocytosis may involve one, two, or all three of these proteins.

Steroid Hormones

Nomenclature and Chemistry. The steroids represent a broad class of lipophilic substances, all of which contain the ring structure illustrated in Figure 1–2 for the compound cholesterol. Each of the rings is given a letter designation as noted in the figure. Steroid hormones also share a common numbering system for their constituent carbon atoms, also illustrated in Figure 1–2. There is a formal chemical nomenclature for steroids based in part on the numbering system, but it is rarely used except by steroid biochemists, and only the common names for steroid hormones are used throughout this text. However, familiarity with the carbon numbering system is advised because many of the common steroid names are based upon structural features or differences at specific carbon atoms. For example, 17-hydroxyprogesterone differs from progesterone in that it contains a hydroxyl function at the 17-carbon position. In addition, the names of many of the enzymatic reactions involved in steroid hormone biosynthesis are based upon the carbon numbering nomenclature. The 21-hydroxylase reaction, for example, introduces a hy-

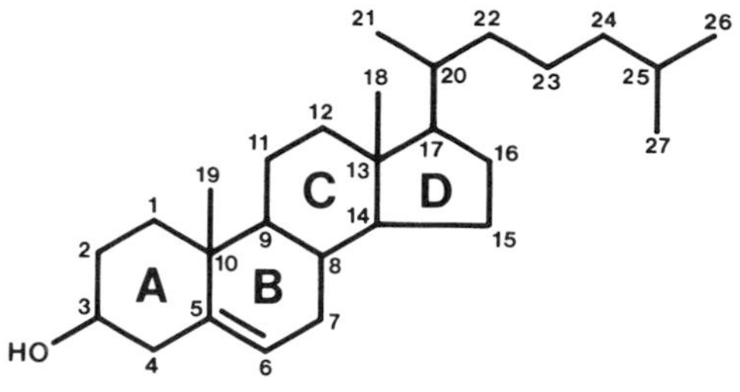

FIGURE 1–2. The ring structure and numbering system of the carbon atoms in steroid hormones, illustrated for the cholesterol molecule.

CHOLESTEROL

droxyl group into the steroid nucleus at the 21-carbon position. Many other examples illustrating the widespread use of the numbering system can be found in various chapters throughout this text.

The steroid hormones are synthesized principally in the adrenal cortex, testis, ovary, and placenta; however, each steroid-producing tissue has its own characteristic profile of secretory products. Steroids differ structurally from one another with respect to the number and position of functional groups, the degree of saturation, the length of the side chain attached to the nucleus, and other chemical characteristics. The structures of several physiologically important steroid hormones are shown in Figure 1–3. Although definitive structure-activity relationships are often difficult to establish, certain structural features seem to be shared by steroids with similar biological activities. For example, steroids with **androgenic** or masculinizing activity, typified by testosterone, contain 19 carbon atoms and do not have a side chain associated with the steroid nucleus (Fig. 1–3). Compounds with **estrogenic** or feminizing activity, such as estradiol, are 18-carbon compounds having an aromatic A-ring. The other physiologically important steroid hormones contain 21 carbons and include the **corticosteroids** and **progestins.**

Corticosteroids are produced exclusively by the adrenal cortex and consist of two types of steroid hormones: glucocorticoids and mineralocorticoids. Glucocorticoids have far-reaching effects on intermediary metabolism and since the most important of the glucocorticoids, cortisol, is hydroxylated at the 17-carbon position (Fig. 1–3), they are sometimes referred to as 17-hydroxy-corticosteroids. By contrast, mineralocorticoids such as aldosterone (Fig. 1–3), which are involved in the regulation of electrolyte balance, lack an oxygen function at the 17-carbon and are therefore 17-deoxycorticosteroids. Progesterone, the most important of the progestins, serves as an intermediate in the synthesis of many other steroid hormones. In addition, it is a major secretory product of the ovary and placenta and has an important function in reproduction. By comparison of structures of the hormones shown in Figure 1–3, it should be evident that relatively minor differences in the structures of steroid hormones can have rather profound effects on the nature of their biological activities.

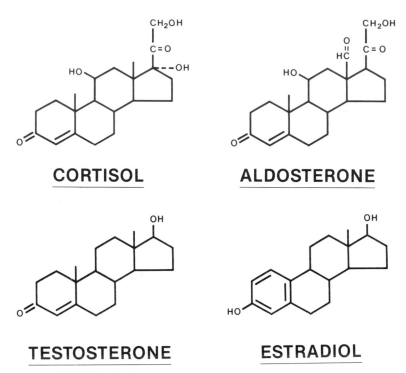

FIGURE 1–3. Structures of representative steroid hormones.

Role of Cholesterol in Steroid Biosynthesis. Cholesterol is the common precursor for all steroid hormones. Accordingly, cholesterol metabolism in steroid-secreting tissues is of major importance in the regulation of steroid hormone biosynthesis. The major processes involved in cholesterol metabolism are illustrated in Figure 1–4. For many years, it was believed that all or most of the cholesterol utilized for steroidogenesis was synthesized from acetate within steroid-producing cells. Although cholesterol synthesis does take place in these cells, plasma lipoproteins that are synthesized in the liver appear to be the major source of cholesterol for steroidogenesis. The relative importance of the different classes of lipoproteins as sources of cholesterol for steroidogenesis seems to be species-dependent, but in humans, low-density lipoproteins (LDL) play the major role. Membrane receptors for lipoproteins have been demonstrated in steroid-producing cells, and binding of lipoproteins to the receptor results in the internalization of the lipoprotein-receptor complex. Once within the steroidogenic cell, the lipoprotein is degraded by lysosomal enzymes, liberating free cholesterol; the receptor may undergo degradation or be recycled to the cell membrane for further use. The uptake and degradation of lipoproteins is hormonally regulated such that at times of in-

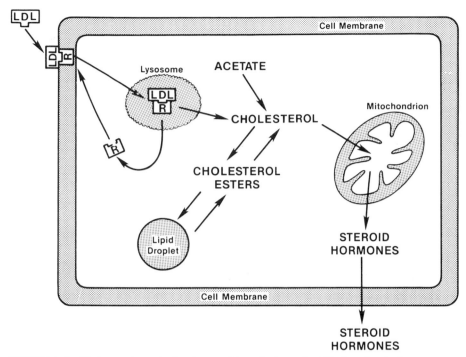

FIGURE 1-4. Cholesterol metabolism in steroid-producing cells. LDL, low-density lipoproteins.

creased need for steroid hormones, increasing amounts of cholesterol are provided as substrate to the steroid-producing cells.

Free cholesterol within steroid-producing cells, whether derived from lipoproteins or synthesized by the cell, may be immediately utilized for steroidogenesis or converted to cholesterol esters. Cells that make steroid hormones contain large amounts of cholesterol esters in structures known as lipid droplets. The cholesterol esters represent the major storage form of cholesterol and must be hydrolyzed to free cholesterol for use in steroidogenesis. The rate of hydrolysis of cholesterol esters, like the uptake and degradation of lipoproteins, is subject to hormonal regulation. Thus, the provision of free cholesterol to the steroid-producing cell can be closely coordinated with the overall activity of the steroidogenic pathway.

Hormone Synthesis and Secretion. Synthesis of the various steroid hormones from cholesterol requires a series of enzymatic reactions that modify the steroid molecule. The major steroidogenic pathways involved in the production of mineralocorticoids, glucocorticoids, androgens, and estrogens are illustrated in Figure 1-5. The figure is organized so that each column represents a distinct functional pathway (mineralocorticoid as opposed to glucocorticoid, and so on), and the same format is consistently used throughout this text.

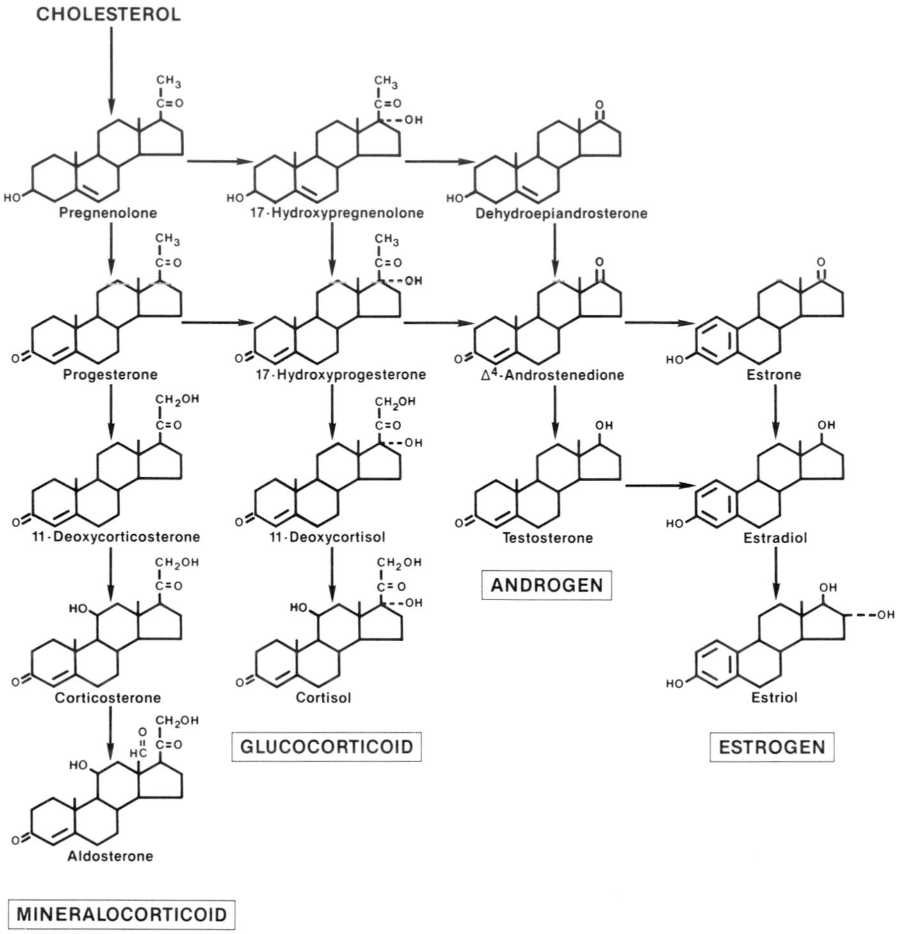

FIGURE 1–5. Pathways involved in the production of the major steroid hormones.

The first step in the pathway, the conversion of cholesterol to pregnenolone, is a reaction that occurs in all steroid-producing tissues and is believed to be the rate-limiting step in steroidogenesis. Accordingly, regulation of steroidogenesis in all tissues occurs principally by modulation of the rate of this enzymatic conversion. The reaction eliminates the side chain from the cholesterol molecule; therefore, it is known as cholesterol side chain cleavage. Since the enzyme catalyzing cholesterol side chain cleavage is highly localized to the mitochondrial fraction of the cell, transport of cholesterol from the cytosol to the mitochondria of the cell is essential for steroidogenesis. Thus, regulation of cholesterol transport plays an important part in the control of steroid hormone synthesis.

Once pregnenolone is formed in steroid-producing cells, its further metabolism is determined by the distribution and relative activities of steroidogenic enzymes within the cell. Some of the enzymatic reactions indicated in Figure 1–5 are limited to certain tissues and the products of those reactions, therefore, are produced in only those tissues. For example, the 11- and 21-hydroxylases are found only in the adrenal cortex and, as a result, the production of glucocorticoids and mineralocorticoids is limited to that gland. The specific enzymatic and secretory profiles of the different steroidogenic organs are discussed in those chapters dealing with each organ system.

As may be seen in Figure 1–5, many of the steps involved in steroidogenesis are hydroxylation reactions, although other types of enzymatic reactions are also required. Each of the enzymes noted tends to be localized to a specific subcellular compartment within the cell. Thus, the step-by-step modification of the steroid molecule during steroidogenesis often requires migration back and forth between different compartments. The intracellular migration necessary for the synthesis of cortisol, for example, is illustrated in Figure 1–6. Little is known about the mechanisms involved in the intracellular transport of steroids between compartments and, in particular, what prevents biosynthetic intermediates from diffusing out of the cell. The involvement of transport proteins has been postulated but not proved. Whatever the mechanism, the intracellular migrations required for hormone synthesis proceed quite efficiently because very little of the intermediate compounds in the

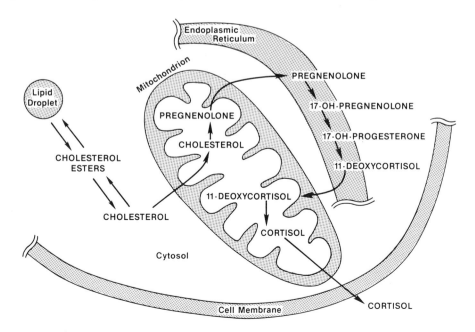

FIGURE 1–6. Subcellular compartmentalization of cortisol biosynthesis.

pathway are normally secreted. Thus, enzymatic modification of the steroid nucleus continues until the final secretory product is formed. Unlike the peptide hormones, there is no mechanism to allow for the storage of steroid hormones after their formation. Only the hormone precursor, in the form of cholesterol esters, is stored in significant quantities within steroid-producing cells. Since steroids are highly lipid-soluble, once the active hormones are produced, they simply diffuse across the cell membrane and into the bloodstream. Thus, for the steroid hormones, biosynthesis and secretion are tightly coupled processes and the rate of hormone secretion is controlled entirely by regulation of the rate of hormone synthesis (steroidogenesis).

HORMONE TRANSPORT IN BLOOD

Although all hormones are, by definition, carried by the blood, they are not all carried in the same way. Depending upon their solubility properties, they may simply be dissolved in plasma or they may be transported in association with certain plasma proteins.

Peptide and Protein Hormones

Peptide and protein hormones are quite hydrophilic, and thus are carried by the blood freely dissolved in plasma. Some hormones of this group may circulate in both monomeric and polymeric forms (e.g., insulin). In other cases, both the intact hormone and dissociated subunits are found in blood (e.g., some pituitary hormones). Nonetheless, all of these forms remain soluble in aqueous media and do not require a specialized transport system.

Steroids and Thyroid Hormones

Given the very limited aqueous solubilities of steroid and thyroid hormones, it is physically impossible for them to exist in free solution at their known plasma concentrations. They circulate at these concentrations only because of a group of plasma proteins that bind these hormones, removing them from free solution, but retaining them in the plasma (Fig. 1–7). Some of these proteins are quite specialized in that they will bind only certain hormones, and they apparently have no other functions. In contrast, others bind virtually all hydrophobic hormones. The extent to which a hormone is protein bound and its distribution among the involved proteins vary from one hormone to another. However, in all cases, the total hormone pool is predominantly in the bound form; in some cases, only 1 per cent or less of the total hormone remains unbound. This is a noteworthy figure since it is generally held that only the pool of free hormone is biologically active. It should be noted that the hormone bound to the carrier protein is in dynamic equilibrium with the free pool, which in turn is in equilibrium with the hormone that is bound to

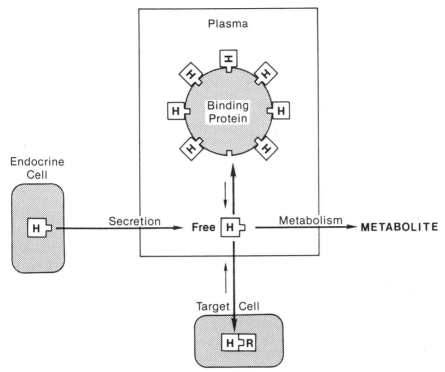

FIGURE 1–7. Production, distribution, and removal of the total plasma pool of a hydrophobic hormone (H). Free hormone may be bound by receptors (R) in target cells or by binding proteins in the plasma.

receptors in the target tissues. Nonetheless, as long as the hormone is bound to the plasma protein, it cannot interact with its receptor and thus it is inactive. It should be apparent, however, that in addition to allowing the dissolution and transportation of hydrophobic hormones, these binding proteins provide for a large hormone reserve that can be called upon to replenish the free pool. It is the magnitude of the free pool rather than the total pool of hormone that is monitored and adjusted to maintain normal endocrine function.

As depicted in Figure 1–7, the size of the free pool, and thus the availability of hormone to its receptors, can be regulated by changes in secretion, metabolism, or protein binding. It is easy to understand that the plasma concentration of a hormone will be a direct function of its secretion rate. The other factors that affect the free hormone concentration may be a bit more subtle, but they are also quite important from both didactic and clinical points of view. For example, the magnitude of the free pool will tend to increase in response to any condition that decreases the rate of hormone metabolism (i.e., degradation). Also, there are both physiological (e.g., pregnancy) and pathological conditions (e.g., liver disease) in which there are changes in the balance between free and bound pools of certain hormones. From a diagnostic standpoint, it is important to recognize that the assays for these hormones in plasma measure the total hormone concentration, i.e., the sum of the protein bound and the free pools. In such cases, it is therefore necessary to also make some determination of the extent of the protein binding of the hormone so that the free hormone concentration can be estimated.

MECHANISM OF HORMONE ACTION

Although hormones elicit a wide variety of biological responses, the molecular mechanisms by which these effects are produced fall into a few general categories. For virtually all hormones, the initial step in this process is binding of the hormone to a receptor in its target tissue. This binding then initiates a sequence of events leading to a change (either increase or decrease) in activity of specific enzymes, which in turn produces the physiological response. The exact nature of these postreceptor events depends on whether the process is initiated by a hydrophilic or lipophilic hormone.

Receptors

Hormone receptors are large proteins capable of noncovalently binding a hormone and are divided into two groups on the basis of the type of hormone bound. Lipophilic hormones (e.g., steroids) that readily pass through the cell membrane bind to receptors located in either the cytoplasm or nucleus of the cell. In contrast, receptors for protein hormones are found on the cell surface, a locale that ensures binding of these hydrophilic hormones that cannot diffuse into cells.

Regardless of their location, receptors have a number of common characteristics. First, they have a **high affinity** for their respective hormone so that significant binding occurs at the quite low hormone concentrations normally found in circulation. Because of this tight binding, hormones often remain bound to receptors for some time, thus prolonging their biological effectiveness. Second, receptors exhibit a high degree of **structural specificity;** receptors for a given hormone will bind only that hormone or very closely related compounds. There is usually a good correlation between the receptor's affinity for a hormone analog and the biological activity of that analog. Third, receptors are **tissue specific** in that significant receptor levels for a hormone are found only in target tissues for that hormone. Tissue and structural specificity of receptors ensures that a hormone acts only at its target tissues. Finally, hormone binding to a receptor causes the appropriate **biological response.** This may seem intuitively obvious, but it distinguishes receptors from a number of other biological proteins capable of binding hormones (e.g., plasma-binding proteins, catabolic enzymes). This property can be assessed by determining if agonists that bind to a hormone receptor mimic the biological activity of that hormone or, conversely, if substances that block hormone binding also disrupt its biological effects.

Since receptor binding is the essential first step by which a hormone produces its effects, it is not surprising that termination of a hormone action usually requires dissociation of that hormone from its receptor. For most hormone-receptor interactions, this dissociation occurs as a natural consequence of a fall in circulating hormone concentrations. Because receptor binding is noncovalent, as free hormone levels decline chemical equilibrium favors dissociation over association. For some protein hormones, however, there is an additional means of terminating hormone binding. After these hormones bind to the receptors on the cell surface, the hormone-receptor complex is internalized by endocytosis much like the LDL-receptor complex (see Fig. 1–4). It was originally thought that internalization was a necessary step in the mechanism of action for these hormones, but it is now generally accepted that internalized hormones are simply degraded after the pyknotic vesicles fuse with lysosomes. The receptors, which are carried in the vesicle membrane, are protected from lysosomal enzymes and recycled to the plasma membrane.

Because receptors are the primary site of interaction between hormone and target tissue, they represent an important means of modulating responsiveness to hormones. Although changes in receptor affinity do occur, changes in receptor number are much more prevalent. Often a hormone will regulate its own receptor, usually by suppressing the number of receptors on target cells. This "down regulation" requires relatively high hormone concentrations so that it is most often associated with pathological, rather than physiological, conditions. From a clinical standpoint, it can play an important role in the development of patient refractoriness to chronic hormone therapy.

The second commonly occurring type of regulation is stimulation of receptors for one hormone by a different hormone. When this occurs, pretreatment, or priming, with the latter hormone is required for the former to exert its full effects. It should be noted that a change in receptor number does not necessarily alter the maximal response of the target tissue. Many types of cells have "spare receptors" in that occupation of a relatively small percentage of the total receptors is sufficient to produce a maximal response. Under these circumstances, the number of receptors needed to be activated to produce a maximal response is not affected by changes in the total number of receptors. However, increases (or decreases) in receptor numbers do increase (or decrease) the probability of hormone binding. Thus, a change in receptor number produces a corresponding shift in sensitivity to, but no change in maximal effectiveness of, the hormone.

Postreceptor Events: Lipophilic Hormones

The first step of hormone action, receptor binding, may be universal, but subsequent events diverge into two general classes based on the chemical nature of the hormone, lipophilic or hydrophilic. The current model for the actions of lipophilic hormones is based largely on studies of the interactions of estrogens with the uterus. According to this model (Fig. 1–8), the hormone enters the cell and binds to a cytosolic receptor. This binding induces a conformational change in the receptor, termed **activation**, that markedly enhances the affinity of the hormone-receptor complex for nuclear chromatin. The activated hormone-receptor complex is then "translocated" to the nucleus where it binds to acceptor sites on chromatin and thereby increases transcription of specific genes. The resulting mRNA, after nuclear processing, is translated on ribosomes into the appropriate protein, which in turn produces the final biological response. This general pathway, or a slightly modified form of it in which free receptors are located in the nucleus, is now thought to account for the actions of all steroid hormones, as well as such other lipophilic substances as thyroid hormones and vitamin D.

While the general scheme of Figure 1–8 is now well established, many of the details remain controversial. The nature of binding-induced activation is obscure since a physical change has been detected in only a few types of receptors. Similarly, little is known about the process of translocation, but

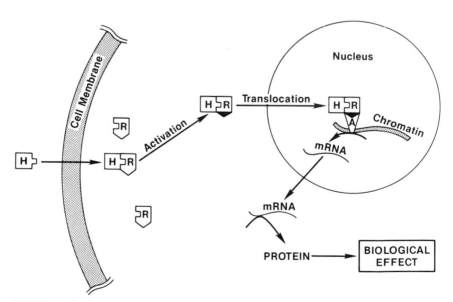

FIGURE 1–8. Subcellular mechanism of action of a lipophilic hormone (H) via an intracellular receptor (R). The H-R complex induces mRNA synthesis by binding to an acceptor site (A) on the chromatin.

perhaps the major unresolved question is the mechanism of gene induction. Some information on this issue is now available for progesterone receptors, which consist of two subunits, one that binds to a specific acidic chromatin protein and the other that then interacts with nearby DNA to induce transcription. However, it seems unlikely that this model can account for the activation of gene transcription by other steroid hormones.

Postreceptor Events: Hydrophilic Hormones

Protein and other hydrophilic hormones cannot enter cells and therefore cannot directly alter intracellular processes the way lipophilic hormones do. Instead, the binding of these hormones to receptors on the cell surface stimulates the synthesis of a second substance within the cell and it is the latter that directly alters enzyme activity. Because of their reliance on an intracellular mediator, these hormones are often said to act via a second messenger, the hormone itself being the first messenger.

Cyclic AMP: The Major Second Messenger. Since its discovery in the 1950s, a plethora of studies have established 3',5' cyclic adenosine monophosphate (cAMP) as the most common second messenger for hydrophilic hormones. Receptor binding of these hormones increases intracellular cAMP by activating an enzyme, adenylate cyclase, that converts ATP to cAMP (Fig. 1–9). The cAMP then stimulates a second enzyme, protein kinase, which phosphorylates a set of proteins. The latter proteins are usually enzymes that exist in active and inactive forms, depending on whether or not they are phosphorylated. Thus, hormones that act via cAMP produce their biological effect by phosphorylating specific enzymes and thereby altering (increasing or decreasing) their activity. Finally, there must be some mechanism for removal of intracellular cAMP once the hormone is no longer present. This is accomplished by the ubiquitous enzyme phosphodiesterase, which converts cAMP to an inactive metabolite, AMP.

Unlike the situation for lipophilic hormones, many of the details of the second messenger concept have been established. It is now known that adenylate cyclase and free receptors are free to move in the plasma membrane, and do so independently rather than being coupled. After hormone binding, the receptor-hormone complex interacts with a regulatory subunit of the enzyme, allowing the subunit to bind guanosine triphosphate (GTP). This binding of GTP in turn activates the catalytic subunit of adenylate cyclase, increasing cAMP production. Activation of protein kinase by cAMP follows a similar pattern in that cAMP binds to a regulatory subunit. However, in this instance, cAMP binding causes dissociation of regulatory and catalytic moieties. Since the former is inhibitory, the free catalytic subunit becomes biologically active.

Other Possible Second Messengers. For some time after its discovery, cAMP was thought to be the second messenger for all hydrophilic hormones.

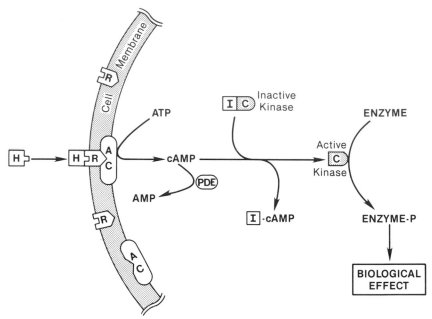

FIGURE 1–9. Subcellular mechanism of action of a hydrophilic hormone (H) via a membrane receptor (R), adenylate cyclase (AC), and cAMP. I and C are inhibitory and catalytic subunits of the kinase, respectively, and PDE is phosphodiesterase.

However, there is now good evidence that other intracellular substances mediate the actions of some hormones. Several possible messengers have been proposed, but few of these are firmly established at this time. One of the first such mediators to be suggested was **cyclic GMP,** which, like cAMP, activates a specific protein kinase. However, attempts to link cGMP with the effects of specific hormones have generally been unsuccessful. It is now thought that while cGMP may modulate tissue responses to hormones it is not a second messenger.

In contrast, cytosolic **Ca^{++}** is clearly a second messenger in some tissues. As already discussed, Ca^{++} plays a key role in initiating protein hormone secretion. In fact, when one protein hormone stimulates release of another, the former acts by increasing intracellular Ca^{++} concentrations.

The **prostaglandins** (PG) are a third possible group of mediators of hormone action. These are a set of structurally related compounds (thromboxane, prostacyclin, PGE, PGF) that are all derived from the same precursor, arachidonic acid. In a variety of tissues, production of arachidonic acid by the breakdown of membrane phospholipid is rate-limiting for prostaglandin production and is under hormonal control. Hormonal stimulation of these tissues produces an increase in prostaglandin synthesis that, in some cases, mediates the endocrine response. In most instances, however, prostaglandins are thought to influence tissue responsiveness to hormones rather than mediate hormone action.

Finally, another potential second messenger, **diacylglycerol,** is also derived from the breakdown of a membrane phospholipid. In this case, hormone treatment causes a rapid breakdown of phosphatidylinositol to diacylglycerol, which in turn stimulates a specific protein kinase. This system may well function similarly to cAMP, although the enzymes regulated by diacylglycerol-responsive protein kinase have yet to be identified. These putative mediators need not be mutually exclusive and two mediators may interact with each other. For example, breakdown of phosphatidylinositol has been proposed to mediate hormone-induced increases in intracellular Ca^{++}, and prostaglandins are often potent stimulators of cAMP production. The relevance of these interactions to the hormonal control of cell function remains obscure, at best.

Features of Hormonal Action

Despite the differences in molecular events induced by lipophilic or hydrophilic hormones, there are several characteristics common to both hormone types that have important implications for hormonal actions. First, the actions of hormones are greatly **amplified** at the target tissue. For example, by activating a gene, one steroid molecule induces formation of many mRNA molecules; each mRNA is used to make many enzymes and each enzyme will produce many end products. A similar cascade occurs with protein hormones, with one hormone producing numerous cAMP molecules and each cAMP activating many latent enzymes. This ability of target tissues to multiply the effect of hormones accounts, in large part, for the ability of the low hormone concentrations normally found in plasma (10^{-11} to 10^{-12} M) to exert profound biological effects.

A second common feature of hormone action is that hormones **regulate rates of existing reactions** rather than initiating new reactions. That is, enzymes under hormonal regulation usually show some activity even in the absence of the hormone. Finally, hormone action is **relatively slow** and **prolonged.** In general, lipophilic hormones that increase protein synthesis take longer to produce an effect than hydrophilic hormones that need only activate a preformed enzyme. Once an enzyme is activated, it is no longer dependent on the presence of hormone. As a consequence, a hormone's effect usually lasts for some time after hormone withdrawal. The length of this period ranges from minutes to days, depending on the cellular processes involved in inactivating the enzyme. This time-course for endocrine events contrasts markedly with that for the central nervous system, which usually operates on time scales of seconds or even milliseconds. Because of these differences, the endocrine system is particularly suited for more tonic types of regulation compared to the very rapid adjustments made by the nervous system.

METABOLISM OF HORMONES

Like all other constituents of the body, the circulating pools of hormones are constantly turning over; this is due to the processes of secretion and metabolism. However, for several reasons, the process of hormone metabolism should not be viewed as simply a mechanism for disposal of used hormones. First, as depicted earlier (see Fig. 1–7), changes in the rate of hormone metabolism can alter plasma hormone concentrations. In addition, metabolic conversion of a hormone is not always associated with a loss of hormonal activity. In some cases, the product of hormone metabolism has greater activity than the original hormone. These conversions, or activations, may take place within target tissues, or in other tissues that then release the more active product for general distribution by the blood. The rate of such hormone activation is itself usually under hormonal control.

The most common site for hormone metabolism (whether it be activation or inactivation) is the liver, but the kidneys are also quite active in this regard. In addition, some hormone metabolism occurs in blood and in target tissues as described in the previous section. The urine is the primary route of excretion of the products of hormone metabolism, and it also contains small quantities of some hormones that have not undergone metabolic transformation. The measurement of urinary concentrations of hormones or their metabolites is often useful as a noninvasive way of assessing endocrine function.

Most hormone metabolism is accomplished by enzyme-catalyzed reactions, but the specific nature of the structural modification differs for different classes of hormones. Steroid hormones generally undergo a series of reduction reactions followed by conjugation with highly charged moieties such as sulfates or glucuronides. The latter process enhances the water solubility of these hydrophobic hormones to facilitate their elimination via the urine. The thyroid hormones, which are iodinated molecules, are metabolized by sequential removal of iodine atoms. This may either increase or decrease the biological activity. Protein hormones are usually metabolized by specific peptidases. For those peptide hormones containing disulfide bonds that are essential for hormonal activity, reduction of these bonds often precedes enzymatic digestion of the peptide chains.

The rate of removal of a hormone from its circulating pool, like the rate of its secretion, can be altered by various conditions. For example, decreased protein binding of a hormone will enhance its removal, liver disease often results in impaired hormone catabolism, and drugs may either increase or decrease the rate of hormone removal. Such factors may be partially responsible for either abnormally high or low plasma hormone levels. Thus, in assessing endocrine dysfunction, it is sometimes necessary to quantify this removal process. (The standard techniques for measuring removal rates and related variables will be presented in Chapter 2.)

REGULATION OF HORMONE SECRETION

As noted earlier, the primary function of endocrine systems is the regulation of various physiological processes. Since the effects of hormones are proportional to their concentrations in blood, it follows that these concentrations must be subject to modulation according to need. Sometimes such modulation prevents change by counteracting disturbing influences and other times it induces appropriate changes from basal concentrations. As illustrated in Figure 1–7, the size of the biologically active pool of certain hormones in blood is determined in part by the rate of hormone removal and by the extent of binding to serum proteins. Of course, the other factor that determines the size of the circulating pool of any hormone is its rate of secretion, and it is changes in this process that are most often responsible for changes in plasma hormone concentrations. The rates of secretion of all hormones are constantly being regulated, often by a combination of several complex mechanisms. The regulatory system for each hormone will be considered in detail in subsequent chapters. However, several principles of regulation will be described now because they are common to the mechanisms that control the secretion of many different hormones. It should be noted at the outset that these control mechanisms are not mutually exclusive, and a given physiological system may include elements of more than one of them.

Feedback Systems

The rate of hormone secretion by any endocrine organ can be varied, and as it varies, it will result in changes in plasma hormone concentrations. However, if this capability is to be useful in maintaining an appropriate hormone concentration, the endocrine organ must constantly be "aware" of the systemic hormone concentration, or some function of it. This awareness is provided in endocrine systems by the existence of **feedback loops** in which information about peripheral hormone concentrations is transmitted back to the secreting organ via the blood.

Before an endocrine example of a feedback loop is presented, it may be helpful to consider a very common example of a physical feedback system, the household heating system. In this case, the controlled variable is the room temperature, and the controlling system includes the furnace, the thermostat, and all connections. The room temperature will be determined by the activity of the heat source (the furnace), which can be varied by turning it on or off.

In order to do this switching appropriately, the system as a whole must know what the desired room temperature is and it must constantly monitor the actual room temperature. The desired temperature (the **set point**) is provided by the thermostat setting, and the actual temperature is provided by a thermometer that transmits, or feeds back, this information to the controlling system. This system includes a mechanism that compares these two temperatures and turns the furnace on as room temperature drops below the desired temperature and off when the temperature is too high. The overall result is that room temperature oscillates somewhat, but this feedback system is still a very effective homeostatic device because it takes corrective action to prevent the controlled variable from drifting too far above or below the set point.

The example of a feedback system just presented is more specifically called a **negative feedback system** because the heat output of the furnace decreases when the room temperature increases, and vice versa. However, there is another type of feedback, called **positive feedback,** in which these two variables change in the same direction. In endocrinology, negative feedback systems are involved in regulating the secretion of virtually every endocrine organ. In contrast, positive feedback is a much less prevalent phenomenon, but it does exist in certain endocrine situations.

In leaving the example of the heating system, it should be emphasized that feedback is entirely an operational concept in that it describes the way in which a system functions without describing the composition of the system. The following endocrine example is also a feedback system, but anatomically it contains both neural and endocrine components, and thus is called a **neuroendocrine** system. Each of the tropic hormones of the anterior pituitary gland is under negative feedback control by the hormones that are secreted by their target organs. The specifics vary somewhat among the tropic hormones, but the principles are similar and can be illustrated by the general diagram in Figure 1–10. The controlled variable is the plasma concentration of the hormone secreted by the target organ (adrenal, gonad, or thyroid). The rate of hormone secretion is regulated by the stimulatory effect of a tropic hormone secreted by the anterior pituitary, which in turn is regulated by a releasing hormone secreted by neurons in the hypothalamus. This region of the brain also contains (1) neurons that can sense the concentration of the target organ hormone in the blood and (2) a set point for the appropriate concentration of this hormone. The hypothalamus compares these two values, and if the circulating concentration of the target organ hormone is less than the set point, it will increase its secretion of the appropriate releasing hormone. This increases tropic hormone secretion, which stimulates secretion by the target organ until the plasma concentration of its hormone returns to the appropriate level. Similarly, if the plasma concentration of the hormone goes above the appropriate level, this cascade of events is reversed and its concentration falls. Thus, target organ hormones are said to exert negative feedback inhibition over the secretion of tropic or releasing hormones or both.

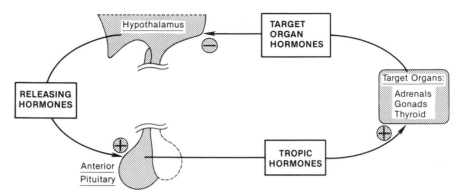

FIGURE 1-10. Negative feedback inhibition of tropic and releasing hormones by target organ hormones. (+) indicates stimulation and (−) indicates inhibition. In some cases, such inhibition occurs at the pituitary.

Such systems maintain relatively constant target hormone levels in much the same way as the heating system maintains room temperature. However, in one sense, the endocrine systems are more sophisticated than the heating system. The latter is referred to as an "on-off" system since the furnace can either be on or off, but not in between. In contrast, the rates of secretion of the tropic and releasing hormones can vary continuously between zero and maximal, and they do so in proportion to how far the plasma concentration of the target organ hormone is from the set point. This is called **proportional feedback,** and it minimizes the oscillation of the controlled variable around the set point. Figure 1–10 illustrates endocrine negative feedback in a general way. It must be noted that there are important exceptions, to be discussed in subsequent chapters.

One final point should be made about endocrine feedback and the nature of the signals throughout the feedback loop. In the example just given, the secretion of the controlling hormones is decreased by an increase in the controlled hormone; this conforms precisely to the definition of negative feedback given earlier. However, in some endocrine feedback systems, such as in the regulation of blood glucose levels, the secretion of the controlling hormones may either increase or decrease as blood glucose rises (Fig. 1–11). In this case, one of the controlling hormones secreted by the pancreas (glucagon) is related to the controlled variable (glucose) in the same way as in the previous examples (i.e., glucagon decreases as glucose rises). However, the secretion of the other hormone depicted (insulin) increases as glucose rises. But, since glucagon causes blood glucose to rise, whereas insulin causes it to fall, both mechanisms result in the same net effect—that of returning blood glucose levels toward normal. Thus, both of these mechanisms are examples of negative

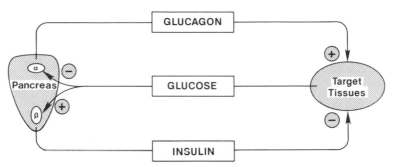

FIGURE 1–11. Two negative feedback loops involved in the hormonal control of plasma glucose levels. (+) and (−) indicate stimulation and inhibition, respectively; α and β identify specific cell types within the pancreas.

feedback even though glucose stimulates the secretion of one hormone and inhibits the release of the other. It should be noted that the overall regulation of blood glucose levels involves many more elements than depicted in Figure 1–11; the complete description of this will be presented in subsequent chapters.

The above example also illustrates that in addition to monitoring and regulating the levels of hormones, negative feedback systems may also monitor and regulate other blood constituents such as glucose, Na^+, and Ca^{++}. In still other endocrine feedback systems it is some consequence of the hormone other than a blood constituent that is regulated. For example, antidiuretic hormone contributes to the regulation of blood volume, and its rate of secretion is regulated in part by a system that responds to changes in blood volume.

Neuroendocrine Reflexes

Many endocrine control systems include neural as well as hormonal components, and thus they are more correctly called **neuroendocrine control systems.** In addition to responding to changes in the controlled variables as described in the previous section, such control systems can elicit hormone release in response to a variety of other stimuli, some of which are exteroceptive. Because of the nature of this response, and recognizing the components of the system, this is referred to as **neuroendocrine reflex activity.** Such reflex arcs ordinarily consist of an afferent limb, which is neural (central or peripheral), and an efferent limb, which is endocrine. A good example of this type of regulation is the increase in oxytocin release caused by suckling (Fig. 1–12). In this reflex, suckling by the infant activates afferent nerves running from the breast to the anterior hypothalamus, and this, in turn, stimulates specific neuroendocrine cells to release oxytocin from the posterior pituitary. The oxytocin is then carried by the blood to the breast, where it causes contraction of the myoepithelial cells in the ducts, which moves the milk toward the nipple, making it accessible to the infant.

Some endocrine control systems include both neuroendocrine reflexes and feedback control. For example, cortisol secretion from the adrenal cortex is subject to negative feedback control, but in addition a neuroendocrine reflex is responsible for mediating the increase in cortisol levels that occurs after exposure to physical or emotional stress. In general, neuroendocrine reflexes are activated only upon demand for a change in hormone secretion, whereas negative feedback loops operate continuously to counteract changes.

Endocrine Rhythms

Although hormone secretion rates are usually regulated by some form of negative feedback, it should not be inferred that they are always maintained at a constant value. Instead, superimposed upon negative feedback control, the secretion rates of virtually all hormones vary as a function of time, resulting in oscillations in plasma hormone concentrations. One quite common type of endocrine oscillation is referred to as a **diurnal** or **circadian** rhythm. These rhythms are characterized by repeating fluctuations in hormone levels that are very regular and have a frequency of one cycle every 24 hours. As depicted in Figure 1–13, cortisol is one of the many hormones that undergoes this type of fluctuation (in addition to being regulated by feedback and stress). This regularity is a result of the hormone secretion being set, or "entrained," by some external oscillation having a period of 24 hours. Most endocrine diurnal rhythms are entrained to the light–dark cycle, but other factors such as activity cycles can also have some influence. It should be noted that such external cues, or "zeitgebers," are necessary for the endocrine rhythm to keep time accurately, but they are not responsible for the rhythmicity itself. If a person is removed from the influence of the zeitgeber, for example by exposure to constant darkness, then the circadian rhythms will continue but they will do

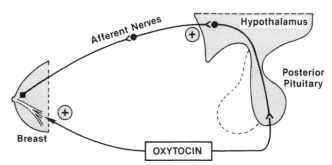

FIGURE 1–12. The neuroendocrine reflex mediating milk ejection in response to suckling. (+) indicates stimulation.

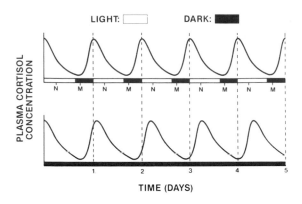

FIGURE 1–13. Diurnal variation in plasma cortisol levels in the presence of a normal light–dark cycle (top), and the slower, "free running" rhythm in constant dark (bottom). N and M, noon and midnight.

so at their own inherent frequency, which is usually slightly slower than the light–dark cycle (Fig. 1–13).

In addition to diurnal rhythms, there are more rapid oscillations in plasma hormone concentrations referred to as **ultradian** rhythms. As implied by the term rhythm, these oscillations show temporal regularity and thus are not simply due to random fluctuations in secretion. Such high-frequency rhythms have only recently been recognized and their significance is still being evaluated.

As noted earlier, the rhythmicity of hormone secretion is not simply a response to external rhythms but rather appears to be due to endogenous oscillators, analogous to the centers producing the rhythmic motions of breathing. The mechanisms responsible for this inherent rhythmicity of endocrine systems have been investigated for years but are still poorly understood. Although some have suggested that several endocrine organs themselves are capable of rhythmic secretion, most investigators believe that the basic rhythmicity, as well as the entrainment to zeitgebers, are functions of the central nervous system. However, the neural and chemical mechanisms by which time is kept and rhythmic activity is generated have yet to be discovered.

PARAENDOCRINOLOGY

This introductory chapter will be closed by returning to the definition of endocrinology, this time to provide some perspective of the bounds of the discipline, how it is advancing, and how it relates to its neighboring (and sometimes overlapping) disciplines. These considerations of the "surroundings" of endocrinology are referred to as **paraendocrinology.** Endocrinology is expanding quite rapidly both in terms of its depth and its breadth. The deepening of the field is provided by the identification of new substances that, on the basis of the circumstantial evidence leading to their discoveries, are quite readily accepted as being hormones. In contrast to this clearly defined frontier, the "lateral" borders of endocrinology are not very sharply demarcated. Many biologically active substances in the body have certain characteristics in common with classical hormones, but for one reason or another they do not completely qualify as hormones. Some of these are recently discovered substances about which our information is simply not yet complete enough to make this judgment. Other substances have been recognized for decades, but their characteristics strain the classical definition of a hormone. Such substances are sometimes referred to as "candidate" hormones, or "potential" hormones. Before we consider examples of these, it will be helpful to describe several mechanisms of humoral communication that are related to, but distinguishable from, endocrine mechanisms. This perspective should help abate the confusion about whether a given substance should or should not be considered a hormone.

Types of Intercellular Communication

As defined at the beginning of this chapter, true endocrine communication involves the release of a humoral messenger into the blood, which carries this hormone to a distant target tissue (Fig. 1–14). The other two types of humoral communication depicted in this figure differ from the endocrine mechanism in that the products released by these cells act locally and they are distributed by simple diffusion. In one of these (**paracrine**), the effect is exerted on neighboring cells, whereas in the other (**autocrine**), the target cell is the same cell that releases the messenger substance. Part of the confusion in classifying these humoral communication systems is because a given substance may function in one manner at one location in the body and by another manner at a different site. For example, somatostatin is known to be a true hormone in that it is delivered by the blood to the pituitary gland where it inhibits growth hormone secretion. However, it is also involved in a paracrine

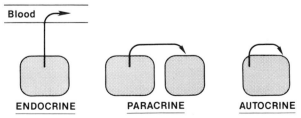

FIGURE 1–14. Types of intercellular communication via chemical mediators.

TABLE 1–1. Some Nonclassical and Candidate Hormones

"Hormone"	Primary Source	Primary Target
Specific Substances		
Melatonin	Pineal	Hypothalamus/pituitary
Thymosin	Thymus	Lymphocytes
Renin	Kidney	Angiotensinogen
Erythropoietin	Kidney	Bone marrow
Atrial natriuretic factor	Heart	Kidney
Classes of Substances		
Growth factors	Multiple	Multiple
Prostaglandins	Multiple	Multiple
Opioid peptides	Multiple	Multiple

mechanism in the GI tract, where it is released by certain cells in the lining of the stomach and acts on neighboring cells to inhibit secretion of the hormone gastrin. In addition to such paracrine communication, the GI tract relies heavily on endocrine mechanisms in regulating both secretion and motility, but since this branch of endocrinology is more logically presented in gastrointestinal textbooks, it will not be dealt with here.

Nonclassical and Candidate Hormones

Some of the substances considered in this section (Table 1–1) can certainly be classified as hormones, but they are not secreted by a classical endocrine organ, and thus they are not described in subsequent chapters dealing with the major endocrine systems. Others of those listed in Table 1–1 are known to be involved in endocrine processes, but they appear to act in an ancillary fashion rather than as hormones *per se*.

Melatonin. The pineal gland produces and releases the indoleamine melatonin; this process is under the stimulatory control of noradrenergic nerves. Melatonin release is controlled primarily by the light–dark cycle with most of the secretion occurring during darkness. Under many circumstances melatonin has an antigonadotropic effect, but the physiological significance of this mechanism is not yet established. Perhaps the most intriguing connection between pineal function and human endocrinology concerns the possibility of a role for melatonin in initiating puberty. Pineal tumors have long been associated with abnormalities in the onset of puberty, and it has been proposed by some that puberty begins because of a decrease in melatonin levels, particularly during the night when the diurnal peaks occur.

Thymosin. There is a long history to the potential endocrine activity of the thymus gland, but still relatively little is known with certainty about this.

Thymosin is a term applied to several substances produced by the thymus that are important as growth factors in lymphocyte maturation, both in the thymus and at remote sites. However, there is also evidence that thymosin is involved in the interaction between the immune system and the hypothalamo-pituitary-gonadal axis. Thymosin may contribute to the negative feedback regulation of gonadotropin secretion exerted by sex steroids, because it enhances gonado-tropin secretion and its own release from the thymus is inhibited by sex steroids.

Renin. This protein is produced in the juxtaglomerular cells of the kidney, and it is classified as a hormone because it is secreted by these cells into the blood. Once released, renin initiates a cascade of events, the result of which is stimulation of the secretion of a steroid hormone by the adrenal cortex; the details of this well-established endocrine mechanism will be presented in Chapter 7. However, renin is also mentioned here because it is a rather unusual hormone in several ways. First, instead of having a specific organ or tissue as its target, it acts upon a protein circulating in the blood, angiotensinogen. Second, the nature of its action is rather unusual; whereas many hormones act by inducing certain enzymes, renin itself is an enzyme. It is a proteolytic enzyme that cleaves the angiotensinogen to give rise to a decapeptide, angiotensin I. Thus, renin is an enzyme by virtue of its action, and it is a hormone because of its means of transport from its cells of origin. As will be seen later, the secretion of renin is in large part controlled by a traditional endocrine feedback loop.

Erythropoietin. The kidneys are also the primary source of a hormone, erythropoietin, which stimulates the development and release of erythrocytes from bone marrow. Erythropoietin release varies inversely with the hematocrit, and it has been shown to be altered by numerous hormones.

Atrial Natriuretic Factor. The hormone-dependent retention of sodium by the kidneys is now well established. In contrast, there has been much discussion but little agreement regarding a hormone that promotes sodium loss, a so-called natriuretic factor. Recent advances in this field are resolving this controversy by confirming that there is, indeed, a natriuretic hormone and that it is a peptide secreted by a rather surprising endocrine organ, the heart. Since this hormone is produced and released by the atria (but not the ventricles), it is specifically referred to as atrial natriuretic factor. It is now known that there are several homologous forms of this factor.

Growth Factors. As will be described in Chapter 14, at least some of the effects of pituitary growth hormone are mediated by several hepatic growth factors called somatomedins. Recent studies in other areas have revealed the existence of a variety of analogous growth factors. Some of the most widely recognized of these are **epidermal growth factor, nerve growth factor,** and **insulin-like growth factor.** As the names indicate, these peptides have mitogenic effects on a variety of tissues, but some of these also enhance somatic growth and some have insulin-like activity. Although this is a rapidly advancing area of endocrinology, many questions remain unanswered about the effects and the endocrine control of these circulating growth factors.

Prostaglandins. The prostaglandins have been of great interest to endocrinologists since their discovery because they were originally isolated from semen, and they have been implicated in many reproductive processes since then. These 20 carbon fatty acids were named in the belief that the seminal prostaglandins were derived from the prostate gland, but they are in fact primarily derived from the seminal vesicles. Also, they are by no means restricted to the semen or even to the reproductive system; prostaglandins are now known to be produced in virtually all tissues. There was considerable early interest in the possible endocrine effects of prostaglandins, but there are very few cases in which they are thought to act as true hormones. Instead, they are most often involved in endocrine systems as intracellular modulators of hormone action as described earlier. As might be expected from their ubiquity, the prostaglandins have been shown to influence a wide variety of endocrine processes, but it is sometimes difficult to determine whether these are physiological or pharmacological effects. It should also be noted that although the prostaglandins have attracted much attention in endocrinology, they are of equal interest in other areas of physiology. They have a variety of cardiovascular effects including the modulation of platelet aggregation and plaque formation, and they also have profound effects in the respiratory, renal, gastrointestinal, and nervous systems.

Endogenous Opioids. The analgesic effect of morphine, an alkaloid extracted from plants, has been shown to be mediated by specific receptors in the brain. Until recently, it has been rather puzzling that receptors should exist for this exogenous substance with no apparent endogenous counterparts. However, it is now clear that there are several classes of endogenous peptides that bind to these same receptors and have morphine-like effects. These are called **endogenous opioid peptides,** and there are several structural families of them, including the enkephalins and the endorphins. These peptides are widely distributed in the nervous system and they are thought to act as neurotransmitters and/or neuromodulators involved in numerous processes in addition to the abatement of pain. The endocrine interest in the endogenous opioid peptides is substantial and multifaceted. They are present in many endocrine organs, they can modulate both the secretion and the actions of various hormones, and they can be derived, at least in part, from a large precursor peptide that is also the precursor of some pituitary hormones.

Thus the growth factors, the prostaglandins, and the endogenous opioids are families of substances that have only recently been characterized and are now being actively investigated. Their distribution and range of biological activities extend well beyond the bounds of endocrinology. Even if they do not meet all of the criteria to be called hormones, it is quite clear that they play important supportive roles in normal endocrine function.

REFERENCES

Jensen, E.V., Greene, G.L., Closs, L.E., DeSombre, E.R., and Nadji, M.: Receptors reconsidered: A 20-year perspective. Rec. Prog. Horm. Res. 38:1, 1982.

Lingappa, V.R., and Blobel, G.: Early events in the biosynthesis of secretory and membrane proteins: The signal hypothesis. Rec. Prog. Horm. Res. 36:451, 1980.

Makin, H.L.J. (ed.): Biochemistry of the Steroid Hormones. Blackwell Scientific Publications, London, 1975.

2

CLINICAL AND DIAGNOSTIC ENDOCRINOLOGY

INTRODUCTION

Chapter 1 has presented an overview of the characteristics of the normal function of endocrine systems. The present chapter will also be general in scope, but it will provide an introduction to abnormal endocrine function. More specific information on endocrine diseases will be presented at the end of each of the subsequent chapters dealing with the individual endocrine systems.

Impact of Endocrine Diseases on Public Health

A large part of a general medical practice is usually devoted to the diagnosis and treatment of endocrine diseases, the most prevalent of which are diabetes, thyroid diseases, and reproductive disorders. In addition, since hormones affect virtually all tissues, endocrine factors are often involved in many other major diseases not primarily classified as endocrine diseases (e.g., psychiatric disorders, atherosclerosis, cancer). Diabetes can be cited as one example of an endocrine disease that has major impact on society. It is estimated that there are over 5 million diabetics in the United States and that another 5 million are borderline diabetics whose disease will subsequently be diagnosed and require treatment. As with many other endocrine diseases, it is not the hormonal imbalance itself but the complications of diabetes (e.g., cardiovascular, neural, and renal) that are responsible for much of the morbidity and mortality of this disease. Because of these complications, diabetes is the fifth leading cause of death by disease in the United States, and the annual cost of providing care for diabetics is estimated to be about $4 billion.

TYPES OF ENDOCRINE PATHOLOGY

Most endocrine disorders can be attributed to one of the following general categories of problems: (1) too little hormone, (2) too much hormone, or (3) an abnormal tissue response to a hormone. Within each of these categories, however, any of a number of specific factors may be responsible for the abnormality.

Hyposecretion

Types of Hyposecretion. An endocrine organ that is secreting too little of its hormone may be doing so because of an abnormality within that organ; this condition is referred to as **primary** hyposecretion. On the other hand, if the organ is not abnormal but is secreting too little hormone simply because it is receiving too little of its tropic hormone, then the condition is called **secondary** hyposecretion. These conditions are illustrated in Figure 2–1 for those target organs (adrenals, gonads, and thyroid) that are regulated by tropic hormones from the anterior pituitary. Note that in both cases secretion of the target organ hormone is, by definition, less than normal, whereas secretion of the tropic hormone may be abnormally high or low depending upon the site of the defect. If there is secondary hyposecretion, secretion of the tropic hormone is low by definition. If there is a primary defect, the tropic hormone is elevated because the reduced target organ hormone levels exert less negative feedback inhibition of tropic hormone secretion.

Causes of Hyposecretion. Many different factors may act singly or in combination to cause hyposecretion of a hormone. Among these are the following (each listed with an example): (1) **genetic**–congenital absence of a steroidogenic enzyme; (2) **dietary**–hypothyroidism due to iodine deficiency; (3) **chemical or toxic**–certain insecticide derivatives may cause necrosis of the

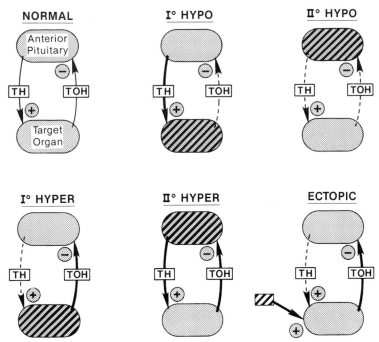

FIGURE 2–1. Various types of abnormal secretion of a target organ hormone (TOH), which is normally regulated by a tropic hormone (TH) from the anterior pituitary. Bold and broken arrows depict greater and less than normal rates of secretion, respectively. Cross-hatching indicates the location of the defect. Stimulation and inhibition are signified by (+) and (−), respectively.

adrenal cortex; (4) **immunologic**–in a common type of thyroiditis, antibodies cause destruction of thyroid tissue leading to hypothyroidism; and (5) **other disease processes**–destruction of endocrine organs by cancer or tuberculosis. In addition to these factors, there are some **idiopathic** endocrine disorders, meaning that the causes are not known. Finally, some cases of endocrine hyposecretion may be **iatrogenic,** i.e., caused by the physician. For example, treatment of hyperthyroidism by thyroidectomy may result in hypoparathyroidism unless care is taken to spare the parathyroid glands.

Treatment of Hyposecretion. The most common means of treating hormone hyposecretion is to administer a hormone preparation that is the same as, or similar to, the one that is missing or inadequate. Such replacement therapy is straightforward in theory, but there are some practical problems associated with it regarding the source and means of administration of the hormone. Although the structures of some hormones are rather constant among mammalian species, others (namely proteins) vary considerably from one species to another. Because of this, it is preferable to replace a missing hormone with the identical compound, either derived biologically from the same species or chemically synthesized. For thyroid and steroid hormones this has not been difficult since these hormones are relatively easy to synthesize and the active forms are common to many species.

In contrast, protein hormones are quite difficult to synthesize, and thus large quantities of human protein hormones are not yet readily available. Fortunately, there is usually considerable overlap in biological activity of mammalian protein hormones even though their structures may vary. Because of this, it has been common to rely on extracts of animal tissues for the treatment of human hyposecretory disorders. Even though problems are sometimes caused by the antigenicity of these "foreign" proteins, this type of replacement therapy is common and in some instances has been life saving (e.g., insulin for diabetics).

On the other hand, growth hormone (GH) is an example of a hormone that has enough species specificity so that the subprimate versions of this protein are not active in humans. Thus, until recently, the only feasible approach for GH replacement was the collection of cadaver pituitaries for the extraction and purification of the human GH. Unfortunately, this source has been inadequate to meet the need for this hormone in the treatment of growth disorders, and in any case the product has now been removed from the market because of possible viral contamination. Human GH has been synthesized chemically, but the procedure is too complex for mass production, so this source of the hormone is also inadequate. However, a solution to this supply problem has recently been derived through genetic engineering. The human GH gene has been synthesized from its mRNA and inserted into bacterial DNA, which was then introduced into bacteria, causing them to mass produce this human hormone. More recently, a hypothalamic hormone that causes the anterior pituitary to secrete GH has been isolated and synthesized. Since it has a much simpler structure than GH (only 44 amino acids), it can be synthesized in large amounts and can be used to treat those patients in whom GH secretion is low because of inadequate secretion of the hypothalamic stimulatory hormone.

Even when there is an appropriate hormonal preparation available, other potential problems in replacement therapy are associated with the manner in which the hormone is administered. Ideally, the hormone should be given in exactly the same manner (route, dose, and timing) as it is normally provided by the endocrine organ. This would require continuous intravenous infusion, a procedure that is not feasible for the chronic treatment usually necessary in endocrine diseases. Instead, most endocrine replacement therapy consists of the periodic administration of doses of a hormone chosen to approximate the amount that would normally be secreted during the interval between treatments. This can sometimes be accomplished by oral administration, but because many native hormones would be digested in the gastrointestinal tract, they must be given by injection. In some cases, portable infusion pumps are now available for long-term treatment. Their use avoids the transient oscillations in hormone levels associated with intermittent injections. Some of the pumps now being developed for insulin administration to diabetics are actually complete feedback systems that monitor blood glucose levels and infuse insulin as needed. It should be noted that neither periodic injections nor constant infusion will mimic the normal secretory pattern of hormones. This is an important issue in the case of some hormones such as the gonadotropin-releasing hormone, which is effective only if given in a pulsatile manner that mimics its endogenous secretory pattern.

The temporal pattern of hormone administration is also important at the time of withdrawal of therapy. For example, during a period of treatment with high doses of glucocorticoids, the adrenal glands will stop producing endogenous glucocorticoids because of the inhibitory effect of the exogenous hormone on the secretion of the tropic hormone regulating adrenocortical secretion. After a prolonged period of such inactivity, the adrenal glands cannot immediately begin secreting again, and the abrupt withdrawal of exogenous glucocorticoids can result in a state of adrenal insufficiency. To avoid such problems, the exogenous hormone treatment is normally withdrawn gradually to allow the adrenal glands to regain their secretory capacity.

There is another type of endocrine therapy that may become feasible as more is learned about the neurotransmitters that regulate both neural and neuroendocrine systems. The manipulation of neurotransmitter pools is already used in the treatment of certain neurological diseases (e.g., dopamine in Parkinson's disease), and the same principle is applicable to the treatment of neuroendocrine disorders. However, as this approach becomes more common, it is important that a crucial difference between hormones and neurotransmitters be kept in mind. Hormones are normally distributed throughout the body, and thus one can administer hormonal preparations systemically with some degree of impunity knowing that they will encounter the same receptors and induce the same effects as the endogenous hormone would. In contrast, endogenous pools of neurotransmitters are normally quite restricted in their distribution. Because of this, the same transmitters can be used in many different synapses throughout the central nervous system without a loss in specificity of information transfer. Thus, systemic administration of neurotransmitters would eliminate that specificity and is likely to elicit many more side effects than would be seen with classical endocrine therapy.

The replacement of human endocrine organs by transplantation is not common even though it is surgically feasible and is done routinely in experimental animals. The reason for this is that, in contrast to a heart or a kidney, the function of an endocrine organ (hormone secretion) can be replaced quite readily by the less radical approach of hormone administration. Nonetheless, there have been attempts to reverse diabetes by transplanting a pancreas, a portion of a pancreas, or just the islets of Langerhans (the endocrine portion of the pancreas). This approach has met with only limited success because of both rejection problems and recurrence of the diabetes. Therefore, it must still be considered an experimental procedure.

Hypersecretion

Types of Hypersecretion. Like hyposecretion, hypersecretion by a particular organ is designated as **primary** or **secondary** depending upon whether the defect is within that organ or is due to excessive stimulation from outside. These conditions are illustrated in Figure 2–1.

Causes of Hypersecretion. There are many types of tumors that may occur in endocrine tissues, and they are responsible for a large proportion of endocrine disease. Some such tumors secrete hormones, often in excess, and thus are referred to as **functional tumors.** In these cases, the hormone being secreted is appropriate to that organ, but it is secreted at too high a rate and it is often not under the control of normal regulatory factors. In contrast, an **ectopic tumor** secretes large amounts of a hormone that ordinarily would not be secreted by the tissue harboring the tumor; this secretion is also not subject to normal control mechanisms. For example, it is not uncommon for tumors in the lung to secrete hormones such as adrenocorticotropin and antidiuretic hormone. In spite of their unusual source, these hormones are fully active and will cause the same symptoms as would be seen as if they were hypersecreted from their normal sources (the anterior and posterior pituitary, respectively).

Another cause for hypersecretion, and one that is being recognized more and more frequently, is **immunologic.** For example, the most common type of hyperthyroidism (Graves' disease) is caused by excessive stimulation of thyroid secretion, not by its normal tropic hormone, but by an immunoglobulin that can mimic the action of the tropic hormone. Finally, a source of endocrine excess that cannot be dismissed is **substance abuse.** Some individuals take thyroid hormones unnecessarily because this "makes them feel more energetic," and certain anabolic hormones (e.g., androgens and growth hormone) are widely abused in athletics. Of course, these instances do not involve hypersecretion by an endocrine organ, but the result is the same since receptors do not distinguish between exogenous and endogenous sources of hormones.

Treatment of Hypersecretion. When an endocrine tumor is detected, it is most often removed surgically or destroyed with radiation treatment. These procedures can also be used to partially ablate or to limit the secretion of a hypersecreting endocrine organ. However, hypersecretion can also be limited in some instances by drugs that block hormone synthesis or inhibit hormone secretion. Finally, some hypersecretory conditions can be treated without actually reducing hormone secretion by giving drugs that inhibit the action of the hormone.

Reduced Responsiveness to Hormones

In this category of endocrine disease, there are adequate amounts of hormone being secreted, but the target tissues are not able to respond normally. This may be caused by a congenital lack of receptors or by a deficiency in an enzyme that is required for activation of the hormone. Both of these cases can be illustrated for the primary male reproductive hormone testosterone. In the testicular femininization syndrome, there are no functional testosterone receptors and in spite of adequate testosterone availability, the symptoms are the same as if no testosterone were present. Similarly, in patients with a 5α-reductase deficiency, adequate testosterone is present in the circulation. However, in many tissues there is no response to the testosterone since this reductase is required for the intracellular conversion of testosterone to an active metabolite, dihydrotestosterone.

ASSESSMENT OF ENDOCRINE FUNCTION

Hormone Measurement

In assessing endocrine function, the most basic determination to be made is the measurement of hormone activity or hormone concentration in body fluids such as blood or urine. Urinary measurements of hormones or their metabolites have historically provided a convenient and noninvasive means of assessing endocrine activity. Also, such measurements have been practical from an analytical standpoint since there are fewer substances in urine than in blood that may interfere with many assays. However, hormone measurements in blood are a more direct index of endocrine activity since it is this pool of hormones that is available to the receptors in target tissues. Also, hormone levels must be measured in blood if it is necessary to have any detailed information about the temporal pattern of changes in hormone levels. As a corollary to this, for those hormones whose plasma concentrations normally vary with time (e.g., diurnally), one must know the time of day that any single assay sample was collected in order to interpret the results correctly—a result that is normal for one time of day may be abnormal for another time. Finally, it should be pointed out that measurements of hormone concentration in plasma are usually taken as an index of the rate of secretion of that hormone. While this is usually true, it must constantly be borne in mind that plasma hormone concentration is determined by both secretion and other factors, such as rate of removal.

Bioassay. The earliest form of endocrine assay is that in which the hormone is administered to an experimental animal and then some biological response is measured. Such assays are called bioassays, and for each hormone there are many possible versions depending upon factors such as the species used, the route of administration, and the response measured. In spite of this variety of approaches, all bioassays require the availability of a **standard** preparation of the hormone (to compare the assay sample to) and the generation of a **standard curve** to allow this comparison. For example, one could assay the amount of androgen activity in a solution by injecting it into mice and then determining the change in weight of an androgen-sensitive organ (e.g., seminal vesicles) as the biological response. In order to quantitatively state the amount of activity in this unknown sample, other mice would have to receive injections of various amounts of a known or standard androgen preparation; this could be synthetic androgen or a crude extract of testicular tissue.

In either case, the results and the method of analysis would be as depicted in Figure 2–2. The biological response is plotted as a function of the amount of hormone administered. The dots represent the mean responses in those mice receiving known amounts of the standard preparation as indicated on the abscissa. The best fit line drawn through these dots is the standard curve, which will typically have a linear portion when the response is plotted as a function of the log of hormone dose (as in Fig. 2–2). This line allows one

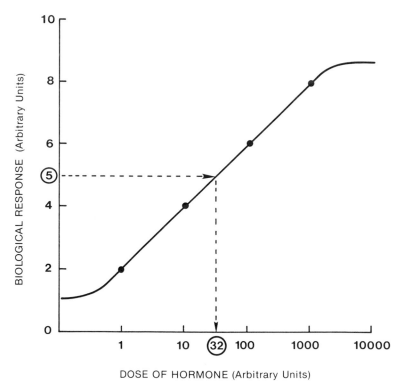

FIGURE 2–2. Idealized results from a bioassay depicting the way in which the standard curve is used to determine the amount of hormone in an unknown sample giving a biological response of 5 units.

to determine the amount of hormone contained in any unknown sample by measuring the biological response it induces. This procedure is illustrated on Figure 2–2 for a sample that caused a response of five units. By projecting to the right as far as the standard curve and then downward to the abscissa, it can be seen that this sample contained 32 units of the hormone being assayed.

The principle of a bioassay is quite simple and (unlike some other assays) there can be no doubt that the results are biologically relevant. However, there are some limitations to this approach that have resulted in its being used less and less as newer techniques are developed. The primary disadvantages to bioassays are that they are (1) not especially sensitive, (2) often rather cumbersome, and (3) generally quite expensive because biological variability demands the inclusion of many animals in the assay. Nonetheless, any other type of assay relies on an end point other than a biological response, and it is often necessary to return to a bioassay to ensure that what the newer and simpler assays are measuring is in fact correlated with biological activity.

Chemical Assay. Chemical assays for a number of hormones were developed after the bioassays, but before the radioimmunoassays that are described in succeeding paragraphs. Most chemical assays involve extraction of the hormone from a biological sample (e.g., plasma), followed by the initiation of some reaction converting the hormone to a product that can be detected by spectrophotometry or fluorometry. The major disadvantages of chemical assays are that they are generally not very sensitive or specific. The latter problem is caused by the presence in plasma of a variety of substances (in addition to the hormone of interest) that may produce the reaction product being measured. Thus, the problems in developing such assays are usually associated with the separation of the hormone from other constituents of plasma rather than with the means of detecting the extracted hormone. Since the hydrophobic hormones are easier to extract from plasma than the hydrophilic ones are, chemical assays have been used much more for measurement of the former than the latter.

Competitive Binding Assays. There are several specific types of competitive binding assays, all of which are based on the same principle to be described here for one of these types, the **radioimmunoassay (RIA)**. The necessary reagents for an RIA are: (1) a preparation of the hormone (H) of interest to use as a standard; (2) a preparation of the same hormone that has been labeled with radioactivity (*H); and (3) an antibody (AB) that will bind H and *H without being able to distinguish between them. The RIA is performed *in vitro*, and all tubes in the assay contain *H and AB. Some tubes (the standards) will contain a known amount of H, whereas the others (the unknowns) will contain a volume of fluid (e.g., plasma, urine, or tissue extract) whose concentration of H is to be determined. All tubes, containing fixed amounts of *H and AB, are incubated under appropriate conditions and the reaction depicted in Figure 2–3 is allowed to proceed. The reaction mixtures are then subjected to one of several possible separation procedures to segregate all free

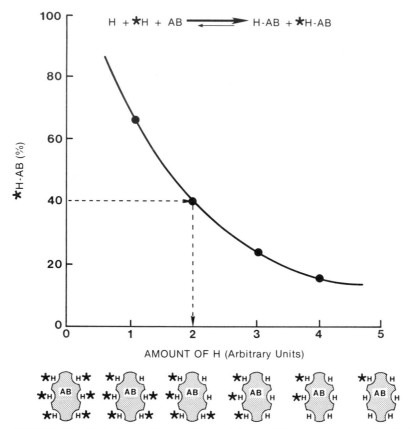

FIGURE 2–3. Illustration of the reaction and the analytical principles involved in RIA. The structures at the bottom represent antibodies (AB) binding various ratios of labeled hormone (*H) and unlabeled hormone (H) corresponding to the abscissa of the graph.

hormones (H and *H) from all bound hormones (H-AB and *H-AB). The latter fraction is retained and the amount of radioactivity in it is determined for each tube. Note that even though both labeled and unlabeled hormones are left in the tubes, the radiation counter can only "see" the radioactive product (*H-AB). The amount of *H-AB in each of the standard tubes is then plotted as a function of H concentration, yielding the standard curve depicted in Figure 2–3.

It should be emphasized that the amount of AB is chosen to be small enough to ensure competition between H and *H for a limited number of binding sites. As a result, if H is relatively low, then the AB will bind little of it and much of the *H. Conversely, with high H, the AB will bind much of it and little of the *H.

The crucial relationship that emerges from the standard curve (Fig. 2–3) is that *H-AB varies inversely with H and thus H can be determined by measuring *H-AB. Then, for each unknown sample in the assay, the amount of *H-AB is determined and read from the ordinate, across to the standard curve, and then down to the abscissa. Figure 2–3 illustrates that an unknown with 40% binding of *H-AB will contain two units of the native hormone, H. Note that the procedure for this analysis is the same as depicted for the bioassay described earlier in that a standard curve is generated from the results of samples with known hormone concentrations, and this curve converts the measured response in an unknown sample to a hormone concentration. The primary difference between the two cases is that the standard curve in the RIA has a negative slope because the two plotted variables (*H-AB and H) are inversely rather than directly related.

Protein-binding assays and **radioreceptor assays** are based on the same principle as just described for RIA. The only difference is that, in place of an antibody, one uses either a serum binding protein or a hormone receptor to bind the H and *H. Thus, the same type of competition is present and the procedures and the analysis are the same for all three of these assays. In practice, the standard curve generation, its linearization, and the calculation of potencies for unknowns are now usually done by a computer rather than the graphic procedure described.

The reason that competitive binding assays have been such a technological triumph for endocrinology is that they circumvent the problems of separating the hydrophilic protein hormones from other plasma proteins. This is a result of the fact that the antibody (or the specific binding protein) binds only the hormone it recognizes and does not interact with any of the other constituents that might interfere with a conventional chemical assay. Another advantage of competitive binding assays is that they are generally much more sensitive than bioassays or chemical assays. Such binding assays are also relatively inexpensive and easy to perform, which allows large numbers of samples to be assayed if necessary.

On the other hand, one must constantly be aware of the fact that an RIA measures immunological activity of the hormone, and this is not always highly correlated with biological activity. However, most RIAs have been demonstrated to agree with standard bioassays, and they have now become the most widely used assays. RIAs have been particularly valuable for protein hormones, but they are also readily available for steroid and thyroid hormones as well as a variety of other substances of medical importance.

Endocrine Kinetics

In addition to the commonly used methods of endocrine function assessment based on measurement of hormones in body fluids, it is sometimes necessary to measure the rate of removal of a hormone from blood. This can be accomplished by injecting a bolus of a trace amount of the hormone of interest (H) labeled with radioactivity (*H) and then collecting a series of timed blood samples for the measurement of the amount of *H in each. It is important to recognize that the difference between these two pools (H and *H) is that the plasma concentration of H does not decrease because it is constantly being replaced by secretion, whereas the plasma concentration of *H will decrease after the injection. Since the H and the *H are being degraded by the same mechanism and at the same rate, the analysis of the disappearance of *H allows calculation of the removal rate of H even though its concentration is not decreasing.

The rate of removal of most hormones from plasma is directly proportional to the plasma concentration of the hormone. Such a removal process is described as **first order** because it proceeds according to the following first order differential equation:

$$\frac{d[*H]}{dt} = -k[*H]$$

Equation 2–1

where t = time, and k is a constant

The solution to this equation yields the following equation, which is an expression of hormone concentration as a function of time:

$$[*H] = [*H_o]e^{-kt}$$

Equation 2–2

where $[*H_o]$ is the plasma concentration of *H at time 0

According to this equation, the plasma concentration of *H will decrease as an exponential function of time as depicted in Figure 2–4, Panel A. However, another version of the solution to equation 2–1 yields the following equation, which is that of a straight line:

$$\ln[*H] = -kt + \ln[*H_o]$$

Equation 2–3

Thus, from an analytical standpoint, it is much more convenient to plot the natural log (ln) of the plasma concentration of *H as a function of time as depicted in Figure 2–4, Panel B. The analysis of this linear plot of decreasing *H concentrations yields two factors that can be used along with the plasma concentration of the unlabeled hormone (H) to calculate its removal rate. First, the slope of the line is equal to the removal constant (k), which is directly related to the removal rate. Second, the y-intercept of the extrapolated straight line can be used to calculate the volume of distribution (V_d), which is the volume into which the total pool of *H (or H) is distributed assuming a constant concentration throughout the volume. This intercept equals the ln[*H] at time zero (i.e., the natural log of the concentration of *H that would have occurred if the total amount of *H injected had been instantaneously distributed throughout its V_d). The V_d can be calculated from this intercept and

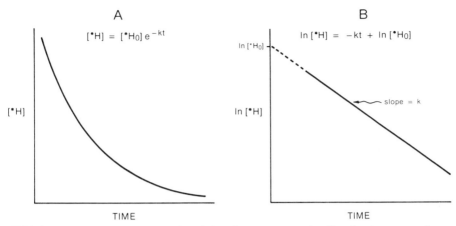

A

$$[^\bullet H] = [^\bullet H_0] e^{-kt}$$

$[^\bullet H]$

TIME

B

$$\ln [^\bullet H] = -kt + \ln [^\bullet H_0]$$

$\ln [^\bullet H_0]$

$\ln [^\bullet H]$

slope = k

TIME

FIGURE 2–4. Equations and graphs of the disappearance of radioactive hormone after a single bolus injection. This example is valid for those hormones, such as protein hormones, that do not readily enter cells. Note that plotting this disappearance as a logarithmic function of time linearizes the data.

the total pool of *H, which of course is simply the amount of *H contained in the bolus injection:

$$[^*H_o] = \frac{^*H \text{ Injected}}{V_d \text{ of } ^*H} \qquad \text{Equation 2–4}$$

This equation is simply a specific application of the general equation:

$$[H] = \frac{Pool}{V_d} \qquad \text{Equation 2–5}$$

that holds for both H and *H. Since both hormone preparations are being removed by the same mechanism, the V_d that is obtained is equally valid for H and *H.

Thus, our graphical analysis has yielded two variables (k and V_d), each of which describes one aspect of the removal process. However, a much more useful description of this process is provided by the metabolic clearance rate (MCR), which is equal to the product of k and V_d:

$$\begin{aligned} MCR &= V_d \times K \\ (\text{vol/time}) &= (\text{vol}) \times (1/\text{time}) \end{aligned} \qquad \text{Equation 2–6}$$

It should be noted that the concept of the metabolic clearance of a hormone is exactly analogous to that of a renal clearance used to describe the removal of a substance by the kidneys. It can be thought of as the volume of blood from which the substance of interest is completely removed (or cleared) per unit of time by the removal process. Continuing with the renal analogy, the actual removal rate (RR) of the substance can be obtained by multiplying the

MCR by the plasma concentration of the substance of interest, in this case the hormone H:

$$RR = MCR \times [H]$$
$$(\text{mass/time}) = (\text{vol/time}) \times (\text{mass/vol})$$

Equation 2–7

The clearance concept is as useful in quantifying the degree of activity of a hormone removal system as it is in assessing renal function. The advantage to using the clearance rate for these purposes is that it is not a function of the hormone concentration. In contrast, the removal rate is determined both by the efficiency of the removal system and the load against which it is working, namely the hormone concentration. Finally, it should be noted that, in the steady state in which [H] is not changing, the removal rate is equal to the production rate of H; if this hormone is secreted by only one organ, then RR provides an index of the rate of secretion of H by this organ.

The plasma half-life $(T_{\frac{1}{2}})$ of a hormone is often used as an index of the rate of its removal. The definition of $T_{\frac{1}{2}}$ in this context is the length of the time interval required for the plasma concentration of H to decrease to one half of what it was at the beginning of the time interval. As long as the removal process is first order, the disappearance curve will be of the form seen in Figure 2–4, and the value for $T_{\frac{1}{2}}$ will be the same no matter at what location along the curve this time interval begins. The $T_{\frac{1}{2}}$ conveys the same information as the k does, but they are inversely related by a constant as follows:

$$T_{\frac{1}{2}} = \frac{0.69}{k}$$

Equation 2–8

The specific value for this constant comes directly from the application of equation 2–2 to the specific case in which $t = T_{\frac{1}{2}}$; when t has this value, $[*H]$ must be one half of $[*H_o]$, and $\frac{1}{2} = e^{-0.69}$. Although the $T_{\frac{1}{2}}$ (or the k) is conceptually simple and widely used, it is not always sufficient. There are situations in which the V_d of a hormone may change and this would not be apparent from the $T_{\frac{1}{2}}$ or the k alone. Once again, we are led to the conclusion that MCR, which accounts for both $T_{\frac{1}{2}}$ and V_d, is the index of choice for quantifying hormone removal processes.

It is important to note that the preceding kinetic analysis characterizes, but it does not identify, the physiological processes actually responsible for the removal of a hormone from the circulation. Physically, the hormone may be biochemically degraded or transported across a membrane to another compartment. In either case, the kinetics of disappearance and the method of analysis would be the same. Finally, it must be recognized that the example presented in this section is the simplest type of analysis because the disappearance of the hormone was characterized by an equation with a single exponential term. Some hormones are cleared from the blood by several different biological processes that are governed by different rate constants. In these cases, the disappearance curve of the labeled hormone is more complex than the one in Figure 2–4. However, techniques available for the analysis of such data will yield an estimate of the MCR.

Diagnostic Procedures

The assays just described form an important part of diagnosing an endocrine abnormality. However, it must be recognized that these assays are essentially an endocrine "snapshot" that reflects the condition at the time the blood sample was obtained, but it is not especially informative about the dynamic function of the endocrine system. To obtain this information, it is often necessary to perturb the system in some way and then determine whether its response is normal. The two most common types of perturbations used are **stimulation** and **suppression** of the endocrine organ whose function is in question. These procedures will be described here only briefly since specific examples are presented in subsequent chapters.

Stimulation (or challenge) tests are performed by administering a hormone (or some other substance) known to elicit a secretory response from the organ of interest and then determining the magnitude of this response by measuring plasma concentrations of the secreted hormone before and after giving the stimulatory agent. Such tests determine whether the responsiveness of an endocrine organ is normal or not, and this information can indicate whether an endocrine defect is primary or secondary (see Fig. 2–1). For example, in the case of hyposecretion, the result of a target organ stimulation test will be less than normal if the condition is primary, but a normal response will be obtained if the hyposecretion is secondary to a pituitary defect.

Similarly, suppression tests can help determine the site of the defect in hypersecretory conditions (Fig. 2–1). In this case, a dose of the target organ hormone (or an analog) is administered, and some index of secretion by this organ is measured before and after the treatment. If the target organ is being driven by a hypersecreting pituitary (except for some pituitary tumors), this procedure will suppress target organ function. Failure to suppress indicates that the abnormality is independent of the pituitary and may either be primary hypersecretion or be caused by stimulation from an ectopic source.

REFERENCES

Griffin, J.E.: Dynamic tests of endocrine function. *In* Williams' Textbook of Endocrinology, 7th ed. J.D. Wilson and D.W. Foster, editors, W.B. Saunders Company, Philadelphia, p. 147, 1985.

Herschman, J.M. (ed.): Endocrine Pathophysiology: A Patient-Oriented Approach, 2nd ed. Lea & Febiger, Philadelphia, 1982.

Yalow, R.S.: Radioimmunoassay of hormones. *In* Williams' Textbook of Endocrinology, 7th ed. J.D. Wilson and D.W. Foster, editors, W.B. Saunders Company, Philadelphia, p. 123, 1985.

PART II

THE BRAIN-PITUITARY INTERFACE

3

NEUROENDOCRINOLOGY AND THE NEUROHYPOPHYSIS

GENERAL NEUROENDOCRINOLOGY

The two major systems in the body that regulate overall bodily functions are the nervous system and the endocrine system. Historically, these systems were viewed as separate entities, each operating independently of the other. However, it is now known that these two systems are intimately interconnected and normally work in close concert. This interaction was first recognized in lower animals, some of which rely on the brain and ganglia as the primary organs of hormone secretion. In humans, the functional relationship between the nervous and endocrine systems has been fully appreciated only over the past few decades. Thus the study of this relationship, **neuroendocrinology,** is a relatively new discipline.

Neuroendocrinology consists of two general divisions or directions. One

53

of these concerns endocrine effects on the nervous system. For example, an essential component of some of the negative feedback loops that regulate pituitary tropic hormone secretion is an inhibitory action of a target organ hormone on certain hypothalamic neurons. In addition, hormones can affect synaptic transmission and neuronal conductance of action potentials as evidenced by the abnormal reflex activity and the behavioral changes that accompany certain endocrine diseases. The other major division of neuroendocrinology consists of the effects of the nervous system on endocrine function. In some cases, there is direct innervation of endocrine cells so that such effects are mediated by the local actions of neurotransmitters. However, the more common type of interface between the nervous and endocrine systems involves a special type of neuron called a **neurosecretory neuron.** As implied by their name, these neurons are capable of secreting substances from their terminals called **neurosecretions** or **neurohormones.**

Characteristics of Neurosecretory Neurons

In many respects, neurosecretory neurons are similar to ordinary neurons; they have axonal and dendritic processes, they have polarized cell membranes that conduct action potentials, they exhibit tonic electrical activity, they release chemical messengers from their terminals, and they are regulated by other neurons that impinge upon them. However, there are several important ways in which neurosecretory neurons can be distinguished from other neurons (Fig. 3–1). First, neurosecretory neurons are **innervated, but they do not innervate.** That is, terminals from other neurons end on these neurons, but their own terminals end on blood vessels rather than on other nerve cells. Second, the product of a neurosecretory neuron is **released directly into the blood,** and for this reason is referred to as a neurohormone. In contrast, the product of an ordinary neuron, a neurotransmitter, is released into a synaptic cleft or neuromuscular junction. Finally, as a direct result of the previous distinction, neurosecretory neurons are unique in that their **products act over**

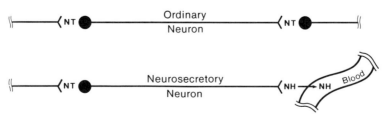

FIGURE 3–1. Comparison of functional arrangements of an ordinary neuron releasing its neurotransmitter (NT) into a synapse and a neurosecretory neuron releasing its neurohormone (NH) into a blood vessel.

long distances relative to the distance across which neurotransmitters act (e.g., a synaptic cleft of less than 50 nm). Some investigators consider neurotransmitter release to be "secretion"; therefore, they believe that all neurons should be classified as neurosecretory. However, we will use this term as in its original context to connote the release of a substance into blood by a neuron.

Based on this description of neurosecretory neurons, it can be seen that they form a crucial interface between the nervous and endocrine systems. Functionally, they can be viewed as transducers that convert the mode of information transmission from neural to endocrine. Such neuroendocrine transduction is often an integral part of all three of the major types of endocrine regulatory systems described in Chapter 1, namely negative feedback, neuroendocrine reflexes, and diurnal rhythms.

Neuroendocrine Systems

Although many endocrine systems contain some element of neuroendocrine regulation, there are three systems that are usually classified primarily as neuroendocrine systems in that their central elements are neurosecretory neurons. The first of these is the **hypothalamo-neurohypophyseal system** to be described in the rest of this chapter. The second is a population of neurons that both originate and terminate within the hypothalamus; these produce and release the **neurohormones that regulate the secretion of the anterior pituitary hormones.** These neurons and their hormones are still being investigated and much of their physiology is not yet known; this is the topic of Chapter 5. Finally, the cells of the **adrenal medulla** (Chapter 13) can be considered part of a neuroendocrine system because they are essentially differentiated postganglionic cells of the sympathetic nervous system. They release their products (epinephrine and norepinephrine) into the blood upon being stimulated by preganglionic nerve fibers.

A recent discovery in neuroendocrinology that adds both excitement and complexity to the field is that there are no longer clear boundaries among hormones, neurohormones, and neurotransmitters. Instead, a given substance may function in more than one of these ways within different systems. For example, norepinephrine is a neurotransmitter that is released into synapses by many sympathetic nerve terminals, but it is also a neurohormone in that it is secreted into the blood by the adrenal medulla. Similarly, many hormones secreted by classical endocrine organs are now known to occur within the neurons of the central nervous system. Many investigators believe that these "hormones" may also function as neurotransmitters or neuromodulators. Table 3–1 contains a partial list of substances found in both neural and endocrine cells. In some cases, neurohormones are now known to be "co-localized" with classical neurotransmitters or neuromodulators—that is, they are contained within the same neurons.

TABLE 3–1.   Some Biologically Active Substances Found in Both Neural and Endocrine Tissues

Neurotensin	Prolactin
Substance P	Growth hormone
Norepinephrine	β-Endorphin
Epinephrine	α-MSH
Somatostatin	ACTH
Calcitonin	TSH

THE HYPOTHALAMO-NEUROHYPOPHYSEAL NEURONS

Given the extensive regulatory influences of the brain and pituitary, it should not be surprising that a primary focus of neuroendocrine interest is the interface between these two organs. Also, most of the neurosecretory neurons of the body are located at this interface. The nature of the connection between the hypothalamus and the posterior lobe of the pituitary (the neurohypophysis) is straightforward and was first recognized long ago. This neuroendocrine system consists of a population of neurosecretory neurons whose cell bodies are in the anterior hypothalamus (supraoptic and paraventricular nuclei), and whose axons course through the median eminence of the hypothalamus, emerge to form the pituitary stalk, and terminate in the posterior lobe (Fig. 3–2). This portion of the pituitary also contains some supportive cells called **pituicytes.** However, from an endocrine standpoint, it is the nerve terminals that are the important part of the posterior pituitary. Thus, functionally and anatomically, the posterior lobe is simply an extension of the hypothalamus.

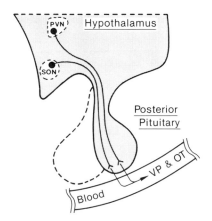

FIGURE   3–2. The hypothalamo-neurohypophyseal system, which secretes vasopressin (VP) and oxytocin (OT).

The cell bodies of the neurosecretory neurons comprising this system are relatively large, and thus the supraoptic and paraventricular nuclei are called **magnocellular** nuclei. These cells are large enough to have been characterized electrophysiologically. They display a bursting pattern of ongoing electrical activity, and such activity increases under those conditions that cause increased hormone release. Specialized staining techniques have also allowed the histological characterization of these neurons; this has led to much of our understanding of their physiology. For example, such staining has revealed granules of "neurosecretory material" within these neurons. These granules are distributed throughout the cell, but they are normally found in highest concentration within the nerve terminal. The observations that the granules in the terminals are depleted when hormone release is stimulated and that they accumulate when hormone release is inhibited led to the conclusion that this neurosecretory material contains the hormones. Similar histological studies revealed that the granules accumulate on the proximal side of an axonal constriction and are depleted on the distal side. These findings indicated that the hormone containing granules are synthesized in the cell body, move down the axon by axoplasmic streaming, and are stored in the nerve terminal until being released into the blood.

NEUROHYPOPHYSEAL HORMONES

In the human, there are two important hormones that are secreted by the posterior pituitary. These are **vasopressin (or antidiuretic hormone, ADH)** and **oxytocin.**

Structures

Vasopressin and oxytocin are cyclic nonapeptides whose structures are given in Figure 3–3. In both cases, the ring structure is formed by a disulfide

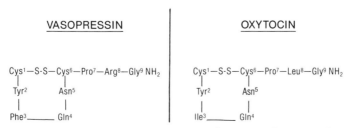

FIGURE 3–3. Structures of vasopressin and oxytocin.

bond between the two half-cystine residues; this bond is essential for biological activity. As a result of the structural homology between these two hormones there is some degree of overlap in their biological activities, but this is not great enough to be of much physiological importance. In addition to vasopressin and oxytocin, varying amounts of other peptides of this structural family are found in the posterior pituitaries of many species. For example, arginine vasotocin (the ring of oxytocin connected to the tail of vasopressin) is found in many species, including the human, but its physiological importance has not yet been established. Another analog, 8-lysine vasopressin, is the physiological antidiuretic hormone in only a few species, but it is just as active as the human hormone (8-arginine vasopressin). It has often been used in clinical testing and as replacement therapy.

Biosynthesis

The synthesis of vasopressin and oxytocin occurs in two stages, the assembly of amino acids into large precursors called **preprohormones,** followed by their post-translational cleavage to release the hormones (Fig. 3–4). The synthesis and packaging of these precursors into granules occurs by the usual mechanisms involving the ribosomes, rough endoplasmic reticulum, and Golgi

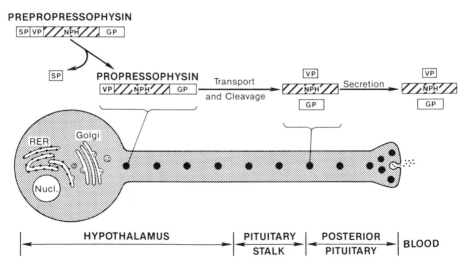

FIGURE 3–4. Diagram of a vasopressin-secreting neuron illustrating the subcellular components involved in synthesis and secretion. This process begins with the synthesis of prepropressophysin, which consists of (1) a signal peptide (SP); (2) vasopressin (VP); (3) neurophysin (NPH); and (4) a glycoprotein (GP). The production and release of oxytocin is identical except that no glycoprotein is involved.

apparatus (Chapter 1). The precursor for vasopressin is called **prepropresso-physin,** and that for oxytocin is called **preprooxyphysin.** The first step in the processing of the precursors is the removal of the signal peptide. This process, which converts the preprohormone to a prohormone, occurs in the endoplasmic reticulum. The subsequent cleavage of the prohormone to release the active hormone occurs in the granules as they move down the axon toward the nerve terminal. Each molecule of prohormone yields one molecule of hormone (approximately 1100 MW) plus one molecule of a large protein (approximately 10,000 MW) called **neurophysin.** The neurophysins associated with oxytocin and vasopressin differ slightly and are referred to as neurophysins I and II, respectively. The vasopressin prohormone also contains a glycoprotein that is released during this cleavage process. The neurophysins were discovered before the larger precursors and were initially thought to play some role in binding and transporting the hormones within the axons. It now seems more likely that these are simply cleavage products that arise as a consequence of hormone production. Since precursor cleavage is virtually complete by the time the secretory granules arrive at the nerve terminal, the mature secretory granules contain all of the cleavage products but essentially none of the intact precursors.

Within a given neurosecretory neuron, only one of the preprohormones is synthesized, and thus a given neuron secretes only vasopressin or oxytocin. However, in contrast to earlier beliefs, neurons producing vasopressin are located in both the supraoptic and paraventricular nuclei, and the same is true for oxytocin-producing cells. It should also be noted that in addition to the classical vasopressin- and oxytocin-producing neurons that terminate in the posterior pituitary, other fibers containing these hormones have recently been found to terminate in the median eminence of the hypothalamus and at numerous extrahypothalamic sites in the central nervous system. However, the physiological function of these peptides in systems other than the neurohypophysis is not yet known.

HORMONE SECRETION BY THE NEUROHYPOPHYSIS

The nerve terminals in which the neurohypophyseal hormones are stored abut on the capillaries of the posterior pituitary, and the hormones are released into blood by exocytosis of the secretory granules. As described in Chapter 1 (Fig. 1–1), this process involves the fusion of the membrane of the secretory granule with the cell membrane in such a way that the contents of the granule are released from the cell at the point of fusion (Fig. 3–4). The rate of hormone release at the nerve terminals is determined by the information received at the cell bodies of these neurons. The mechanism that couples these events involves membrane depolarization and Ca^{++} influx. Thus, it is referred to as **stimulus–secretion coupling,** in analogy to excitation–contraction coupling in muscle. This whole process is initiated by depolarization of the neurosecretory neurons in response to neural afferents in the anterior hypothalamus. When the membrane potential of the neurosecretory neurons reaches its threshold voltage, an action potential is generated that sweeps down the axon. The depolarization of the nerve terminal increases its permeability to calcium, allowing this ion to enter the cell down electrical and chemical gradients. The calcium then interacts with the secretory granules to induce exocytosis. However, the details of this interaction are not yet known.

NEUROHYPOPHYSEAL HORMONE DISTRIBUTION

The hormones of the posterior lobe are released into the systemic circulation and, like other hydrophilic hormones, are dissolved in the plasma rather than being transported in association with binding proteins. Because of the nonspecific nature of exocytosis, anything contained in the secretory granules is released. Thus, both of the neurophysins, and the glycoprotein derived from propressophysin, are released from nerve terminals with vasopressin and oxytocin. Neurophysin levels in blood can be measured and are known to fluctuate (with the corresponding hormone), but there is no known function for these proteins in blood. Some vasopressin is also released into the hypothalamo-hypophyseal portal vessels from those neurons terminating in the median eminence of the hypothalamus (Chapter 5). Vasopressin and oxytocin are also found in cerebrospinal fluid, where their concentrations vary diurnally, apparently independently of their plasma concentrations.

EFFECTS OF NEUROHYPOPHYSEAL HORMONES

Oxytocin

Oxytocin stimulates the contraction of the myometrium of the uterus and the myoepithelial cells surrounding the alveoli in the breasts. The details of these effects are presented in Chapter 10.

Vasopressin

Vasopressin, or antidiuretic hormone, has two major effects corresponding to its two names; it causes **contraction of vascular smooth muscle** (i.e., a pressor effect), and it enhances the **retention of water by the kidneys** (i.e., antidiuresis). The latter effect is of greater physiological importance, and under normal conditions, vasopressin is the primary endocrine factor regulating renal water loss and overall water balance. In contrast, the pressor effect of basal plasma levels of vasopressin plays only a minor role in regulating blood pressure. The pressor effect becomes substantial only under conditions that elicit extreme increases in circulating vasopressin levels (see below).

The antidiuretic and pressor effects just described are caused by the vasopressin that is released into the general circulation by the classical magnocellular system of neurons. In addition, the vasopressin released into the hypothalamo-hypophyseal portal circulation is thought to play a modulatory role in regulation of the secretion of certain anterior pituitary hormones. The function of the vasopressin recently found in extrahypothalamic areas of the central nervous system is unknown. However, evidence exists that this peptide can affect learning, memory, and behavior.

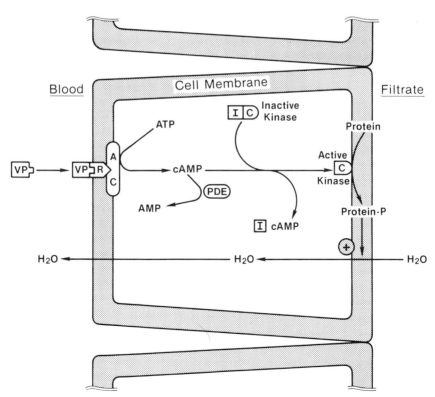

FIGURE 3–5. Antidiuretic mechanism of action of vasopressin (VP) on cells of the distal tubule and collecting ducts. R, receptor; AC, adenylate cyclase; PDE, phosphodiesterase.

MECHANISM OF ACTION OF VASOPRESSIN

The two primary effects of vasopressin are mediated by two different types of receptors referred to as V_1 (pressor effect) and V_2 (antidiuretic effect) receptors. It has been suggested that a third type of receptor is involved in vasopressin's action on anterior pituitary hormone secretion. Like the classical adrenergic receptors, these receptor types are distinguished according to the effects of various vasopressin agonists and antagonists.

The most completely understood action of vasopressin is the one that mediates its antidiuretic effect via V_2 receptors. Vasopressin decreases the free water clearance by the kidneys by increasing the permeability to water of the distal tubule and collecting ducts (Fig. 3–5). The first step in this action is the binding of vasopressin to the V_2 receptor on the target cell membranes. This binding occurs on the serosal, or peritubular, side of the cell, where it activates adenylate cyclase located on the inner surface of the cell membrane. As a result of this activation, ATP is converted to **cyclic AMP,** which is the intracellular second messenger. Cyclic AMP activates a protein kinase that phosphorylates certain membrane proteins; this results in an increase in the permeability of the luminal membrane to water. Thus, there is an increase in water movement down its concentration gradient from the dilute renal filtrate, across the tubular cell, and into the hyperosmolar extracellular fluid of the medullary region.

The mechanism of V_1 receptor-mediated effects is less well defined, but it apparently involves calcium rather than cyclic AMP as an intracellular mediator.

METABOLISM OF NEUROHYPOPHYSEAL HORMONES

Some intact vasopressin and oxytocin is cleared from the circulation by the kidneys, but most is first metabolized in liver and kidney by reduction of disulfide bonds and cleavage of the peptide chain. The plasma half-life of vasopressin is 15 to 20 minutes.

REGULATION OF HORMONE SECRETION

Oxytocin

The rate of secretion of oxytocin is regulated by several classical neuroendocrine reflexes as described in Chapter 10.

Vasopressin

Osmotic Regulation. The most important mechanism for the continuous regulation of vasopressin secretion is one in which secretion is modulated in response to changes in plasma osmolality. Like most negative feedback systems, this one is easy to understand when one knows what the action of vasopressin is and how this action would be expected to affect plasma osmolality. Clearly, the time that the body should enter a stage of antidiuresis is when the total amount of body water is less than optimal relative to total solute. Under such conditions the osmolality of body fluids increases, and this provides the stimulus to the secretion of vasopressin (Fig. 3–6). Osmosensitive cells located in the anterior hypothalamus monitor the osmolality of blood perfusing this area. These cells have not been identified with certainty, but, in contrast to the original proposal, it is probably not the vasopressin-secreting cells themselves that monitor the osmolality. The operation of this mechanism can best be illustrated by an example given in Figure 3–6. Elevated blood osmolality induces action potentials in the osmoreceptors, which activate the magnocellular neurons, producing vasopressin release from their terminals through stimulus–secretion coupling. The increase in the circulating vasopressin levels decreases the free water clearance by the kidney, resulting in a dilu-

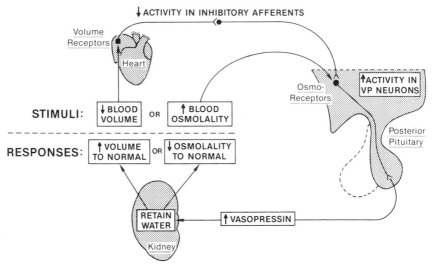

FIGURE 3–6. The major mechanisms regulating vasopressin (VP) secretion. A perturbation in either blood volume or osmolality will modify vasopressin secretion to contribute to the restoration of these parameters to their normal values. However, this restoration requires appropriate adjustments in water intake by thirst as well as the modulation of water retention depicted. Also, the two responses indicated may be affected by simultaneous changes in sodium balance.

tion of the hyperosmolar body fluids. As this process returns the osmolality to normal, the stimulus to vasopressin secretion is reduced, and its secretion returns to the basal rate. If water is retained in excess of solute and the osmolality of blood falls below normal, the mechanism just described is reversed to reduce vasopressin secretion, causing water loss until osmolality returns to normal. This is an extraordinarily sensitive neuroendocrine control system in that a change in osmolality of as little as 1 to 2 per cent will induce significant changes in vasopressin secretion.

Blood Volume Regulation. The mechanism of secondary importance in regulating ongoing vasopressin secretion is based on the maintenance of appropriate blood volume (Fig. 3–6). This mechanism relies primarily on the detection of changes in blood volume by stretch receptors in the atria of the heart. Decreased stretch (i.e., decreased volume) will decrease the rate of firing in these receptors. This information is conveyed over an inhibitory vagal pathway to the vasopressin-secreting cells in the anterior hypothalamus. These neurosecretory cells are activated (by the reduction of inhibitory input), and the result is an increase in vasopressin secretion, leading to conservation of water. This contributes to the restitution of blood volume. Similarly, increases in blood volume will inhibit vasopressin secretion. Changes in blood volume large enough to alter blood pressure will also affect the carotid sinus and aortic arch baroreceptors that contribute to the modulation of vasopressin secretion. Severe hemorrhage is the most potent stimulus known for vasopressin secretion, and it can result in plasma concentrations of vasopressin that are sufficient to invoke its pressor effect.

Other Factors. The mechanisms just described provide for the continuous regulation of vasopressin secretion. Since they function as negative feedback systems, they tend to resist changes in volume or osmolality by causing "corrective" changes in hormone secretion. In addition to this ongoing kind of control, vasopressin secretion can be altered by various more acute conditions (Table 3–2). For example, vasopressin secretion is increased by certain types of stress, pain, and a number of drugs (e.g., opiates). In contrast, some other drugs (e.g., α-adrenergic agents) and ethanol will inhibit vasopressin secretion. The physiological rationale for these factors in modulating vasopressin

TABLE 3–2. Factors That Affect Vasopressin Secretion

Increase	Decrease
Increased plasma osmolality	Decreased plasma osmolality
Decreased blood volume	Increased blood volume
Some stresses	Ethanol
Pain	α-Adrenergic drugs
Opiates	Opiate antagonists
Barbiturates	

secretion is not as obvious as for the blood volume and osmolality mechanisms. However, the effects of some of the drugs have been exploited in treating certain abnormalities in vasopressin secretion. The effect of ethanol on vasopressin secretion partially accounts for the copious flow of urine after the ingestion of beer. In addition to containing a large volume of water for the kidneys to excrete, beer contains ethanol, which reduces vasopressin secretion and thus impairs the kidneys' ability to retain water.

CLINICAL APPLICATION

Hyposecretion of Vasopressin

The primary symptom of vasopressin deficiency is the production of large volumes of urine, sometimes many liters per day. This condition is called **diabetes insipidus** because the urine is very dilute and "tasteless" (i.e., insipid). Diabetes insipidus is distinct from the more common diabetes mellitus, which is caused by an insulin deficiency. In the latter case, the large urine volume (diabetes) is caused by the renal loss of glucose, and thus the urine is "sweet." There are two types of diabetes insipidus; the one caused by inadequate vasopressin secretion is called **pituitary (or hypothalamic) diabetes insipidus.** There is also a **nephrogenic diabetes insipidus.** In this disease vasopressin is secreted, but the kidneys cannot respond to it normally, and thus they produce large volumes of urine. In addition, a psychiatric problem called **primary polydipsia,** or compulsive water drinking, causes polyuria or "diabetes."

Of course, one must be able to distinguish among these possibilities for a given patient in order to choose appropriate treatment. The measurement of plasma vasopressin concentrations is valuable in this process, but the availability of this assay is still somewhat limited. However, it is also possible to diagnose such problems with simple procedures by applying one's knowledge of the effects of vasopressin and the mechanisms controlling its secretion. For example, this system can be challenged by a brief period of dehydration followed by the measurement of urine osmolality (Table 3–3). In response to a period of fluid deprivation, a normal individual (or a compulsive water drinker) can conserve water by secreting extra vasopressin; in such cases, urine osmolality will increase in order to maintain normal plasma osmolality. In contrast, a patient with pituitary diabetes insipidus will not be able to increase vasopressin secretion, and one with nephrogenic diabetes insipidus will not respond to the vasopressin secreted, so that urine osmolality will not increase in either case.

Pituitary and nephrogenic diabetes insipidus can be distinguished from each other by administering exogenous vasopressin, which will correct the problem if it is of pituitary origin but not if it is nephrogenic. Note that the

TABLE 3–3.   Differential Diagnosis of Primary Polydipsia and Two Types of Diabetes Insipidus (DI)

Condition	Urine Osmolality After:	
	Dehydration	*ADH Administration*
Normal	Increase	Increase*
Pituitary DI	No change	Increase
Nephrogenic DI	No change	No change
Primary Polydipsia	Increase	Increase*

*If ADH is given to an individual who has just been dehydrated (as is often the case in such diagnostic testing), urine osmolality will show little if any further increase after the ADH since it may already be maximal because of dehydration.

deficiency of vasopressin is often referred to as hypothalamic, rather than pituitary, diabetes insipidus. This is because damage, or even removal, of the neurohypophysis causes only a transient diabetes because vasopressin production in the hypothalamus can continue. After a recovery period of several days hormone release resumes, even from the severed neurons of the pituitary stalk. Hypothalamic diabetes insipidus has many causes; one of the more common is tissue destruction by a hypothalamic tumor.

Hypersecretion of Vasopressin

The elevation of vasopressin secretion in the absence of the usual osmotic or volumetric stimuli is usually referred to as the **syndrome of inappropriate ADH secretion, or SIADH.** This condition is most often caused by a vasopressin secreting tumor, resulting in hyponatremia and low plasma osmolality. Such tumors are usually ectopic, with the lung being a relatively common site for vasopressin secreting tumors. Of course, if the cause of SIADH is a tumor, its removal should correct the abnormal water balance. SIADH from other causes can be treated by simply restricting water intake or by drugs that will increase free water clearance by the kidneys or reduce vasopressin secretion.

REFERENCES

Culpepper, R.M., Hebert, S.C., and Andreoli, T.E.: The posterior pituitary and water metabolism. In Williams' Textbook of Endocrinology, 7th ed. J.D. Wilson and D.W. Foster, editors, W.B. Saunders Company, Philadelphia, p. 614, 1985.

Ivell, R., Schmale, H., and Richter, D.: Vasopressin and oxytocin precursors as model prepro-hormones. Neuroendocrinology 37:235, 1983.

Kleeman, C.R., and Berl, T.: The neurohypophysial hormones: Vasopressin. *In* Endocrinology, Vol. 1, L.J. DeGroot, et al., editors. Grune and Stratton, New York, p. 253, 1979.

Krieger, D.T.: Brain peptides: What, where, and why? Science 222:975, 1983.

Reichlin, S.: Neuroendocrinology. *In* Williams' Textbook of Endocrinology, 7th ed. J.D. Wilson and D.W. Foster, editors, W.B. Saunders Company, Philadelphia, p. 492, 1985.

4

ADENOHYPOPHYSIS

INTRODUCTON

Anatomy and Development

The adenohypophysis includes both the **anterior lobe** and **intermediate lobe** of the pituitary. However, since the intermediate lobe in humans is rudimentary both structurally and functionally, this chapter will focus on the anterior lobe and its hormones. Anatomically, the anterior lobe is different from the other major portion of the pituitary, the posterior lobe. The latter is predominantly neural tissue that arises developmentally as an evagination of the diencephalon. In contrast, the anterior lobe is glandular tissue that arises from **Rathke's pouch** (oral epithelium) and migrates during development to the base of the brain to join the developing posterior lobe.

Historically, the functional relationship between the brain and the posterior pituitary was readily apparent because of the direct anatomical connection. In contrast, even though it was known in the 1940s that the secretion of anterior pituitary hormones was influenced by the brain, the mechanism of this regulation was not immediately apparent. Attempts to demonstrate neural connections between the hypothalamus and the anterior lobe were largely unsuccessful. Then, around 1950, it was proposed (primarily by Sir Geoffrey Harris) that the **functional link between the brain and the anterior pituitary is vascular, not neural.**

Blood Supply

Most of the blood supply to the anterior pituitary is derived, not from a direct arterial source, but from a portal system called the **hypothalamo-hypophyseal portal vessels** (Fig. 4–1). These vessels arise from a capillary plexus in the median eminence of the hypothalamus, course down the pituitary stalk, and then disperse to become the vascular sinusoids of the anterior lobe. These blood vessels were discovered as early as the 1930s, but they were described as "veins" and were originally thought to be the venous drainage of the anterior pituitary. Their role as the functional connection between the brain and anterior pituitary was proposed and confirmed only after establishment of the correct direction of blood flow. As implied by the term portal, a vascular arrangement such as this moves blood from one capillary bed to another without passing through the systemic circulation. This specialization allows for the local delivery of substances at relatively high concentrations. In the case of the hypothalamo-hypophyseal portal system, the blood flows from the hypothalamus to the pituitary, delivering hypothalamic factors that regu-

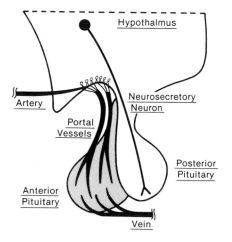

FIGURE 4–1. Diagram of the hypothalamo-pituitary unit contrasting the vascular connection between the brain and the anterior pituitary to the neuronal connection between the brain and the posterior pituitary.

late pituitary hormone secretion. The details of the hypothalamic regulation of the anterior pituitary are presented in Chapter 5.

ADENOHYPOPHYSEAL HORMONES

There are six protein hormones secreted by the anterior pituitary that have clearly established functions in humans. These hormones are listed in Table 4–1, in which they are grouped according to their structural families.

Names and Actions of Major Hormones

The actions of each of the major anterior pituitary hormones will be dealt with in detail in subsequent chapters (Chapters 6 through 10, and 14). However, a brief statement of their primary effects will be given now to provide the rationale for their nomenclature. **Follicle-stimulating hormone (FSH)** stimulates the growth and development of the ovarian follicles in females and is required for spermatogenesis in the male. **Luteinizing hormone (LH)** is responsible for ovulation, luteinization (i.e., formation of a corpus luteum), and regulation of ovarian steroid secretion in the female. In the male, this hormone regulates testicular steroid secretion by the interstitial (or Leydig) cells, and thus it has also been called interstitial cell–stimulating hormone (ICSH). In both sexes, **thyroid-stimulating hormone (TSH)** causes secretion of thyroid hormones and growth of the thyroid gland. **Growth hormone (GH)** is the primary hormone responsible for the regulation of overall growth of the body,

TABLE 4–1.   Six Major Hormones Secreted by the Anterior Pituitary Gland*

Hormone	Abbreviation	Size
Glycoprotein Family		
Follicle-stimulating hormone	FSH	96 (α)
		115 (β)
Luteinizing hormone	LH	96 (α)
(or interstitial cell–stimulating hormone)	(or ICSH)	115 (β)
Thyroid-stimulating hormone	TSH	96 (α)
(or thyrotropin)		112 (β)
Somatomammotropin Family		
Growth hormone	GH	191
(or somatotropin)		
Prolactin	PRL	198
Pro-Opiomelanocortin Family		
Adrenocorticotropin	ACTH	39
(or corticotropin)		

*Their sizes are given as the number of amino acids in the whole molecule or in the α- and β-subunits of the glycoprotein hormones.

and it influences both bone and soft tissues. **Prolactin (PRL)** enhances milk production in females but has no known function in males. **Adrenocorticotropin (ACTH)** regulates glucocorticoid secretion by the adrenal cortex and promotes adrenal growth. Because they each regulate the function of another specific endocrine organ, FSH, LH, TSH, and ACTH are called **tropic hormones,** and FSH and LH are more specifically referred to as **gonadotropins.** With the recent recognition that GH causes some of its effects by stimulating the release of other hormones (somatomedins) from the liver (see Chapter 14), it too is sometimes categorized as a tropic hormone.

Secondary Actions

In addition to the primary actions just listed, all of the anterior pituitary hormones exert a variety of other effects as well. For example, three of them (GH, ACTH, and TSH) have lipolytic activity. In addition to the primary roles of the gonadotropins described above, LH also plays some role in follicular development and FSH participates in the regulation of ovarian steroid secretion. Finally, in some species, prolactin plays an important role in modulating salt and water balance and it also has behavioral effects. However, these effects have not been established in humans.

Other Adenohypophyseal Hormones

β-Lipotropin. It has long been known that extracts of the anterior pituitary have lipolytic activity. Some of this activity can certainly be attributed to the lipolytic effects of known pituitary hormones, but there has also been speculation that there is an additional pituitary hormone whose only action is to stimulate lipolysis. Such a hormone has been identified; it is a 91–amino acid peptide called β-lipotropin. It undeniably has lipolytic activity and it is secreted by the anterior pituitary, but its importance in the physiological regulation of lipolysis has not yet been firmly established. Nonetheless, the interest in this peptide has been sustained because it was found to be a key intermediate in the post-translational processing of the preprohormone for ACTH and related peptides (see below).

Endogenous Opiates. There has been widespread interest in the recent discovery that the central nervous system contains several types of endogenous opiates, namely the **endorphins** and **enkephalins.** Like the opiate drugs (e.g., morphine), these peptides induce analgesia by binding to specific receptors in the brain. The endogenous opiates are not restricted to the central nervous system, and at least one of them (β-**endorphin**) is produced and released by both the anterior and intermediate lobes of the pituitary. In addition, some of these naturally occurring opiates have been shown to modulate the secretion of certain major adenohypophyseal hormones, either by acting on the pituitary itself or on hypothalamic neurons that regulate the secretion of anterior lobe hormones (Chapter 5).

Melanocyte-Stimulating Hormones. In many vertebrate species the intermediate lobe is more prominent than it is in the human, and it secretes several melanocyte-stimulating hormones (MSHs). In some of these animals, the MSHs play very important roles in regulating skin coloration by controlling the dispersion of melanin-containing granules called **melanophores.** Even though the intermediate lobe is rudimentary in humans, it does contain and may secrete two MSHs; these are α-MSH, which is a fragment of ACTH, and β-MSH, which is also part of the ACTH family (see next section).

STRUCTURAL FAMILIES

All of the adenohypophyseal hormones are proteins or peptides. However, on the basis of more detailed information about their structures, they can be subdivided into three separate families. This classification is convenient didactically, and it also helps one to understand the rationale for overlapping biological activities, cross-reactivities in assays, and the secretion of more than one of the hormones by a single cell.

Glycoprotein Family

The two gonadotropins (**LH** and **FSH**) and **TSH** are structurally similar glycoproteins, each consisting of two subunits (α and β). The subunits are held together by noncovalent binding, and each is itself a glycoprotein. However, neither type of subunit has biological activity when separated from the other. The α-subunit is virtually identical for each of the three hormones whereas the structure of each of the β-subunits is unique. Thus, the type of activity exerted by the whole hormone (e.g., TSH-like activity) is determined by the β-subunit. This has been demonstrated by recombination experiments. These show, for example, that β-TSH can be combined with an α-subunit from either FSH or LH to yield biologically active TSH. These subunits were discovered in extracts of pituitary tissue, but they are now known also to be present in blood. This is a result of their being secreted with the intact hormones from the pituitary rather than their being formed by systemic dissociation of the parent hormones. Even though the plasma concentrations of some subunits normally vary in proportion to the concentrations of the whole hormones, this ratio can change in some disease states. The physiological significance of these subunits, if any, is not yet known. Although not a pituitary hormone, chorionic gonadotropin is also a member of this glycoprotein family and is composed of α- and β-subunits that are similar to those of LH (Chapter 10).

Somatomammotropin Family

As implied by the name of this family, it contains **GH** and **PRL.** These are both single chain proteins with several disulfide bonds (two in GH and three in PRL). There is approximately 50 per cent homology between the structures of human GH and PRL. Among the pituitary hormones, GH is unique in that it is highly species specific. All pituitary hormones show some structural variation among species, but in most cases this variation is not great enough to cause significant functional species specificity. However, with GH, the extensive structural variation causes GH from most animals to be ineffective in humans, and this has had considerable clinical impact.

Pro-opiomelanocortin (POMC) Family

The members of this family are not only structurally related, but they are also derived from the same large precursor molecule. Thus they provide an excellent example of a process by which several peptide hormones with different biological activities can be derived from the selective cleavage of a large precursor rather than from the *de novo* synthesis of individual peptides. Furthermore, different cell types can make use of the same precursor and yet can specialize in the production of different cleavage products (hormones) depending upon their specific enzymatic composition. This is analogous to the widely known situation in which various steroidogenic tissues use the same general pathway of cholesterol metabolism to produce a variety of different steroid hormones.

The parent molecule (POMC) and the general cleavage cascade for this peptide hormone family are diagrammed in Figure 4–2. Although we will restrict our attention to the cells of the adenohypophysis, it should be noted that the same pathway exists in cells of numerous other tissues, including the central nervous system. It has also been proposed that some cells may take up an intermediate peptide of this cascade from the circulation and use it as substrate to generate other fragments rather than generating them from the parent compound, POMC.

The initial processing of POMC occurs in both the anterior and intermediate lobes and gives rise to **ACTH, β-lipotropin,** and an N-terminal fragment. Of all of the peptides in this cascade, ACTH (secreted by the anterior lobe) is the one of greatest physiological importance. ACTH is the simplest of the six primary hormones of the anterior lobe (see Table 4–1), having only 39 amino acids. Intermediate lobe cells also produce ACTH, but they use it primarily as substrate to produce α-**MSH** and the **corticotropin-like intermediate lobe peptide (CLIP).** α-MSH is simply the first 13 amino acids of ACTH, and the remaining fragment, CLIP, can be found in the circulation but has no known function. Both lobes of the adenohypophysis can cleave β-lipotropin to yield β-**endorphin** and γ-**lipotropin** (Fig. 4–2); the former includes the amino acid sequence of **metenkephalin,** and the latter contains β-**MSH,** but the pitu-

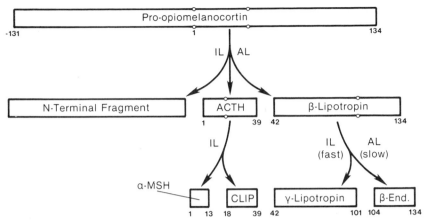

FIGURE 4–2. Cleavage of pro-opiomelanocortin to yield ACTH and related peptides. By convention, the numbering of the amino acids begins with the first one of ACTH and then increases positively toward the C-terminal and negatively toward the N-terminal. Cleavage occurs at pairs of basic amino acids indicated by the circles. Abbreviations not defined in the text are: IL, intermediate lobe; AL, anterior lobe; and β-End, β-endorphin.

itary appears not to secrete appreciable quantities of these two peptides under normal conditions.

ADENOHYPOPHYSEAL HORMONE STORAGE AND SECRETION

Cells of Origin

With one exception, there is a unique cell type that secretes each of the six major hormones of the anterior pituitary; the exception is the **gonadotropes,** which apparently secrete both FSH and LH. A good correlation exists between the staining characteristics of the pituitary cells and the structural categories of the hormones they secrete. The gonadotropes and **thyrotropes** (which secrete TSH) are **basophilic,** and the hormones they secrete are all glycoproteins. GH and PRL are secreted by **somatotropes** and **lactotropes,** respectively, both of which are **acidophilic.** Some uncertainty still exists about the classification of the **corticotropes,** which secrete ACTH (and probably some other POMC derivatives), but it seems most likely that they are basophilic. Some pituitary cells ("chromophobes") do not stain with common dyes. Among those that do ("chromophils"), there is a ratio of acidophils to basophils of approximately 3:1. As is true for other protein hormones, the anterior pituitary hormones are stored in membrane bounded secretory granules, the sizes and shapes of which can be used to distinguish specific cell types (e.g., somatotropes) within a general staining category (e.g., acidophils).

Hormone Release

The pituitary hormones are released by exocytosis, the process by which the membrane of a secretory granule fuses with the cell membrane in such a way that the hormone is extruded through an opening at the point of membrane fusion (Fig. 1–1). This process requires Ca^{++} and is regulated by hormones from the hypothalamus (Chapter 5). Estimates of daily secretion rates of the pituitary hormones are given in Table 4–2. Note that some of these rates are expressed in terms of "units," rather than mass, per day. This is not uncommon if a hormone's precise structure is not known or if the pure hormone is in extremely short supply. The units refer to an amount of biological activity compared to a standardized reference preparation that has been partially purified and widely distributed.

DISTRIBUTION OF ADENOHYPOPHYSEAL HORMONES

The anterior pituitary hormones are quite hydrophilic and thus are freely dissolved in the blood without being associated with carrier proteins. Approximate plasma concentrations are given in Table 4–2. Since all of these hormones are distributed throughout the body, it is worth reiterating that hormones can have quite specific sites of action in spite of this nonspecific distribution because the receptors for a given hormone are located only in those tissues that are target tissues for that hormone. For example, ACTH and LH are both delivered to the adrenal cortex, and both are steroidogenic hor-

TABLE 4–2.   Approximate Daily Secretion Rates, Basal Plasma Concentrations, and Half-Lives for the Six Major Anterior Pituitary Hormones

Hormone	Secretion Rate	Plasma Concentration	Plasma Half-Life
Glycoprotein Family			
Follicle-stimulating hormone	200 IU/day	1–12 mIU/ml	180 min
Luteinizing hormone	1000 IU/day	5–15 mIU/ml	30 min
Thyroid-stimulating hormone	50–200 μg/day	1.8 μU/ml	50 min
Somatomammotropin Family			
Growth hormone	1–2 mg/day	2–4 ng/ml	20–25 min
Prolactin	200 μg/day	6–10 ng/ml	20–30 min
Pro-Opiomelanocortin Family			
Adrenocorticotropin	25–30 μg/day	20–50 pg/ml	20–25 min

Data collected primarily from Daughaday, W.H.: The anterior pituitary. *In* Williams' Textbook of Endocrinology, 7th ed. J.D. Wilson and D.W. Foster, editors, W.B. Saunders Company, Philadelphia, 1985.

mones, but only ACTH increases adrenal steroidogenesis because this gland contains receptors for ACTH but not for LH.

It has recently been discovered that the "anterior pituitary" hormones are also located in extrapituitary sites, most notably the brain. It was initially suggested that these hormones were released from the pituitary and simply taken up by the brain from the circulation. However, it is now clear that certain regions of the brain can synthesize pituitary hormones (e.g., GH and ACTH). There is considerable speculation, but as of yet no proof, about what roles these hormones may play in brain function.

MECHANISM OF ADENOHYPOPHYSEAL HORMONE ACTION

The details of the mechanisms of action of the anterior pituitary hormones will be presented later in the appropriate chapters. However, it may be noted here that more is known of the mechanisms of action of the classical tropic hormones than of the mechanisms for GH and PRL. ACTH, TSH, and both gonadotropins act by binding to cell membrane receptors and activating adenylate cyclase. Beyond this common step, there is considerable divergence in the mechanisms of action because the processes of hormone secretion are quite different in, for example, the thyroid and adrenal cortex. The mechanisms of GH and PRL action are not well understood, but they appear not to involve activation of adenylate cyclase.

ADENOHYPOPHYSEAL HORMONE METABOLISM

Like other protein hormones, the anterior lobe hormones are enzymatically degraded in the liver and kidneys. In addition, significant quantities of the glycoprotein hormones are removed from the blood by the kidneys and appear in the urine. They may be modified somewhat in the process, but they retain both biological and immunological activity when excreted. The metabolic clearance rates of these glycoprotein hormones are inversely related to their sialic acid content. Thus, FSH, which contains the greatest amount of sialic acid, has a longer half-life than does LH or TSH. (The half-lives of the established anterior pituitary hormones are given in Table 4–2.)

In addition to systemic degradation, it appears that PRL is catabolized to some extent within the lactotropes. The contents of some of the secretory granules in these cells are released by exocytosis in the usual manner, but under conditions of low hormone release, some granules are degraded intracellularly by lysosomal enzymes. No physiological role for this autodigestive process has as yet been established.

REGULATION OF ADENOHYPOPHYSEAL HORMONE SECRETION

Types of Regulation

The two most important factors that regulate anterior pituitary hormone secretion are **hypothalamic hormones** and **feedback by target organ hormones** (Fig. 4–3). The release of each of the anterior lobe hormones is stimulated or inhibited by one or more of the neurohormones released into the hypothalamo-hypophyseal portal vessels by hypothalamic neurons. (This type of regulation will be presented in detail in the next chapter.) In addition, the secretion of each of the classical tropic hormones (FSH, LH, TSH, and ACTH) is influenced by the plasma levels of the corresponding target organ hormones. This is usually a negative feedback relationship in that increases (or decreases) in target organ hormone levels will decrease (or increase) the secretion of the tropic hormone (Fig. 4–3). The one exception to this is the positive feedback effect of estrogen on LH secretion, which causes an extremely dramatic rise in LH levels at one particular stage of the female menstrual cycle (Chapter 9). Some endocrinologists now consider GH also to be a tropic hormone since some of its effects are mediated by peptides (somatomedins) that are released from the liver in response to GH. Since somatomedins have been shown to inhibit GH secretion, it can now be said that GH also is regulated

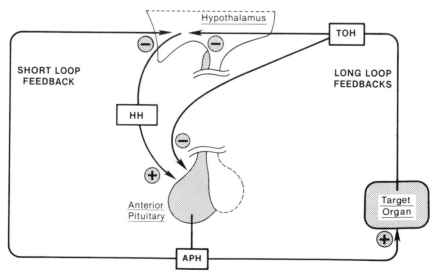

FIGURE 4–3. Regulation of anterior pituitary hormone (APH) secretion by hypophysiotropic hormones (HH), short loop negative feedback, and long loop negative feedback by target organ hormones (TOH).

by the negative feedback effect of a target organ hormone. These feedback effects of target organ hormones may be exerted directly on the pituitary or on the release of hypothalamic hormones, which in turn regulate pituitary function.

In addition to the traditional "long loop" feedback just described, some evidence exists for "short loop" feedback of the pituitary hormones. Short loop negative feedback refers to a pituitary hormone's suppression of its own secretion by acting at the hypothalamus to inhibit the release of a stimulatory neurohormone (Fig. 4–3). Of course, the same result could be achieved by enhancing the release of an inhibitory hypothalamic hormone. Most of the evidence for short loop feedback comes from animal studies, and the importance of such mechanisms in humans is not yet known.

Patterns of Secretion

In spite of the fact that negative feedback mechanisms tend to stabilize hormone secretion, none of the pituitary hormones is secreted at a constant rate. Thus, their plasma concentrations vary with time, and they often do so in a regular and predictable way. For example, the gonadotropins are released in short secretory episodes (in response to bursts of secretion of a hypothalamic hormone), which are then followed by more prolonged periods of little or no secretion. The gonadotropins also show a much slower type of secretory cyclicity in that a large "surge" of hormone release occurs approximately every 28 days in association with the menstrual cycle. As described in Chapter 9, these two secretory rhythms are controlled by separate mechanisms.

The plasma levels of the other anterior pituitary hormones all show diurnal variation, i.e., regular oscillations with a period of 24 hours. These rhythms are secondary to hypothalamic rhythms and they are particularly apparent for ACTH and GH. ACTH levels (like the glucocorticoid levels they drive) are highest around 6 AM and lowest around midnight. In contrast, GH levels are very low for most of the 24-hour period, with nearly all of its secretion occurring during the few hours after the onset of deep sleep. Frequent blood sampling throughout the day and night reveals that the diurnal rhythms in pituitary hormone levels are not smooth sinusoidal curves. Rather, they are characterized by a spiking pattern indicating that hormone secretion is occurring in discrete bursts separated by "silent" periods of little or no secretion. Although a bolus of hormone can be released into the blood almost instantaneously, it is cleared from the blood more slowly, as determined by its half-life. Thus, each burst of secretion causes a plasma concentration profile that has a steep rise but a more gradual fall (Fig. 4–4). As the frequency of these bursts is increased, they will begin occurring before the hormone from the previous burst has been cleared from the circulation, and thus they will combine to increase the mean plasma concentration. Therefore, a rhythm in mean concentration can be generated by varying the frequency of bursts of secretion.

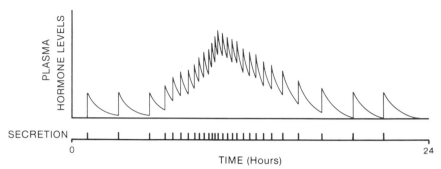

FIGURE 4–4. Hypothetical diurnal rhythm in plasma hormone levels due to changes in frequency of bursts of secretion.

One important consequence of these diurnal rhythms to the physician is that, when monitoring these hormones, he must know the time of day at which the sample was obtained in order to know whether the result is normal or not.

CLINICAL APPLICATION

Abnormalities in Pituitary Hormone Secretion

Hypersecretion or hyposecretion of the anterior pituitary hormones may be caused by many different factors, including developmental anomalies, autoimmune disorders, trauma, or, more commonly, pituitary adenomas. In some cases the abnormal secretion is a direct result of a pituitary disorder, but in others it is a consequence of either hypothalamic or target organ dysfunction. There may be simultaneous involvement of all anterior pituitary hormones (e.g., "panhypopituitarism"), "isolated" malfunction in which the secretion of only one hormone is abnormal, or any combination of disorders. The most common of the isolated secretory problems is excess prolactin secretion from an acidophilic adenoma.

Target Organ Abnormalities

Often, a normal anterior pituitary will secrete too much or too little of a tropic hormone because of abnormal secretion by the corresponding target organ. Thus, because of the feedback relationship between these two organs, some symptoms of target organ disease may result from secondary changes in pituitary hormone secretion rather than a direct effect of the abnormal target organ hormone levels. For example, primary hypothyroidism is characterized by a reduction in plasma levels of thyroid hormones, which stimulates TSH secretion. The elevated TSH levels cause one symptom of this disorder, namely hypertrophy of the thyroid gland (goiter). Even though the high TSH can elicit this growth response, it may or may not be able to induce an adequate secretory response from the diseased thyroid. Similarly, the hyperpigmentation in patients with primary hypoadrenocorticism is partially due to increased ACTH secretion, caused by the low cortisol levels. Recall that ACTH is structurally related to the MSHs. Because of this, it has slight MSH-like activity that can become apparent when the blood levels of ACTH are very high. In addition, low cortisol levels also increase MSH release, which contributes to the hyperpigmentation.

Assessment of Pituitary Disorders

The recent availability of radioimmunoassays for all of the anterior pituitary hormones has done much to enhance assessment of pituitary disease. Useful information can sometimes be obtained by simply measuring plasma hormone levels, although the interpretations of single measurements must take into account the temporal patterns of secretion described earlier. Often pituitary function can best be assessed under the more dynamic conditions of determining whether hormone secretion changes appropriately in response to suppression or stimulation. A suppression test is usually an attempt to reduce pituitary hormone secretion by giving a target organ hormone; these tests are straight forward and will be dealt with in subsequent chapters.

There are several types of stimulation tests (also called challenge or provocative tests) to assess the secretory capacity of the pituitary; this is often referred to as testing pituitary secretory "reserve." One common way of accomplishing this is to reduce the plasma levels of the appropriate target organ hormone by blocking its secretion pharmacologically. For example, the inhibition of adrenal cortisol synthesis (and thus secretion) reduces the negative feedback signal to the pituitary, and if the pituitary is normal, it will respond by increasing its ACTH secretion. The magnitude of this response (and thus the status of pituitary function) can be assessed in several different ways. Some other means of challenging the pituitary are not as closely related to normal physiology but have nonetheless been of clinical value. For example, ACTH reserve can also be tested by administering vasopressin or by inducing hypoglycemia by injecting insulin. The latter procedure, or the infusion of arginine, has also been used as a provocative test for GH secretion. Finally, as the hypothalamic hormones that stimulate the pituitary are becoming available (Chapter 5), they are being used to test pituitary function because they are the hormones that exert the physiological control over pituitary secretion.

Treatment of Pituitary Disorders

If a pituitary disorder is secondary to target organ dysfunction, it will, of course, be corrected by treatment of the primary disorder. Pituitary tumors are quite common causes of pituitary hypersecretion and they are usually treated by surgery or radiation therapy. Pituitary hyposecretion is treated by hormone replacement, the details of which depend upon the specific hormone involved. The sources of pituitary hormone preparations for clinical use include (1) pituitaries from domestic livestock, (2) cadaver pituitaries, (3) placental tissue and urine of pregnant women, (4) chemical synthesis, and (5) bacteria into which genes for human hormones have been introduced.

The method of choice for producing a given hormone is determined largely by its structural complexity and degree of species specificity. For the discussion of specific examples, it is again useful to divide the pituitary hormones into their structural classes.

Pro-opiomelanocortin Family. ACTH is the hormone that has been of primary interest in this family, and it has been available from animal pituitaries for many years. There is essentially no functional species specificity for this hormone; that is, ACTH from any of the mammalian species is active in all of the other species, including humans. There is some structural variation among the species, but the first 24 amino acids are the same in all types of ACTH. Of the six primary pituitary hormones, ACTH has the simplest structure (only 39 amino acids), and thus it was the first to have its structure determined and to be synthesized. Since the first 24 amino acids possess full biological activity, some synthetic preparations for clinical use consist of only these 24 (or the first 25) amino acids.

Glycoprotein Family. TSH, FSH, and LH are all available from animal sources. In addition, gonadotropin replacement is often achieved by treatment with a placental gonadotropin (human chorionic gonadotropin), which is closely related to LH both structurally and functionally. However, this hormone is much more readily available than LH since it can be extracted from placentas or from the urine of pregnant women. Similarly, urine from postmenopausal women is used as a source of a gonadotropin preparation with high FSH activity (human menopausal gonadotropin, HMG).

Somatomammotropin Family. In contrast to PRL for which there is little clinical need, GH has been in great demand but limited supply. The primary reason for the limited supply of GH is its species specificity. GH extracted from animal pituitaries was found to be ineffective in the treatment of pituitary dwarfs because the structure of human GH (and those of some other primates) is quite different from those of other mammals. The primary structure and synthesis of human GH was reported in about 1970, but because of its large size, the synthesis was not commercially feasible to meet the demand. Thus, the only source of this hormone continued to be human cadaver pituitaries, but, as noted earlier, the supply from this source has never been adequate and fear of viral contamination has caused its removal from the market. Recently, large quantities of human GH have been produced by bacteria that have received plasmids containing the human GH gene; the supply from this source is virtually unlimited. GH is the only pituitary hormone so produced, but this is also the only case in which there was any great need for this technology.

The technological problem of an adequate GH supply now appears to be solved, but this solution is giving rise to ethical problems for the medical community concerning the appropriate indications for GH treatment. The availability of GH offers the potential for much abuse by individuals who have no GH deficiency. The target for some of this concern is organized athletics, since GH has anabolic effects. In addition, there is a large "gray zone" regarding GH treatment for children within, but at the low end of, the normal growth range. Even more complicated is the anticipated demand for "cosmetic" GH treatment to increase the stature of children whose height is already absolutely normal. Such problems have not been encountered with most other types of hormone treatment. For example, many individuals with diabetes mellitus must receive insulin to survive, but a person without diabetes has no need for insulin treatment and no reason to request such treatment. The concerns about "hormonal substance abuse" in the past have centered largely on the anabolic steroids (e.g., androgens) and to a lesser extent on thyroid hormones, but GH can now be added to this list.

REFERENCES

Chappel, S.C., Ulloa-Aguirre, A., and Coutifaris, C.: Biosynthesis and secretion of follicle-stimulating hormone. Endocrine Rev. 4:179, 1983.

Daughaday, W.H.: The anterior pituitary. *In* Williams' Textbook of Endocrinology, 7th ed. J.D. Wilson and D.W. Foster, editors, W.B. Saunders Company, Philadelphia, p. 568, 1985.

Eipper, B.A., and Mains, R.E.: Structure and biosynthesis of pro-adrenocorticotropin/endorphin and related peptides. Endocrine Rev. 1:1, 1980.

Frasier, S.D.: Human pituitary growth hormone (hGH) therapy in growth hormone deficiency. Endocrine Rev. 4:155, 1983.

Keller-Wood, M.E., and Dallman, M.F.: Corticosteroid inhibition of ACTH secretion. Endocrine Rev. 5:1, 1984.

Morley, J.E.: Neuroendocrine control of thyrotropin secretion. Endocrine Rev. 2:396, 1981.

Refetoff, S., Frank, P.H., Roubebush, C., and DeGroot, L.J.: Clinical Endocrine Disorders of Hypothalamus and Pituitary: Evaluation of Pituitary Function. *In* Endocrinology, Vol. 1, L.J. DeGroot, et al., editors. Grune and Stratton, Inc., New York, p. 175, 1979.

**THE HYPOTHALAMO-
ADENOHYPOPHYSEAL INTERFACE**

**THE HYPOPHYSIOTROPIC
HORMONES**
Nomenclature
Actions
Structures

**DISTRIBUTION OF
HYPOPHYSIOTROPIC HORMONES**
Hormones in Blood
Cells of Origin

**HYPOPHYSIOTROPIC HORMONE
SYNTHESIS AND SECRETION**

**MECHANISM OF
HYPOPHYSIOTROPIC HORMONE
ACTION**

HORMONE METABOLISM

**REGULATION OF
HYPOPHYSIOTROPIC HORMONE
SECRETION**
Hypophysiotropic Neurochemistry
Hormone Feedback
Exteroceptive Factors
Enteroceptive Factors

CLINICAL APPLICATION
Hypothalamic Dysfunction
Differentiation Between Hypothalamic
and Pituitary Disorders
Hypophysiotropic Hormone
Replacement Therapy

5

ENDOCRINE HYPOTHALAMUS

THE HYPOTHALAMO-ADENOHYPOPHYSEAL INTERFACE

The physical connection between the hypothalamus and the anterior pituitary is the **hypothalamo-hypophyseal portal system** introduced in Chapter 4 (Fig. 5–1). The importance of these blood vessels as the **functional link between the brain and the anterior pituitary** has been established only over the last several decades. It is now clear that the secretion of all of the anterior lobe hormones is regulated by neurohormones that are delivered from the hypothalamus to the pituitary by these blood vessels. These neurohormones are secreted by neurosecretory neurons that arise in several different regions of the hypothalamus (see below), but the site of termination for all of these neurons is the **median eminence** of the hypothalamus. The median eminence is also the site at which the portal vessels originate. The nerve terminals end in close contact with the primary capillary plexus of these vessels, into which

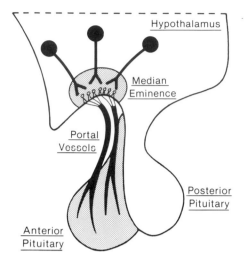

FIGURE 5–1. Hypothalamic neurosecretory neurons and hypothalamo-hypophyseal portal vessels.

they release their hormones. The anatomical convergence of these hypothalamic neurons at the median eminence has a functional correlate in that the hypothalamus receives diverse input from many brain areas. After integrating this information, it sends a simple signal to the anterior pituitary via the portal vessels to either stimulate or inhibit the secretion of a specific pituitary hormone. Because of this convergence, the median eminence is sometimes called the **final common pathway** for regulating adenohypophyseal secretion.

The vascular nature of the connection between the hypothalamus and the anterior pituitary is in marked contrast with the neuronal connection between the hypothalamus and the posterior pituitary described in Chapter 3. Although the physiology of the neurosecretory neurons controlling the anterior lobe is not as completely defined as that of the hypothalamo-neurohypophyseal neurons, it appears thus far that many functional similarities exist between these two groups of secretory neurons (described later). However, a major difference between them is that the posterior lobe hormones are released into the general circulation whereas the hypothalamic hormones are released into the pituitary portal vessels.

THE HYPOPHYSIOTROPIC HORMONES

Nomenclature

Since the neurohormones just described are "tropic" to the anterior pituitary, they are often called **hypophysiotropic hormones.** Depending upon the nature of their actions, they are also called **releasing hormones** or **inhibiting**

hormones. Before their identities were established, these substances were generally referred to as releasing or inhibiting "factors" rather than hormones. Because some but not all of these hormones have been identified, both terms are still in use, but "hormone" is generally reserved for those substances whose structures are known.

For more than 20 years before the identification of the first hypophysiotropic hormone in 1970, there was overwhelming evidence for the existence of these hormones. For example, upon transplantation to a remote site in the body, the anterior pituitary will revascularize and remain viable, but its function is dramatically altered. Such transplanted pituitaries secrete all of their hormones except one at greatly reduced rates; the exception is prolactin, which is hypersecreted. These findings indicated that (1) the normal location of the anterior pituitary has functional importance (even though this is not true for most endocrine organs), and (2) prolactin is normally under some tonic inhibitory control whereas the other anterior lobe hormones are normally regulated by stimulatory factors. Similar results were obtained when the portal vessels were transected with the pituitary remaining *in situ;* secretion of all anterior pituitary hormones except prolactin decreased, and hormone secretion returned to normal only when the vessels regenerated. This led to the conclusion that the vascular connection between the hypothalamus and the anterior pituitary was responsible for conveying the stimulatory and inhibitory signals to the pituitary.

Actions

The names and abbreviations of the seven generally accepted hypophysiotropic hormones are listed in Table 5–1; in each case, the primary action of the hormone is apparent from its name. It should be noted that although these hormones were named according to the function originally attributed to them,

TABLE 5–1. Major Hypophysiotropic Hormones*

Hormone	Abbreviation	Size	Site of Origin
Thyrotropin-releasing hormone	TRH	3	PVN
Gonadotropin-releasing hormone	GnRH	10	POA
Growth hormone-inhibiting hormone (or somatostatin)	GHIH	14	AHA
Growth hormone-releasing hormone	GHRH	44	ARC
Corticotropin-releasing hormone	CRH	41	PVN
Prolactin-releasing factor	PRF	?	?
Prolactin-inhibiting hormone (or dopamine)	PIH	—	ARC

*Except for dopamine (a catecholamine), their sizes are given as the number of amino acids in each. The abbreviations for their primary sites of origin are given in the text.

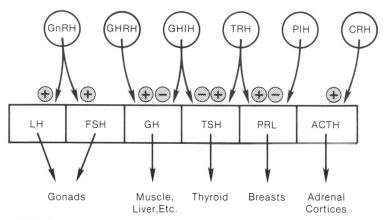

FIGURE 5–2. Overlapping functions of hypophysiotropic hormones (circles) in regulating secretion of anterior pituitary hormones (rectangles).

most of them have more than one effect. In contrast to the original proposal of one hypothalamic regulatory factor for each anterior pituitary hormone, it is now clear that there is both divergence and convergence in hypothalamo-pituitary regulation. That is, some hypothalamic hormones regulate the secretion of more than one pituitary hormone, and a given pituitary hormone may be controlled by more than one hypothalamic hormone (Fig. 5–2). For example, the hormone that was first found to stimulate LH secretion was initially called LHRH but is now generally called GnRH because it causes secretion of both gonadotropins. In other cases, a hormone's name is appropriate for one, but not for another, of its actions (e.g., TRH releases both thyrotropin and prolactin).

Structures

Of the hypophysiotropic hormones identified as of this writing, all except one are peptides; the exception is the prolactin-inhibiting hormone, which is dopamine. Perhaps it is not surprising that the first of these peptides to be identified is the one whose structure is much simpler than those of the other known hypophysiotropic hormones. TRH, which was identified in 1970, consists of only three amino acids as illustrated in Figure 5–3. The next two hypophysiotropic hormones to be identified were GnRH and somatostatin (GHIH) consisting of 10 and 14 amino acids, respectively (Fig. 5–3). Note that GnRH, like TRH, has a cyclic glutamic acid at its N-terminal and an amide at the C-terminal. Somatostatin is rather unique among these hormones in that it has a disulfide bond forming a ring structure. Also, there are several larger forms of somatostatin, but these are of unknown significance in humans. CRH and GHRH have only recently been identified and are somewhat larger than the

TRH

(pyro)Glu - His - Pro - NH$_2$

GnRH

(pyro)Glu - His - Trp - Ser - Tyr - Gly - Leu - Arg - Pro - Gly - NH$_2$

Somatostatin

Ala - Gly - Cys ————————————————— S - S ————————————————— Cys

Lys - Asn - Phe - Phe - Trp - Lys - Thr - Phe - Thr - Ser

FIGURE 5–3. Structures of the first three hypophysiotropic hormones to be identified.

three peptides noted earlier (Table 5–1). One major hypophysiotropic hormone still to be identified is PRF. TRH certainly can stimulate prolactin release, but its physiological importance in this regard has not yet been firmly established. There is also some evidence that PRF may be the substance known as "vasoactive intestinal peptide," a 28–amino acid peptide found in the hypothalamus and in many peripheral nerves.

The hypophysiotropic hormones have already been characterized in numerous vertebrate species and in some nonvertebrates. These studies have revealed very little structural, and virtually no functional, species specificity among these hormones.

DISTRIBUTION OF HYPOPHYSIOTROPIC HORMONES

Hormones in Blood

Like all hormones, the hypophysiotropic hormones are released into blood and thereby are distributed throughout the body. However, these hormones differ from most other hormones in that they are secreted into a portal circulation. As a result, they reach their target cells (in the anterior pituitary) in much higher concentrations than occur in the systemic circulation. This type of distribution is intermediate between a classical endocrine system in which the hormone is released into the general circulation and a neuronal system in which the neurotransmitter is released into a confined space (i.e., a synapse).

Cells of Origin

Even before the chemical identification of any of the hypophysiotropic hormones, it was known from stimulation and lesion experiments, as well as from studies of hypothalamic extracts, that these hormones were not homogeneously distributed within the hypothalamus. This suggested that the various hormones were secreted by different groups of neurons that arise from different regions of the hypothalamus. However, since the anatomical discrimination of these techniques was very poor, this functional zonation was rather gross. More recent immunocytochemical methods have allowed the identification and anatomical tracking of individual neurons on the basis of the specific hormones they contain. These studies have confirmed the earlier notion that the various types of hormone-producing neurons arise from selected nuclei and form reasonably discrete tracts *en route* to the median eminence. Because all of the hypophysiotropic hormones are transported to their nerve terminals and stored there until their release, the median eminence contains extraordinarily high concentrations of all of these neurohormones. As listed in Table 5–1, the paraventricular nuclei (PVN) contain the cell bodies of most of the TRH- and CRH-secreting neurons, whereas the arcuate nuclei (ARC) give rise to most of the cells that secrete GHRH and PIH (dopamine). Somatostatin- and GnRH-containing cells arise primarily in the anterior (AHA) and preoptic (POA) areas of the hypothalamus, respectively. The immunocytochemical studies that have allowed this mapping of the hypothalamus have also revealed that some of these hormones are contained in the same neurons as other neuropeptides or neurotransmitters. For example, certain hypothalamic neurons contain both CRH and the neurohypophyseal hormone, vasopressin. This phenomenon is generally referred to as **co-localization.**

The hypophysiotropic hormones are often called hypothalamic hormones because they were discovered in this region of the brain and they are clearly of physiological importance there. However, this term is a misnomer since nerves containing these hormones are now known to occur in many areas of the brain outside of the hypothalamus. The extrahypothalamic pools of these hormones are synthesized locally rather than being transported to these sites from the hypothalamus. Although the concentration of these hormones is highest in the hypothalamus, the total amount of hormone is greater outside the hypothalamus than it is within. It appears that these "hormones" are not released into the blood at these extrahypothalamic sites, but rather they are acting locally as neurotransmitters or neuromodulators. Their precise roles are unknown, but collectively they are thought to modulate a wide variety of functions ranging from motor activity,(TRH) to libido (GnRH).

Shortly after the discovery that the hypophysiotropic hormones were not restricted to the hypothalamus, it was found that they are even located outside of the brain. In fact, these peptides are widely distributed in nerves and endocrine cells along the gastrointestinal tract. Conversely, many peptide hormones first identified in the gut are now known to also occur in the brain. Examples of both of these groups of peptides are given in Table 5–2. Although the functions of these peptides in their "alternate" locations are not always apparent, it has been noted that their dual distribution may be related to simi-

TABLE 5–2. Selected Peptides Found in Both Brain and Gastrointestinal Tract

"Brain" Peptides Found Later in Gut	"Gut" Peptides Found Later in Brain
Somatostatin	Vasoactive intestinal peptide
TRH	Secretin
GHRH (in tumors)	Glucagon
Enkephalins	Gastrin
Neurotensin	Cholecystokinin

larities in embryological origin of the tissues involved. Somatostatin is present at numerous sites along the gastrointestinal tract; its function in the pancreas and gastrointestinal tract are described in detail in Chapter 12.

HYPOPHYSIOTROPIC HORMONE SYNTHESIS AND SECRETION

With the exception of dopamine, which is a catecholamine, all of the known hypophysiotropic hormones are peptides that are synthesized as large precursors, which then undergo post-translational cleavage to produce the hormones. These hormones are packaged in secretory granules that are transported to the nerve terminals where they are stored until released. Although the release process has not yet been studied extensively, all that is known is analogous to the stimulus-secretion coupling that occurs in the neurosecretory neurons of the posterior pituitary (Chapter 3). Thus, depolarization of the neurons in the presence of Ca^{++} causes exocytosis of the stored granules into the perivascular space. The hormones then rapidly diffuse into the fenestrated capillaries and are transported to the anterior pituitary.

MECHANISM OF HYPOPHYSIOTROPIC HORMONE ACTION

The effects of the hypophysiotropic hormones, like those of other peptide hormones, are initiated by their binding to receptors on the membranes of target cells. The intracellular coupling between this binding and the subsequent release of pituitary hormones is a subject of current investigation, but little is known with certainty. It appears that the mechanisms may differ among the hypophysiotropic hormones, and that they may even differ for a given hormone (e.g., TRH) that affects the secretion of more than one pituitary hormone (i.e., TSH and PRL). Some of the earlier studies on the intracellular mechanism of action of these hormones suggested that cyclic AMP was involved as a second messenger, but this view is no longer widely held. Instead, much of the current work indicates that the effects of at least some of the hypophysiotropic hormones (e.g., TRH and GnRH) are mediated by intracellular Ca^{++} and the **polyphosphoinositide system.** This second messenger system is thought to mediate the actions of various neurotransmitters and hormones. Since the Ca^{++}-polyphosphoinositide system has been most completely characterized for α_1-adrenergic receptor mediated effects, it is described in detail in the chapter on adrenal medullary hormones (Chapter 13). The system is somewhat unusual in that it involves two intracellular second messengers, both of which are derived from a membrane polyphosphoinositide called **phosphatidylinositol 4,5-bisphosphate (PIP$_2$).** The binding of a hormone to its receptor induces very rapid hydrolysis of PIP$_2$ by phospholipase C to yield the two messengers, **inositol triphosphate (IP$_3$)** and **diacylglycerol.** IP$_3$ causes an increase in intracellular Ca^{++}, initially from an intracellular store (probably the endoplasmic reticulum) and later from extracellular Ca^{++}. The other product of PIP$_2$ hydrolysis, diacylglycerol, mediates hormone action by activating protein kinase C. This kinase then phosphorylates certain enzymes that, along with the elevated intracellular calcium, are responsible for the final biological effects of the hormone (see Fig. 13–4).

HORMONE METABOLISM

Since the hypophysiotropic hormones have only recently been discovered, not much is known yet about their metabolism. Not surprisingly, most of what is known concerns those hormones discovered first, such as TRH and GnRH. In general, these hormones have short half-lives, on the order of several minutes.

TRH is enzymatically degraded in various tissues, including plasma, pituitary, brain, liver, and kidney. One pathway for TRH degradation is deamidation, and another is cleavage of the pyroglutamyl residue by a peptidase.

REGULATION OF HYPOPHYSIOTROPIC HORMONE SECRETION

This section will consider the regulation of hypophysiotropic hormone secretion from several perspectives. First, the biochemical inputs to the neurosecretory neurons, both neurotransmitters and circulating hormones, will be examined. Then the influences of various conditions, both exteroceptive and enteroceptive, on the hypothalamo-pituitary unit will be considered.

Hypophysiotropic Neurochemistry

Like other neurons, those secreting the hypophysiotropic hormones receive synaptic input from many other neurons (Fig. 5–4). Even before the identification of these neurohormones, attempts were made to determine which neurotransmitters were responsible for exerting control over the secre-

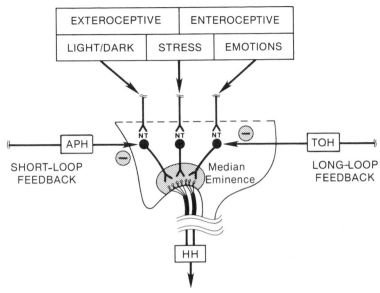

FIGURE 5–4. Regulation of hypophysiotropic hormone (HH) secretion by various factors via neurotransmitters (NT), and by negative feedback effects of anterior pituitary hormones (APH) and target organ hormones (TOH).

tion of the hypophysiotropic hormones. Such studies are still in progress, and the results to date are so complex that no simple summary can be given. Nonetheless, there is now reasonable evidence that most of the known neurotransmitters can act at various hypothalamic sites to modulate hypophysiotropic hormone secretion. For example, norepinephrine has been shown to affect the secretion of all of the major anterior pituitary hormones by modulating hypophysiotropic hormone release. Depending upon the hormone involved and on the precise hypothalamic location, the effects of norepinephrine may be either stimulatory or inhibitory.

In addition to the classical neurotransmitters, there are many neuropeptides (such as those listed in Table 5–2) that are now being investigated for their possible importance in regulating hypophysiotropic hormone secretion. Among the neuropeptides investigated, the endogenous opioids have perhaps been of most interest, and have been shown to affect the secretion of all of the major anterior pituitary hormones by modulating the secretion of the corresponding hypophysiotropic hormones.

Hormone Feedback

In addition to being regulated by neurotransmitters, the hypophysiotropic neurons are controlled by various hormones that reach the hypothalamus via the blood (Fig. 5–4). Most of these effects are negative feedback effects of either anterior pituitary or target organ hormones (Chapter 4). The latter type of feedback (long loop) is of greater physiological importance and may be exerted either at the pituitary or at the hypothalamus. It is generally accepted that the thyroid hormones feed back primarily at the anterior pituitary, whereas the other target organ hormones (glucocorticoids and sex steroids) act primarily at the hypothalamus, and thus regulate pituitary tropic hormone secretion by regulating hypophysiotropic hormone release. On the other hand, short loop feedback by anterior pituitary hormones is exerted only at the hypothalamus and may be involved in regulating the secretion of both tropic and nontropic hormones. Thus, the biochemical inputs to the hypophysiotropic neurons consist of both neurotransmitters and hormones. As a result of these various factors acting at both levels of the hypothalamo-pituitary unit, both stimulatory and inhibitory elements contribute to the overall regulation of each of the major anterior pituitary hormones.

Exteroceptive Factors

The hypophysiotropic neurons receive neuronal input from many different areas of the brain, which can provide information related to a wide variety of environmental conditions. The example of endocrine diurnal rhythms being entrained by light–dark cycles has already been described. In addition, in many species, certain visual and tactile stimuli associated with courting rituals and copulation act through the central nervous system to stimulate gonadotropin secretion. Also prevalent in lower animals, and perhaps operative in humans, are the olfactory signals called **pheromones.** These are also called "exohormones" because they transmit information between individuals within a species. Many pheromones are associated with reproductive function in species ranging from insects to primates; they may function in various ways such as communicating sexual attraction, modulating gonadotropin secretion, and even terminating pregnancy. The role of pheromones in human reproduction is thought to be limited, but they may be responsible for the fact that women who live together sometimes have synchronous menstrual cycles. It is thought that pheromonal communication can occur without the recipient being consciously aware that a signal has been received.

Physical stress or trauma affects the secretion of all of the hypophysiotropic hormones in one way or another. The secretion of CRH (and thus ACTH) is increased by all types of stress, and in fact a common endocrine definition of stress is "any condition that will elicit ACTH secretion." The effects of physical stress on the secretion of the other anterior pituitary hormones are somewhat variable, but as a general rule, TSH secretion is inhibited and GH secretion is stimulated. As noted earlier, both TSH and GH are under the influences of both stimulatory and inhibitory hormones from the hypothalamus. However, it is not yet known which particular hypophysio-tropic hormones mediate the effects of stress on their secretion.

Enteroceptive Factors

There are numerous neuroanatomical connections between the hypothal-amus and the portions of the brain that are concerned with emotions (i.e., the limbic system). Thus, hypophysiotropic hormone secretion is greatly influ-enced by the emotions. From an endocrine standpoint, an emotional distur-bance is as much a "stress" as is physical trauma; CRH and ACTH secretion are increased, and the other hormones of the hypothalamo-pituitary unit are affected in various ways. A common clinical manifestation of this phenomenon is the menstrual irregularities in women who are emotionally upset. Similarly, failure to lactate is often due to psychological factors.

Finally, it should be noted that continuous interaction occurs among the various factors that regulate hypophysiotropic hormone secretion. For exam-ple, negative feedback loops strive to maintain relatively constant hormone levels, but superimposed on this type of regulation are the diurnal rhythms. Similarly, stress mechanisms may "break through" the negative feedback mechanisms to alter hormone secretion at times of special need.

CLINICAL APPLICATION

Hypothalamic Dysfunction

Only those hypothalamic neurons that secrete the hypophysiotropic hor-mones have been described in this chapter, but of course there are also many other cells in the hypothalamus and they regulate a wide variety of other func-tions. Thus, the symptoms of hypothalamic dysfunction may or may not in-clude endocrine symptoms. For example, psychological disturbances, prob-lems with food and water intake, abnormal thermoregulation, and a variety of other neurological symptoms such as headaches and eye signs may be caused by hypothalamic disease. A variety of pituitary abnormalities may also be caused by hypothalamic disease; these are manifested as hypersecretion or hy-posecretion depending upon whether the affected hypothalamic hormone is stimulatory or inhibitory and whether its secretion is increased or decreased. Hypothalamic hyposecretion will increase prolactin release (because of its tonic inhibitory control by the hypothalamus), whereas this condition will re-duce the secretion of the other anterior pituitary hormones. Like intrinsic pi-tuitary disease, hypothalamic disease may involve only one or numerous pitu-itary hormones. Reproductive disorders, particularly precocious puberty, are among the more common endocrine symptoms of hypothalamic disease. How-ever, it should be noted that hypothalamic dysfunction is actually not very common.

Differentiation Between Hypothalamic and Pituitary Disorders

The endocrine manifestations of hypothalamic disease are the same as those of pituitary disease. Because of this, and because assays for the hypophysiotropic hormones are not generally available in clinical laboratories, it is not always easy to distinguish hypothalamic from pituitary disease. With the recent availability of several hypophysiotropic hormones and of reliable assays for anterior pituitary hormones, it is now sometimes possible to make this distinction by doing a "pituitary stimulation test." For example, if the pituitary is hyposecreting one of its tropic hormones, this could be caused by an intrinsic pituitary problem or it could be secondary to hypothalamic hyposecretion of the corresponding releasing hormone. In the latter situation the pituitary is essentially normal and will give a normal (or exaggerated) secretory response when stimulated with exogenous releasing hormone. In contrast, a subnormal response would indicate pituitary disease. This procedure is analogous to the more common procedure for distinguishing pituitary from target organ disease described in Chapter 2. The application of this approach to the diagnosis of hypothalamic disease is certainly sound in theory and it has been of some value in practice. However, because of the relatively wide variation in pituitary responses among individuals, it is sometimes difficult to classify the response in a given patient as normal or abnormal. Consistent with the description of target organ disease as "primary" and pituitary disease as "secondary" disorders, hypothalamic disease is often referred to as "tertiary" endocrine dysfunction.

Hypophysiotropic Hormone Replacement Therapy

Although the hypothalamic releasing and inhibiting hormones have only recently been discovered, they are already being used for a variety of purposes in the diagnosis and treatment of endocrine diseases. Also, because of recent advances in peptide chemistry, many analogs (i.e., thousands) of these hormones have been synthesized. Somatostatin may be unique among the hypophysiotropic hormones in that it has been used for several therapeutic purposes even though no specific endocrine disease has yet been attributed to its absence. In addition to inhibiting growth hormone secretion, somatostatin has a wide variety of other inhibitory effects. Thus, it has been used to treat diabetes mellitus (Chapter 12) and gastrointestinal disorders as well as acromegaly (excess growth hormone secretion).

Temporal Considerations. Even before the clinical testing of certain hypophysiotropic hormones, the results of animal studies suggested that the temporal pattern of treatment with these hormones might be important. As described earlier, many of the hypophysiotropic (and thus anterior pituitary) hormones are secreted in a pulsatile or episodic pattern rather than at a constant rate. Thus, it was not surprising to find that these hormones are most effective therapeutically when administered in a pulsatile fashion that mimics the pattern of their secretion *in vivo*. An example of this phenomenon is the treatment of hypogonadotropic hypogonadism with GnRH. This disease is characterized by gonadal hypofunction in spite of relatively normal overall plasma levels of gonadotropins (Chapter 8). However, when examined in greater temporal detail, it appears that the **secretory pattern** of gonadotropins in such patients is abnormal and may in fact be responsible for the disease. This is supported by the finding that reproductive function can be normalized by treating these patients with GnRH in a pulsatile pattern that mimics the endogenous GnRH pattern of secretion.

Neuroendocrine Pharmacology. Physiologically, the modulation of hypophysiotropic hormone release is provided by neurotransmitters from the neurons impinging upon hypophysiotropic neurons (see Fig. 5–4.). As more is learned about the identities of these neurotransmitters, one can envision the use of neurotransmitter agonists or antagonists in the treatment of hypothalamic endocrine dysfunction. This would be analogous to the current use of a dopamine precursor to treat parkinsonism, which is caused by inadequate dopamine in a specific region of the brain. However, with such therapy, one must bear in mind a basic difference between neurotransmitters and hormones. Hormones are normally distributed throughout the body, but their receptors occur only in specific (target) tissues. Thus, with classical (i.e., systemic) endocrine therapy one can be assured that the exogenous hormone will be distributed as is the endogenous hormone and will act only at target tissues. In contrast, systemic treatment with a neurotransmitter (or a drug that alters neurotransmitters) does not mimic the distribution of endogenous neurotransmitters. Thus, various side effects may result because the same neurotransmitter is used in many synapses other than the ones of interest involving the hypophysiotropic neurons. The reproductive dysfunction that occurs in individuals receiving drugs that alter catecholamine economy may be an example of such a complication.

REFERENCES

Ben-Jonathan, J.: Dopamine: A prolactin-inhibiting hormone. Endocrine Rev. 6:564, 1985.

Bex, F.J., and Corbin, A.: LHRH and analogs: Reproductive pharmacology and contraceptive and therapeutic utility. *In* Frontiers in Neuroendocrinology, L. Martini and W.F. Ganong, editors, Raven Press, New York, p. 85, 1984.

Conn, P.M.: The molecular basis of gonadotropin-releasing hormone action. Endocrine Rev. 7:3, 1986.

Gershengorn, M.C.: Thyrotropin releasing hormone: A review of the mechanisms of acute stimulation of pituitary hormone release. Molec. Cell. Biochem. 45:163, 1982.

Hokin, L.E.: Receptors and phosphoinositide-generated second messengers. Ann. Rev. Biochem. 54:205, 1985.

Ramirez, V.D., Feder, H.H., and Sawyer, C.H.: The role of brain catecholamines in the regulation of LH secretion: A critical inquiry. *In* Frontiers in Neuroendocrinology, L. Martini and W.F. Ganong, editors. Raven Press, New York, p. 27, 1984.

Reichlin, S.: Medical progress: Somatostatin—Parts I and II. N. Engl. J. Med., 309:1495 and 1556, 1983.

Reichlin, S.: Neuroendocrinology. *In* Williams' Textbook of Endocrinology, 7th ed. J.D. Wilson and D.W. Foster, editors, W.B. Saunders Company, Philadelphia, p. 492, 1985.

Santoro, N., Filicori, M., and Crowley, Jr.,W.F.: Hypogonadotropic disorders in men and women: Diagnosis and therapy with pulsatile gonadotropin-releasing hormone. Endocrine Rev. 7:11, 1986.

Vale, W., and Greer, M. (eds): Corticotropin-Releasing Factor. Fed. Proc., Vol. 44, 1985.

PART III

ENDOCRINE SYSTEMS

6

THYROID PHYSIOLOGY

THE THYROID GLAND

The thyroid gland consists of two lobes of endocrine tissue located just below the larynx on each side of the trachea; these lobes are attached to each other ventrally by a narrow portion of the gland called the **isthmus**. The function of this organ is to secrete thyroid hormones, which are important regulators of overall metabolism in most tissues. A tropic hormone from the anterior pituitary gland provides the primary means of maintaining both the structure and the function (secretion) of the thyroid. This tropic hormone is, in turn, subject to negative feedback regulation by the thyroid hormones.

101

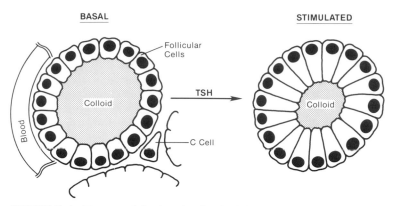

FIGURE 6–1. Diagram of the functional unit of the thyroid, the follicle, in both basal and stimulated states.

Functional Anatomy

The cells that secrete the thyroid hormones are organized into functional units called **follicles** (Fig. 6–1). Each follicle is composed of a layer of cells at its periphery surrounding an inner lumen filled with **colloid,** a substance that contains thyroid hormones and serves as an extracellular storage reservoir for the hormones. Under conditions of basal thyroid hormone secretion, the follicular cells are rather cuboidal or even flattened, and the lumen of the follicle is large. When the cells are stimulated to secrete their hormones, they become larger and more columnar at the expense of the lumen. The latter decreases in size as the colloid is consumed to provide the hormones that are released.

Interspersed among the follicles are the **parafollicular, or C, cells** which have no apparent functional relationship to the follicular cells. These are called C cells because they secrete a hormone, **calcitonin,** which contributes to the endocrine regulation of calcium balance; this hormone will be considered in more detail in Chapter 16.

Also coursing among the follicles are blood vessels and nerves. The basal blood flow to the thyroid is higher than to any other endocrine organ and it may increase even further with certain types of thyroid disease. Of course, these vascular connections comprise the primary functional connections for the thyroid because its products leave by this route and the tropic hormone that regulates thyroid function arrives via the blood. In addition to this primary (hormonal) mode of regulation, there is some evidence that the thyroid nerves may participate in modulating thyroid function. The thyroid gland receives adrenergic, cholinergic, and peptidergic nerve fibers that terminate on both blood vessels and follicular cells. However, the extent of the involvement of these nerves in regulating thyroid blood flow and hormone secretion is not yet established.

THYROID HORMONES AND THEIR SYNTHESIS

Structural Characteristics

The first thyroid hormone to be discovered was **tetraiodothyronine (T_4 or thyroxine)**. Subsequently it was recognized that the thyroid secretes another hormone as well, **triiodothyronine (T_3)**; this hormone is structurally similar to T_4 but its biological potency is several times greater than that of T_4. There is also a third iodinated thyronine of interest found in blood, **reverse T_3 (rT_3)**. However, in contrast to T_3 and T_4, little if any of this material is secreted by the thyroid, and it has virtually none of the biological effects of T_3 and T_4. As depicted in Figure 6–2, the subscripts in these abbreviations indicate the number of iodine molecules contained in these hormones.

Biosynthesis

Before the specific steps in thyroid hormone biosynthesis are considered, it may be helpful to present an overview of the entire process. The basic ingredients for this process are **iodide** and the amino acid **tyrosine,** both of which must be sequestered from the blood by the follicular cells. Throughout the biosynthetic process, the tyrosine remains incorporated in a large protein.

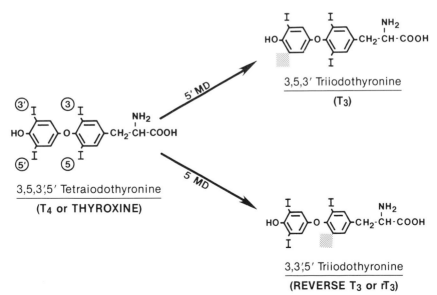

FIGURE 6–2. Structure and nomenclature of thyroxine, and its conversion to the two triiodothyronines by 5'- and 5-monodeiodinase (MD). Shaded squares indicate the sites of deiodination.

The tyrosine residues are first iodinated, then two of them are joined to form the hormones that are finally cleaved from the protein as needed.

Requirement for Iodine. Most of the total body pool of iodine is normally located in the thyroid gland and this is largely organic iodine in the form of stored hormones. Normal thyroid function is dependent upon an adequate dietary intake of iodine, which is approximately 500 µg/day in the United States (Fig. 6–3). Most of this is ingested as organic iodine, and except for the small amount lost in the feces, it is converted to iodide ions and then absorbed from the intestine. Of the amount absorbed, most is lost in the urine.

Most of the remainder is captured by the thyroid as iodide ions by means of its very active iodide "trapping" mechanism. This is an energy-requiring membrane pump that transports iodide from the circulation to the inside of the follicular cells against both electrical and chemical gradients. As a result of this activity, the intracellular iodide concentration is normally about 25 times greater than the extracellular concentration. The ratio of these concentrations is often referred to as the **thyroid/serum (or T/S) ratio**, and it may increase up to tenfold upon stimulation of the thyroid. Several other organs (such as salivary glands) can also trap iodide in this manner but not nearly to the extent that the thyroid can. It should also be noted that the iodide trap is not completely specific for iodide because several other anions can also be trapped by this pump; this is of little physiological significance but it allows for several testing procedures that are clinically useful. Some of the trapped iodide "leaks" back into the circulation, but most of it is utilized in the synthesis of T_3 and T_4. These are ultimately metabolized and the iodide is excreted in both urine and feces (Fig. 6–3).

Thyroglobulin. The tyrosine molecules used for thyroid hormone biosyn-

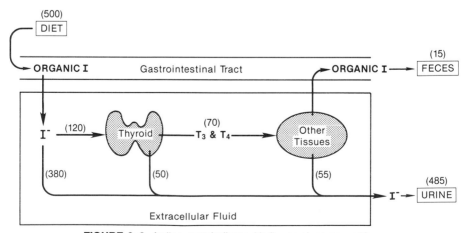

FIGURE 6–3. Iodine metabolism with fluxes given as µg/day.

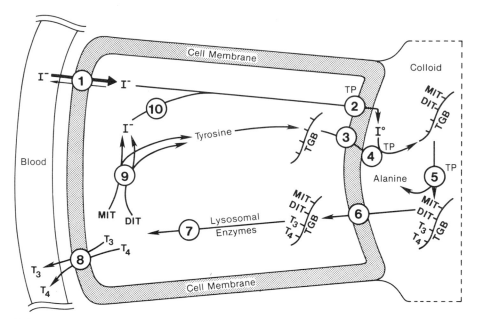

FIGURE 6–4. Follicular cell showing steps in synthesis and release of T_3 and T_4. TP is thyroperoxidase. The numbers identify the major steps: (1) Trapping of iodide; (2) oxidation of iodide; (3) exocytosis of TGB; (4) iodination of TGB; (5) coupling of iodotyrosines; (6) endocytosis of TGB; (7) hydrolysis of TGB; (8) release of T_3 and T_4; (9) deiodination of MIT and DIT; (10) recycling of iodide.

thesis are not present as free amino acids within the follicular cells, but rather they are the tyrosyl residues of a large glycoprotein called **thyroglobulin (TGB).** This protein has a molecular weight of approximately 660,000, and these tyrosyl residues are incorporated in it by the usual peptide linkage. TGB is produced in the rough ER of the follicular cells, it is glycosylated and packaged into secretory vesicles in the Golgi apparatus, and it is released through the apical membranes into the colloid by exocytosis; the colloid consists primarily of TGB. All of the steps of thyroid hormone biosynthesis occur on this protein, and this synthesis seems to happen as the TGB is being released into the colloid. In fact, some investigators believe that synthesis is completed in the lumen of the follicle, which is of course an extracellular site.

   Steps of Biosynthesis. There is a fairly well-defined sequence of steps involved in the conversion of the iodide and tyrosine into the hormones T_3 and T_4 (Fig. 6–4). After iodide has been pumped into the cell, it is transformed to an oxidized form of iodine whose exact identity is not yet known but may be atomic iodine, I^0. This reaction occurs very rapidly and requires an enzyme (**thyroperoxidase**) and an oxidant (**hydrogen peroxide**). The product of the reaction is quickly attached to the ring of a tyrosyl residue of TGB to form **3-monoiodotyrosine (MIT).** This is then iodinated again to yield **3,5-diiodoty-**

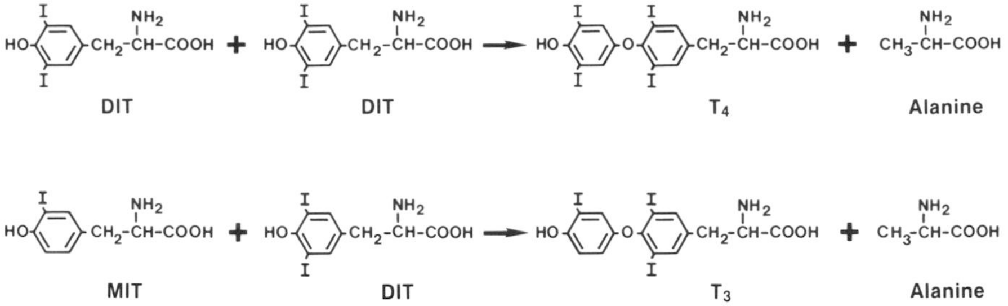

FIGURE 6–5. Production of T_4 and T_3 by the coupling of iodinated tyrosyl residues within the TGB molecule.

rosine (**DIT**). The next step in hormone synthesis is the oxidative coupling of two of these iodo*tyrosines* to form one iodo*thyronine* (Fig. 6–5). The latter will be either a T_3 or a T_4 molecule depending upon which iodotyrosines are coupled, and in each case a molecule of alanine is also produced. Two DITs will combine to form T_4, whereas the ring of MIT attached to DIT will yield T_3. In theory, the ring of DIT coupled to MIT will also yield rT_3, but little if any of this reaction actually occurs in the thyroid. This coupling of iodotyrosines, like their iodination, requires thyroperoxidase, but the specific reactions and intermediates are still open to question.

Storage in Colloid

It should be borne in mind that the hormones synthesized by the steps just presented are still held in peptide linkage within the TGB molecule. Furthermore, until they are secreted, they remain stored in this form in the colloid. It is estimated that the T_3 and T_4 normally stored in the thyroid can supply the body's needs for several months. In addition to containing T_3 and T_4, the TGB also contains considerable amounts of the iodotyrosines MIT and DIT. The proportions of these iodinated compounds may vary, but normally T_4 is in greatest abundance (35 per cent) and T_3 is least prevalent (less than 10 per cent). Most of the remaining 55 per cent of iodine in the colloid is in the form of MIT and DIT with somewhat more than half of this being in the latter.

Extrathyroidal Deiodination of T_4

The metabolism of the thyroid hormones will be considered in detail in a later section of this chapter. However, it should be noted in this discussion of hormone synthesis that approximately 80 per cent of the circulating T_3, and virtually all of the rT_3, are formed by extrathyroidal metabolism of circulating T_4 rather than by thyroid secretion (Fig. 6–2). More specifically, the T_4 is selectively monodeiodinated to give rise to T_3 or rT_3. This occurs in numerous tissues, but liver and kidney are particularly rich in the enzymes for deiodination. Many other tissues have less of these enzymes per unit mass, but if their mass is large (such as muscle), they may contribute significantly to the total deiodinative production of T_3 and rT_3. There are two types of deiodinating enzymes involved in this process. The first of these removes the iodine from the 5' position on the phenolic (or outer) ring of T_4. It is therefore called **5'-monodeiodinase,** or sometimes, outer ring deiodinase. The product of this reaction is T_3, a hormone with greater biological activity than the substrate, T_4. The other type of enzyme is called **5-monodeiodinase** (or inner ring deiodinase), and it generates rT_3 from T_4 by cleavage of the iodine at the 5 position on the inner ring. Thus, when considering overall thyroid hormone biosynthesis, one's attention must go beyond the thyroid gland itself. The final step in the production of most of the circulating T_3 and all of the rT_3 occurs at numerous extrathyroidal sites, even though all of the substrate for these reactions (T_4) is secreted by the thyroid.

Modulation of Deiodination Rates

The degrees of activity of the 5- and 5'-monodeiodinases can be changed by a variety of physiological and experimental conditions. The importance of this modulation should be apparent because one of these enzymes gives rise to the most active thyroid hormone and the other to an inactive compound. It should also be noted that the deiodinases in different tissues may respond differently to a given condition. The most common deviation from normal is seen in a variety of severe (but nonthyroidal) illnesses in which T_3 levels fall, rT_3 levels rise, and T_4 usually remains unchanged. This so-called "low T_3 syndrome" has been attributed to reduced activity of 5'-monodeiodinase, which decreases the conversion of T_4 to T_3. Since this same enzyme is primarily responsible for the degradation of rT_3, this condition increases rT_3 levels by reducing its clearance rather than increasing its production. Very similar changes occur during starvation and after treatment with certain drugs. The modulation of these enzymes may be of physiological importance during the perinatal period at which time there is a transition from the prenatal dominance of rT_3 to the postnatal dominance of T_3.

THYROID HORMONE SECRETION

The release of the thyroid hormones into the blood requires a rather complex process because the hormones are stored at an extracellular site (the follicular lumen) and they are still covalently bound within the TGB molecule. Therefore, the major stages involved in release are (1) internalization of the TGB-hormone complex, (2) cleavage of the hormone from the TGB, and (3) release of the hormones into the blood (Fig. 6–4). Endocytotic activity of the apical membranes is responsible for the transport of the TGB into the cells, resulting in the appearance of globules or droplets of membrane-bounded colloid within the cells. These colloid droplets coalesce with lysosomes whose enzymes hydrolyze the peptide bonds of the TGB, releasing the biologically active iodothyronines (T_3 and T_4) as well as the inactive iodotyrosines (MIT and DIT). The T_3 and T_4, being very lipophilic, pass freely through the basal membranes of the follicular cells and into the blood. Although the thyroid has some deiodinase activity, there is apparently little intrathyroidal conversion of T_4 to T_3 because the ratio in which these two hormones are released is normally similar to their ratio in the colloid. The MIT and DIT released from the TGB are of no endocrine value, and if they were released in large quantities, this would result in wasting of the iodide that was originally sequestered at considerable metabolic expense. To avoid this, the follicular cells contain an enzyme, **iodotyrosine dehalogenase,** that removes iodide from the MIT and DIT, allowing it to be recycled in the synthesis of more hormone. This enzyme is quite specific in that it will not interact with iodothyronines (T_3 and T_4) nor will it deiodinate the iodotyrosines still incorporated in the TGB.

Until recently, it was thought that TGB, being a large protein, could not escape into the circulation. However, with the development of better assays, it has become apparent that small amounts of TGB are present in the circulation of normal individuals, and there is some evidence that it reaches the blood via the lymphatics. The circulating levels of TGB increase in certain thyroid diseases, but nothing is known of the extrathyroidal role of this protein in health or disease. It does not seem to be a significant precursor for thyroid hormone production outside of the thyroid gland.

DISTRIBUTION OF THYROID HORMONES

As described in the previous section, thyroid hormones are cleaved from TGB shortly before their release, and it is this free form of the hormone that actually enters the blood. Once they are released, however, these free hormones are very quickly attached to binding sites both in the blood and in target cells (Fig. 1–7). The latter sites are the receptors through which the hormones exert their effects. Within the blood, there are several proteins that bind both T_3 and T_4 very avidly, resulting in less than 1 per cent of the T_3 and less than 0.1 per cent of the T_4 being left in the unbound form. This is remarkable because only this small fraction of the total hormone pool has access to the receptors in the target cells and thus is able to exert biological activity.

There are three important proteins involved in thyroid hormone binding (Fig. 6–6), and one of the hormones (T_4), is distributed among all three of these proteins. **Thyroxine-binding globulin (TBG)** has the greatest affinity but the lowest capacity for T_4. At the other extreme, **albumin** has a very low affinity but an enormous capacity for T_4. The third protein, **thyroxine-binding pre-**

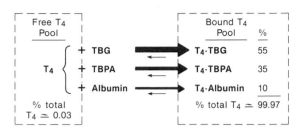

FIGURE 6–6. Binding of T_3 and T_4 to plasma proteins.

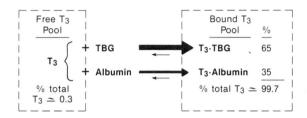

albumin (**TBPA**), has an affinity and a capacity that are intermediate between the other two binding proteins. The name of this protein should not imply that it is a precursor to albumin but simply that it migrates ahead of albumin during electrophoresis. Even though TBG specifies "thyroxine" in its name it also binds T_3, and in this case too its affinity is high but its capacity is low. T_3 is also bound by albumin with a low affinity and a high capacity. TBPA has an affinity for T_3 that is similar to that of albumin, but since there is much less TBPA than albumin in the blood, very little if any T_3 is bound to TBPA. The approximate distribution of T_3 and T_4 among the three binding proteins under normal conditions is given in Figure 6–6.

The bonds between the thyroid hormones and their binding proteins are reversible, and thus the free and bound hormone pools are in a state of dynamic equilibrium. The balance between these two pools may be altered by a variety of conditions, both physiological and pathological. For example, high levels of estrogens (either exogenous or endogenous as during pregnancy) increase the hepatic production of TBG. This makes more binding sites available, which attracts hormones from the free pool and tends to decrease the size of this pool. However, this is a transient situation because the system compensates by reducing the rate of hormone removal, and if the imbalance is severe enough, by activating thyroid hormone secretion via the pituitary (see below). The end result is that a new steady state is established in which the free pool is brought back to normal but the bound pool is greater than normal. Of course, the total hormone pool (bound plus free) will also be elevated. It is important to note that such an individual will be euthyroid since it is the free pool that is active, and this pool is normal. Since thyroid hormone assays measure both bound and free pools, the results of such assays must be combined with some assessment of the degree of protein binding in order to be meaningful diagnostically. These considerations are also important in pharmacotherapeutics since many drugs can displace thyroid hormones from the binding proteins, tending to increase the size of the free pool. However, the same compensatory mechanisms are involved in returning the free pool to normal, resulting in a euthyroid state in the presence of lower than normal total thyroid hormone concentrations.

ACTIONS OF THE THYROID HORMONES

Virtually every tissue in the body is affected in one way or another by the thyroid hormones. The study of these actions has been complicated by several factors. For example, some effects are secondary to others (rather than being a direct result of hormone action), some effects are biphasic with respect to dose of hormone, and numerous other hormones interact with thyroid hormones as they exert their effects. In spite of these complexities, it is reasonably accurate to simply view the thyroid hormones as the primary determinants of the overall metabolic rate of the body. Certainly, the metabolic rate is affected by other factors as well, but it is generally proportional to the availability of thyroid hormones, and its regulation is the primary function of T_3 and T_4. Most, if not all, of the actions to be described can be elicited by either T_3 or T_4. Even though they are qualitatively similar, there is a quantitative difference between them in that T_3 is approximately four times more potent than T_4 on a molar basis. In the following section on mechanism of action, more will be said about the relationship between these two hormones in exerting their effects.

Calorigenic Effect

Long before the recognition of some of the subcellular effects of thyroid hormones, it was observed that whole animals and most tissues respond to thyroid hormones by increasing their oxygen consumption and heat production, a reflection of the increase in overall metabolic rate. This so-called calorigenic effect is not apparent in a few tissues such as brain, anterior pituitary, testes, and spleen, but even these tissues are responsive to thyroid hormones in other ways.

Fuel Metabolism

In addition to exerting these effects on the general metabolic rate, thyroid hormones modulate the rates of many of the specific reactions in intermediatory metabolism. Some of these are probably secondary to the calorigenic effect, but others cannot be since they occur before the calorigenic effect begins. Thyroid hormones increase intestinal glucose absorption and its subsequent entry into fat and muscle, and they further enhance such entry by potentiating the stimulation of glucose uptake by insulin. The conversion of glucose to glycogen is facilitated by small amounts of thyroid hormones, but the reverse (glycogenolysis) occurs with larger amounts, and liver glycogen depletion is often seen in hyperthyroid patients. All aspects of lipid metabolism are stimulated by thyroid hormones, but the net effect favors lipolysis, which tends to deplete fat stores. Thyroid hormones also lower plasma cholesterol levels by enhancing the tissue uptake of low-density lipoproteins, which are particularly rich in cholesterol. The effect of thyroid hormones on protein metabolism is also multifaceted. The synthesis of certain enzymes is enhanced by thyroid hormones, and the protein synthesis needed for normal somatic growth requires adequate amounts of thyroid hormone. Nonetheless, catabolic effects predominate at high doses of thyroid hormones, and hyperthyroidism is often accompanied by protein degradation and muscle wasting. Thus, while the effects of thyroid hormones on carbohydrate, fat, and protein metabolism are complicated by the influence of time and dose, it is of practical importance to note that, under hyperthyroid conditions, the overall effects favor consumption rather than storage of fuel.

Sympathomimetic Effect

Many of the symptoms of hyperthyroidism are similar to those observed with activation of the sympathetic nervous system. Even though the plasma levels of catecholamines (epinephrine and norepinephrine) are not elevated in hyperthyroid patients, it is generally accepted that some kind of interaction exists between these two regulatory systems. A large part of this interaction reflects the ability of thyroid hormones to increase tissue responsiveness to catecholamines, probably by causing a proliferation of β-adrenergic receptors in target tissues. This matter has some practical medical significance in that β-adrenergic blocking drugs (e.g., propranolol) are often useful in the treatment of hyperthyroid patients.

Cardiovascular System

The thyroid hormones increase heart rate and force of contraction because they increase the responsiveness of the heart to circulating catecholamines by the mechanism just described. This is accompanied by an elevated pulse pressure caused by an increased systolic pressure with no change in diastolic pressure. In addition, the heat load generated by the calorigenic effect throughout the body results in peripheral vasodilation, which decreases peripheral resistance. Because of this and the increased heart rate, cardiac output increases.

Nervous System

Even though the calorigenic action of the thyroid hormones is not apparent in brain, thyroid hormone receptors exist in this organ, and some aspects of central nervous system function are affected by these hormones. This is indicated by the behavioral changes associated with thyroid disease; hyperthyroid patients are mentally quick, even anxious and irritable, whereas hypothyroid patients are mentally slow and lethargic. In the hypothyroid neonate, central nervous system development is impeded. This impedance may lead to permanent mental retardation if the condition is not recognized and treated promptly. Peripheral nerves are also affected by thyroid hormones, and their conduction velocity varies directly with the availability of thyroid hormones.

MECHANISM OF THYROID HORMONE ACTION

Biochemical Model

In Chapter 1, two general mechanisms of hormone action were described. Even though the thyroid hormones are amino acid derivatives, they are not very water soluble, and thus their mechanism of action conforms more closely to the "lipophilic model" presented in Figure 1–8. However, the current view of the mechanism of thyroid hormone action differs from that depicted in the figure in one major way: there are apparently no cytosolic receptors for thyroid hormones. Instead, these hormones pass by diffusion through the plasma membrane and from there into the nucleus where specific receptors for the thyroid hormones have been identified (Fig. 6–7). Through interactions with these receptors, the thyroid hormones induce transcription, resulting in the production of mRNA, which leaves the nucleus and is translated on ribosomes to specific proteins. These proteins, many of which are enzymes, are then responsible for inducing the wide variety of metabolic actions of the thyroid hormones.

It was formerly believed that thyroid hormones produced their calorigenic effect by uncoupling oxidation from phosphorylation in the mitochondria. This notion has now been abandoned. Even though there are some thyroid hormone binding sites in mitochondria, it is generally accepted that the primary mechanism of action is via the nuclear receptors and enzyme induction. It has been proposed that the induction of a specific enzyme, Na^+/K^+ –ATPase, might be largely responsible for the calorigenic effects of the thyroid hormones. The synthesis of this enzyme is stimulated in a number of tissues by thyroid hormones. According to this hypothesis, the resulting increase in the work of ion transport causes the elevated oxygen consumption and thermogenesis, i.e., the calorigenic effect of the hormones. However, not all of the experimental evidence is in accord with this proposal and further investigation is needed.

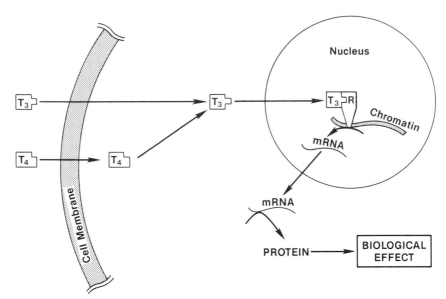

FIGURE 6–7. Proposed subcellular mechanism of thyroid hormone action.

T_3 vs. T_4

Although all of the actions described in the previous section can be observed after the administration of either T_3 or T_4, it has been suggested that T_4 can exert effects only by being converted to T_3 (Fig. 6–7). According to this hypothesis, T_4 is a prohormone rather than a hormone. Certainly T_4 functions as a prohormone when extrathyroidal tissues use it as substrate for the deiodinative production of T_3, which is then released into the blood. However, in some thyroid hormone target cells T_4 is monodeiodinated to T_3 that is retained within the cells, and it is in this case that the classification of T_4 as a hormone as opposed to a prohormone has been debated. A true hormonal role for both T_3 and T_4 is suggested by the fact that the nuclear receptors will bind both of these iodothyronines, although T_3 is bound with a greater affinity than is T_4. Also, even if all of the T_4 entering a target cell is converted to T_3 before exerting an effect, the T_4 still fits the classical definition of a hormone in that it is the humoral messenger carried by the blood to the target cell. It is only during the exertion of its effect within the target cell that it is converted to T_3.

THYROID HORMONE METABOLISM

Deiodination

In most cases, the consideration of hormone metabolism is concerned primarily with the conversion of active hormones to metabolites that are inactive,

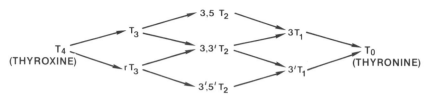

FIGURE 6–8. Stepwise deiodination of iodothyronines by the 5-monodeiodinase (downward arrows) and the 5'-monodeiodinase (upward arrows).

or at least less active than the original hormone. However, thyroid hormones undergo a series of deiodinations to produce substances that may be either more or less active than the parent compound, depending upon which iodine is removed. This cascade of reactions, beginning with the fully iodinated thyronine (T_4), is depicted in Figure 6–8. The deiodination of T_4 by 5'- and 5-monodeiodinase was described in an earlier section (see Fig. 6–2) concerning hormone synthesis because these reactions give rise to most of the circulating T_3 and rT_3, respectively. The T_3 and rT_3 are then degraded to thyronine by the sequential monodeiodinations seen in Figure 6–8; none of the intervening diiodothyronines or monoiodothyronines are thought to have physiologically significant biological activity. Note that since these monodeiodinases do not distinguish between the 3 and 5 (or 3' and 5') positions, only two enzymes are required to accomplish all four of these deiodinations.

Other Routes of Metabolism

The deiodinative cascade is responsible for the removal of most (approximately 75 per cent) of the circulating T_3 and T_4, but these compounds also undergo other metabolic conversions. For example, the alanine portion of T_3 and T_4 can be converted to acetic acid by transamination and decarboxylation to yield **triac** and **tetrac**, respectively. These metabolites can be found in the circulation of normal subjects. Although they have a small amount of biological activity, their importance has not yet been determined. Like other hydrophobic hormones (e.g., steroids), the thyroid hormones and these derivatives are usually conjugated by sulfation or glucuronidation.

Sites of Metabolism

The deiodination of thyroid hormones occurs in many different tissues, but liver and kidney have particularly high deiodinase activity and are thought to make major contributions to the circulating pools of T_3 and rT_3. These two organs are also the primary sites for the production of tetrac and triac. At least

80 per cent of the total thyroid hormone pool undergoes metabolic transformation by either the deiodinative or nondeiodinative routes; the metabolites are excreted primarily in the urine. This leaves up to 20 per cent of the T_3 and T_4 to be excreted without being catabolized. Most of the unmetabolized hormone is excreted in the feces via biliary secretion, leaving only a small amount (approximately 5 per cent of the total) to be excreted in the urine, primarily as sulfates and glucuronides. The liver and kidneys are the primary sites for conjugation of the thyroid hormones and their metabolites.

Clearance Rates

Perhaps the most striking aspect of the metabolic clearance of thyroid hormones from the blood is that it occurs so slowly relative to other hormones. Thyroid hormone half-lives vary considerably among species, but in the human the half-life of T_3 is approximately one day and that of T_4 approximately six and one half days. These extremely long half-lives can be attributed to the fact that such a large proportion of the circulating thyroid hormone pool is protein bound and therefore not subject to the metabolic reactions just described. Protein binding also affects the relative volumes of distribution of the thyroid hormones. T_4, which is more tightly bound to plasma proteins than T_3 is, has a volume of distribution that is approximately one fourth that of T_3 (Table 6–1). This does not mean that there is a difference between the actual physical volumes into which these two hormones are distributed. It does mean that a greater proportion of the total T_3 pool is outside of the plasma compartment. This is consistent with the fact that T_3, relative to T_4, is less tightly bound in the plasma and is more tightly bound by the extravascular receptors within the target cells.

TABLE 6–1.   Approximate Values for Thyroid Hormone Plasma Concentrations and Kinetic Parameters

	Total Plasma Concentration (µg/dl)	Free Plasma Concentration (ng/dl)	Plasma Half-Life (days)	Volume of Distribution (liters)	Metabolic Clearance Rate (l/day)	Total Production Rate (µg/day)
T_4	8.0	2.0	6.5	10	1	80
T_3	0.12	0.3	1.0	40	25	30
rT_3	0.03	0.2	0.7	100	100	30

Production rates for T_3 and rT_3 include thyroidal secretion and extrathyroidal deiodination. Note difference in units for total and free hormone concentrations.

REGULATION OF THYROID HORMONE SECRETION

As described in earlier sections, the primary determinant of thyroid hormone action is the free hormone concentration in blood. It has also been noted earlier that numerous factors can modulate the size of this free hormone pool (e.g., secretion, metabolism, and protein binding). Among these, it is the rate of hormone secretion that is usually most important in causing changes in plasma hormone concentrations. Thus, this section will consider the mechanisms that regulate thyroid hormone secretion and in doing so will describe the function of the entire hypothalamo-pituitary-thyroid axis (Fig. 6–9).

Factors Directly Affecting the Thyroid Gland

Thyrotropin. The pituitary hormone thyrotropin (thyroid-stimulating hormone, TSH) is the most important physiological regulator of thyroid hormone secretion. Thyroid activity is enhanced by TSH, and it is reduced in the absence of TSH. As is usual for peptide hormones, TSH acts by binding to cell membrane receptors and activating adenylate cyclase (see Fig. 1–9). The subsequent formation of cyclic AMP leads to protein kinase activation, and ultimately to the stimulation of all of the steps of thyroid hormone synthesis and release (see Fig. 6–4). Because there are so many different cellular functions involved in the overall process of thyroid hormone secretion, the biochemical pathway for the mechanism of action of TSH must diverge greatly beyond the formation of cyclic AMP. However, the details beyond this step are still not well understood. TSH stimulates the iodide pump in the cell membrane, enhances the biochemical reactions for iodotyrosine production and conjugation,

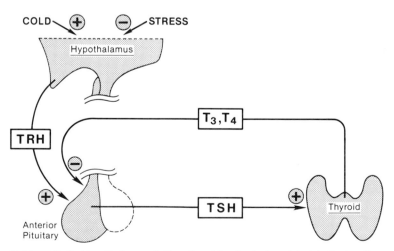

FIGURE 6–9. Hypothalamo-pituitary-thyroid axis. (+) and (−) indicate stimulation and inhibition, respectively.

causes the apical membranes to increase their endocytotic activity, induces the migration of lysosomes from the basal to the apical region, enhances the breakdown of TGB to liberate T_3 and T_4, and as a result increases the release of these hormones into the blood.

Despite the diversity of these actions, it appears that the involvement of cyclic AMP is a crucial and common step because cyclic AMP analogs can mimic TSH in virtually all of these actions. There is also some evidence that the stimulation of thyroidal carbohydrate metabolism by TSH may be involved in mediating many of these actions. TSH stimulates thyroidal glucose oxidation and the production of cofactors which are necessary for the various energy-requiring processes involved in thyroid hormone secretion. Prostaglandins are also thought to be involved in mediating the effects of TSH on hormone secretion, but little is known of their precise roles(s) in this process.

In addition to regulating thyroid hormone secretion, TSH is responsible for maintaining the structural integrity of the thyroid gland. The thyroid will atrophy in the absence of TSH, and it will undergo hypertrophy and hyperplasia in response to excess stimulation by TSH.

Thyroid-Stimulating Immunoglobulins. Under certain abnormal conditions, the thyroid may be stimulated by circulating immunoglobulins. These are antibodies that are thought to be directed against TSH receptors. This topic will be presented in more detail in a subsequent section, but it is worth noting here that, except for the time course of action, the results of such stimulation are essentially the same as those seen upon stimulation by TSH; these antibodies increase both secretion and growth of the thyroid. Moreover, they apparently do so by interacting with the TSH receptors and activating adenylate cyclase as TSH does.

Thyroid Nerves. Although not depicted in Figure 6–9, the thyroid gland receives a neuronal input as well as the hormonal input indicated. There is no doubt that the primary control over thyroid function is exerted by the humoral factors—TSH in health and antibodies in some thyroid diseases. However, there is also evidence that thyroid hormone secretion can be affected by the activity of thyroid nerves, perhaps by their modulation of responsiveness to TSH.

Iodine. As noted before, iodine is an essential component for thyroid hormone synthesis. Thus, iodine deficiency will decrease thyroid hormone secretion. Paradoxically, an excess of iodine will also decrease thyroid hormone secretion. This action of iodine is referred to as the **Wolff-Chaikoff effect,** and it is due to a reduction in the organification of iodide and thus a reduction in hormone synthesis. High doses of iodine will also reduce thyroid hormone release by lessening responsiveness to TSH, and this effect is particularly apparent when the thyroid is secreting at a greater than normal rate. One practical result of these antithyroidal effects is that large doses of iodine are sometimes used to prepare hyperthyroid patients for surgery by reducing thyroid function and causing regression of the hyperplastic gland.

Negative Feedback Effects of Thyroid Hormones

TSH, like the other tropic hormones of the pituitary, is subject to negative feedback inhibition by the target organ hormones—in this case, T_3 and T_4. In the thyroid axis, this inhibition is definitely exerted at the level of the anterior pituitary, but there may also be a secondary inhibitory effect at the hypothalamus (Fig. 6–9). The pituitary site has been demonstrated convincingly by showing that thyroid hormones reduce the TSH secretory response to **thyrotropin-releasing hormone (TRH)**, a hormone that is known to act at the anterior pituitary. This feedback system is bidirectional in that abnormally high thyroid hormone levels will decrease TSH secretion, and low levels of thyroid hormones will cause TSH secretion to increase; both of these situations are frequently encountered in thyroid disease. Both T_3 and T_4 are involved in this feedback mechanism, and it is the free pools rather than the protein-bound ones that exert this inhibition. The pituitary thyrotropes contain nuclear receptors that bind both thyroid hormones, but they bind T_3 more avidly than T_4. Nonetheless, the circulating levels of TSH are more closely correlated (inversely) with T_4 levels than they are with T_3. This apparent contradiction is explained by the fact that the thyrotropes have an active 5'-monodeiodinase that converts much of the T_4 that enters the cell to T_3 (see Fig. 6–7). Although some T_4 may bind to receptors without conversion to T_3, and some of the intracellular T_3 is taken up from the circulation as T_3, a large part of the inhibition of TSH secretion is accomplished by circulating T_4 entering the cell and being converted to T_3. The T_3 then enters the nucleus to exert the final effect. Whether it is T_3 or T_4 that occupies the receptors, the inhibition of TSH is brought about by the induction of an inhibitory protein. Like most other negative feedback loops, this one tends to provide stability to TSH (and thus thyroid hormone) output.

Hypothalamic Regulation of TSH Secretion

In addition to the continuous regulation of TSH secretion by thyroid hormone feedback, the hypothalamus provides neuroendocrine control mechanisms to stimulate or inhibit TSH secretion as needed (Fig. 6–9). The primary mediator of this hypothalamic regulation is TRH, which is a tripeptide produced in certain hypothalamic cells. This neurohormone is released into the hypothalamo-pituitary portal blood vessels. These then deliver it to the anterior pituitary where it stimulates both the synthesis and release of TSH. TRH acts by binding to cell membrane receptors, and it is known to stimulate pituitary adenylate cyclase activity. However, not all findings are in agreement with the proposal that cyclic AMP is the physiological mediator of TRH action.

In addition to TRH, there are two other hypothalamic factors known to affect TSH secretion. **Dopamine** inhibits TSH secretion in both humans and animals, but its physiological importance remains to be demonstrated. The neurohormone **somatostatin** will also inhibit TSH secretion. This may be important physiologically since TSH secretion increases after neutralizing endogenous somatostatin in animals by passive immunization.

These stimulatory and inhibitory hypothalamic hormones are presumably responsible for mediating the changes in TSH secretion induced by certain environmental conditions. For example, various types of stress inhibit TSH secretion, but it is not known whether such actions are mediated by decreased TRH, increased somatostatin, or some other mechanism. Exposure to cold increases TSH (and thyroid hormone) secretion in various types of experimental animals. Even though this type of response makes sense physiologically, it is not present in adult humans. In contrast, the newborn infant has a very dramatic TSH response to exposure to a cold environment. Finally, the diurnal rhythm in plasma TSH levels is thought to be due to variations in hypothalamic TRH release.

Temporal Considerations

Compared to the extremely rapid transmission of information in the nervous system, endocrine communication in general is rather sluggish, and among the endocrine systems, the thyroid axis is one of the slowest in its overall function. The one portion of this system that does respond quickly is its neuroendocrine component, the hypothalamus. Activation of the TRH-secreting neurons results in a very prompt release of this hormone. It reaches its target cells in the pituitary quickly, where it increases TSH release within a few minutes. TRH has a short half-life and its effect does not significantly outlast its presence.

The full secretory response of the thyroid gland to TSH requires several hours, but some of the intervening intracellular events are apparent within several minutes of exposure to TSH. There is a prompt activation of adenylate cyclase after the TSH binds to its receptors. Also, increased organification of iodide, hormone synthesis, and endocytosis of TBG can be detected within minutes. Other aspects of thyroid hormone synthesis and release, such as stimulation of the iodide trapping mechanism, are not apparent until several hours after exposure to TSH.

It is the action of the thyroid hormones themselves in which the "sluggishness" of the thyroid axis is most apparent. The metabolic response to T_3 or T_4 is seen only after a delay of several hours, and the maximal response is not seen until several days after exposure to the hormones. The duration of this response is also quite long, in part because of the long half-lives of these hormones but also because the response can continue after the plasma thyroid hormone concentrations have returned to normal. Although these statements apply to both T_3 and T_4, T_3 has a somewhat shorter delay and duration of action than T_4. The feedback inhibition of TSH secretion by the thyroid hormones does not require as much time as the metabolic effects, but it is seen only after a delay of an hour or two because it requires the synthesis of an inhibitory protein.

Overall, the thyroid axis responds rapidly at the hypothalamo-pituitary unit, but beyond this level, the system is governed by processes that have extremely long time constants. One result of this is that the long half-lives of T_3 and T_4 damp the diurnal rhythm that is quite obvious in TSH levels but not particularly apparent in circulating thyroid hormone concentrations.

CLINICAL APPLICATION

Abnormalities of thyroid function are among the most common of all endocrine disorders. The two major categories of thyroid disease are hyperthyroidism and hypothyroidism. However, in both of these cases, the altered thyroid state may be caused by any of a number of specific abnormalities. In addition to distinguishing normal from abnormal thyroid states, a physician must determine the specific cause of the abnormality in order to choose appropriate treatment. Certainly the signs and symptoms are important in this process, but a final diagnosis will also require certain laboratory measurements, and in some cases testing of the function of the patient's thyroid axis. This section will begin with a brief description of the signs and symptoms of classical hyperthyroidism and hypothyroidism, many of which can be predicted from knowledge of the actions of thyroid hormones. It will then consider the measurements that can currently be made in assessing thyroid function, and finally, several common testing procedures for determining the site of the defect (primary or secondary) will be discussed. Much of this information will serve to reinforce the basic physiology of the previous sections.

Common Thyroid Disorders

Hyperthyroidism. The hyperthyroid patient has an elevated basal metabolic rate, heat intolerance, warm skin, and excessive perspiration. Because of the catabolic effect of the elevated thyroid hormone levels, such patients lose weight in spite of increased food intake, and the associated muscle wasting results in weakness. Involvement of the nervous system is apparent from nervousness, tremor, and emotional lability. Because of both the direct effects of thyroid hormones and their interactions with catecholamines, various cardiovascular abnormalities are present in hyperthyroidism such as tachycardia, arrhythmias, and elevated systemic and pulse pressures. In addition, in response to the excessive heat load, there is peripheral vasodilation that reduces total peripheral resistance and increases cardiac output. In spite of the latter, the heart may fail to meet the metabolic demands of the body in severe cases of hyperthyroidism.

The most common cause of hyperthyroidism is **Graves' disease,** an autoimmune disease in which the thyroid is stimulated by antibodies directed against TSH receptors. Even before the identification of this factor, it was known that its effect on the thyroid was quite similar to that of TSH except for its extended duration of action. Because of this, this factor was originally called the **long-acting thyroid stimulator, or LATS.** However, this IgG is now more commonly referred to as the **thyroid-stimulating immunoglobulin (TSI).** In addition to stimulating thyroid hormone secretion, TSI is responsible for the enlarged thyroid gland (**goiter**) seen in patients with Graves' disease. Another hallmark of Graves' disease is **exophthalmos,** which is a protrusion of the eyeballs caused by edema and deposition of mucopolysaccharides within the retro-orbital space. The etiology of this condition is still being debated.

Hypothyroidism. The hypothyroid patient has a reduced basal metabolic rate, cold intolerance, cool dry skin, coarse hair, and a hoarse voice. Such individuals are easily fatigued, and they have slow reflexes and muscle cramps. They may gain weight and are often constipated. An infiltration of the skin with mucopolysaccharides occurs, leading to a puffy appearance primarily of the face, hands, and feet. This condition is referred to as **myxedema,** but this term is also used as a synonym for hypothyroidism. The central nervous system is affected by the inadequate thyroid hormone levels such that there is slow mentation, slow speech, poor memory, and sometimes personality changes or even frank psychosis. Both the heart rate and contractility are reduced, and because of increased plasma cholesterol levels, there is a propensity for atherosclerosis in hypothyroidism.

Congenital hypothyroidism (cretinism) is characterized by dwarfism, mental retardation, and a puffy face with protruding tongue. This condition is of particular concern because the mental retardation is preventable if treatment is started promptly, but it is not reversible once developed. A vitally important recent development in this area is the establishment of neonatal screening programs in which congenital hypothyroidism can be diagnosed from one drop of blood from a newborn infant. It is usually the compensatory increase in plasma TSH levels that is measured in such screening programs.

Laboratory Tests

Measurement of Hormone Levels. Although it is quite logical to measure some biological effect of the thyroid hormones as an index of the thyroid state, this is not very practical or reliable. The basal metabolic rate (BMR) will of course vary with plasma thyroid hormone concentrations, and its measurement was formerly used in diagnosing thyroid disease. However, the determination of BMR is rather cumbersome and imprecise, and the BMR is affected by numerous factors other than the thyroid hormones. Fortunately, assays are now available for the measurement of thyroid hormones in plasma. The earlier assays were indirect in that they were based on a measurement of **protein-bound iodine (PBI)** in blood. This provides a reasonable index of thyroid hormone concentrations since most of the iodine in blood is that which is incorporated in the thyroid hormones, and most of this is protein bound. Although

PBI determinations are still sometimes done, they are rapidly being replaced by direct assays for thyroid hormones. These are either radioimmunoassays (RIAs) or competitive protein-binding assays (see Chapter 2), and they are readily available for both T_3 and T_4. RIAs for TSH are also routine now, but those for TRH and rT_3 are still primarily research tools.

Assessment of Binding Proteins. Since the thyroid hormones are so extensively bound to plasma proteins, an evaluation of thyroid function should also include some information about these binding proteins. It would be ideal to determine the plasma concentrations of the free thyroid hormones, but even though this is possible, it is not often feasible. There is, however, a very commonly used indirect index of the status of thyroid hormone binding called the **resin T_3 uptake (RT$_3$U)**. It must be emphasized at the outset that the T_3 uptake is *not* a measurement of T_3 levels. This test is an *in vitro* assessment of the degree of protein binding of the thyroid hormones. It is performed by incubating a plasma sample with some radioactive T_3 and a resin, which will bind the T_3 not already bound to the plasma proteins (Fig. 6–10). The amount of the radioactive T_3 that is bound to the resin is determined, and this is expressed as a percentage of the total radioactive T_3 or as a ratio of this uptake to that of a normal plasma pool.

The test is based on the competition for the labeled T_3 between the binding sites on the plasma protein and those on the resin. In hyperthyroidism, the excess thyroid hormone occupies more of the binding protein sites than normal, leaving few sites available for the labeled T_3. Thus, in this case, there is more of the labeled T_3 available for binding to the resin and the value of

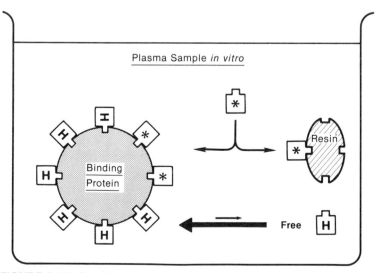

FIGURE 6–10. Principle of resin T_3 uptake test. The radioactive T_3 (*) will bind to the binding protein at those sites not already occupied by endogenous hormone (H) and the remaining * will be absorbed by the resin.

TABLE 6–2. Relative Values of the RT₃U and Related Variables Under Various Conditions

	Normal	Hyperthyroid	Hypothyroid	Pregnant
Total T_4	N	↑	↓	↑
Free T_4	N	↑	↓	N
Protein-binding sites (total)	N	N	N	↑
Protein sites available to *	N	↓	↑	↑
RT₃U	N	↑	↓	↓
FT₄I	N	↑	↓	N

Abbreviations not defined in text are: N, normal; ↑, greater than normal; ↓, less than normal; *, radioactive T_3.

the T_3 uptake will be high (Table 6–2). This reading will also be high if there is a decrease in TBG (with normal thyroid hormone) concentrations because the number of binding sites on the protein will again be low, and there will be more of the labeled T_3 left for binding to the resin. The T_3 uptake will be low if thyroid hormone levels are low (with normal binding proteins) or if the number of protein binding sites is high (as seen in pregnancy or estrogen treatment). Clearly, this test is not a quantitative measure of the available binding sites or of the free thyroid hormone concentrations. Nonetheless, the T_3 uptake test is quite useful, particularly when combined with a measurement of plasma T_4 concentrations. The T_3 uptake ratio is often multiplied by the T_4 concentration to obtain the so-called **free T_4 index (FT₄I).** It should be emphasized that the FT₄I is also not actually a measure of the free T_4 concentration, but it is well correlated with free T_4 levels and thus with thyroid state. The reason that the FT₄I is such a good, yet simple, index of the thyroid state is that it is based on both hormone concentration and the status of the binding proteins.

Functional Tests

Radioactive Iodine Uptake (RAIU) Test. As described earlier, thyroid hormone secretion includes many steps ranging from the trapping of iodide to the actual release of the hormones. Since these interdependent steps are normally operating in unison, there are many different variables that could be measured as an index of the overall process of thyroid hormone secretion. One common test of thyroid function is the RAIU test. This is a noninvasive test in which a trace amount of radioactive iodine is given orally and then the amount of radioactivity taken up by the thyroid gland is determined by an external detector and expressed as a percentage of the administered dose. It is important that only a trace amount of the radioactive iodine be given since large amounts will destroy thyroid tissue and in fact are often used to treat hyperthyroid patients. Of course, this test is most directly related to the function of the iodide-trapping mechanism, but it is also a reasonable indicator of overall thyroid function. Results are usually found to be elevated in hyperthyroidism and reduced in hypothyroidism.

Thyroid Suppression Test. The thyroid suppression test is used to determine whether the thyroid gland is being controlled by TSH (as it should be), or whether it is secreting autonomously. The principle of this test relies on the negative feedback inhibition of TSH by thyroid hormones. In practice, the test consists of administration of a thyroid hormone (usually T_3) and assessment of thyroid gland function (usually by the RAIU or plasma T_4 levels) both before and after the hormone treatment. Under normal conditions, TSH is regulating thyroid function and the T_3 will suppress TSH secretion. Therefore, in this case, the RAIU (or plasma T_4) will be decreased after T_3 treatment. In certain abnormal situations such as Graves' disease, the thyroid is not being regulated by TSH; therefore, the hyperactivity of the thyroid gland will not be suppressible by the T_3.

TSH Stimulation Test. This test has often been used to distinguish primary from secondary hypothyroidism, and its description serves to further illustrate the interactions within the pituitary-thyroid axis. Primary hypothyroidism is due to a failure of the thyroid gland itself, whereas in secondary hypothyroidism the thyroid is normal but it is receiving inadequate stimulation by TSH (Fig. 6–11). In each case, the thyroid hormone concentration will be low, but only in primary hypothyroidism (normal pituitary) will this cause an elevation in TSH levels. The TSH stimulation test is used to distinguish between these two situations, and this is done by administering exogenous TSH and then determining whether the thyroid response to it is normal or not. In secondary hypothyroidism, the thyroid gland is normal and the TSH

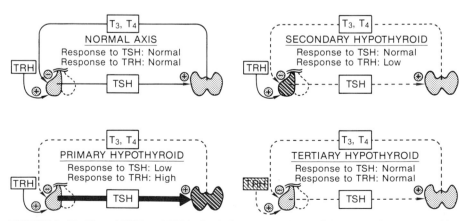

FIGURE 6–11. Use of TSH and TRH stimulation tests to distinguish among three types of hypothyroidism. Pituitary and thyroid are depicted as in Figure 6–9. Broken lines indicate less than normal secretion and the bold line indicates greater than normal secretion. Cross-hatching identifies the organ that is abnormal.

will elicit a normal response. In contrast, the abnormal thyroid gland in primary hypothyroidism will not respond normally to the exogenous TSH just as it does not respond normally to the elevated endogenous TSH levels. Although this test has been used for many years to distinguish between primary and secondary hypothyroidism, it is now being phased out. The recent availability of an RIA for TSH offers a simpler way of making this distinction; TSH levels are high in primary and low in secondary hypothyroidism. In primary hypothyroidism, the elevated TSH cannot elicit a normal secretory response, but it can cause hypertrophy leading to goiter formation. Thus, a goiter may be present in either hypothyroidism or hyperthyroidism (see earlier discussion) depending upon whether or not the abnormality is at the thyroid itself.

TRH Stimulation Test. Now that TSH assays and synthetic TRH are available, a TRH stimulation test has been developed that allows even finer discrimination among the possible types of hypothyroidism. In this test, TRH is administered and the pituitary response to it is determined by measuring plasma TSH levels. The principle of this test is exactly the same as that of the TSH stimulation test. However, in this case one is distinguishing between a hypothalamic and a pituitary abnormality. If the pituitary is failing, the TSH response to the exogenous TRH will be less than normal (Fig. 6–11). On the other hand, if the pituitary is hyposecreting simply because the hypothalamus is releasing inadequate amounts of TRH, then its response to the exogenous TRH will be normal. This finding is indicative of a recently discovered disease referred to as **hypothalamic** (or **tertiary**) **hypothyroidism.** It should be noted, however, that the responses to the TRH stimulation test are quite variable and thus must often be interpreted in conjunction with other diagnostic information.

REFERENCES

DeGroot, L.J.: Thyroid hormone action. In Endocrinology, Vol. 1, L.J. DeGroot, et al., editors. Grune and Stratton, Inc., New York, p. 357, 1979.

DeGroot, L.J.: Thyroid physiology; endocrine and neural relationships. In Endocrinology, Vol. 1, L.J. DeGroot, et al., editors. Grune and Stratton, Inc., New York, p. 373, 1979.

Engler, D., and Butger, A.G.: The deiodination of the iodothyronines and of their derivatives in man. Endocrine Rev. 5:151, 1984.

Ingbar, S.H.: The thyroid gland. In Williams' Textbook of Endocrinology, 7th ed. J.D. Wilson and D.W. Foster, editors, W.B. Saunders Company, Philadelphia, p. 682, 1985.

Kaplan, M.M.: The role of thyroid hormone deiodination in the regulation of hypothalamo-pituitary function. Neuroendocrinology 38:254, 1984.

Larsen, P.R., Silva, J.E., and Kaplan, M.M.: Relationships between circulating and intracellular thyroid hormones: Physiological and clinical implications. Endocrine Rev. 2:87, 1981.

Morley, J.E.: Neuroendocrine control of thyrotropin secretion. Endocrine Rev. 2:396, 1981.

Pittman, C.S.: Hormone metabolism. In Endocrinology, Vol. 1, L.J. DeGroot, et al., editors. Grune and Stratton, Inc., New York, p. 265, 1979.

Refetoff, S.: Thyroid hormone transport. In Endocrinology, Vol. 1, L.J. DeGroot, et al., editors. Grune and Stratton, Inc., New York, p. 347, 1979.

Wartofsky, L., and Burman, K.D.: Alterations in thyroid function in patients with systemic illness: The "euthyroid sick syndrome." Endocrine Rev. 3:164, 1982.

126

7

ADRENAL CORTEX

INTRODUCTION

The adrenal gland is a compound organ composed of two distinct endocrine tissues. The inner portion of the gland, the adrenal medulla, produces catecholamines and is discussed in Chapter 13. The outer portion of the adrenal gland, the cortex, secretes a variety of steroid hormones. The adrenal cortex and medulla are derived from embryologically distinct structures, their hormonal secretions have different actions and mechanisms of action, and regulation of cortical and medullary hormone secretion is each independent of the other. Consequently, despite their anatomical proximity, there is virtually no functional relationship between the adrenal cortex and adrenal medulla.

Anatomy

The cortex constitutes about 80 per cent of the human adrenal gland and consists of three different anatomical zones (Fig. 7–1). The outermost zone of the cortex, which lies immediately beneath the capsule of the gland, is the **zona glomerulosa.** The middle zone, the **zona fasciculata,** is the largest portion of the cortex, and the innermost zone is known as the **zona reticularis.** Histologically, the adrenal cortical cells are characterized by an abundance of lipid droplets, mitochondria, and smooth endoplasmic reticulum. Cholesterol esters, the precursors for steroid hormones, are stored in large amounts in the lipid droplets, and many of the enzymes involved in steroidogenesis are found in the mitochondria or the endoplasmic reticulum, explaining the abundance of these organelles.

The adrenal cortex in the human fetus differs both structurally and functionally from that in the adult. During fetal life the adrenal cortex consists of a thin outer zone of cells that later develops into the permanent adult cortex, and a much larger inner zone, known as the **fetal zone.** The fetal zone begins to involute shortly before birth and completely disappears within a year after birth. The fetal adrenal cortex is proportionately much larger than the adult gland because of the large size of the fetal zone. Because the functions of the fetal adrenal cortex are closely associated with those of the placenta, these two organs are discussed together in Chapter 11.

Hormones Produced

The adrenal cortex produces a number of different steroid hormones, which although they are structurally similar, have a variety of different biological effects. As the sole site of production of **glucocorticoids** and **mineralocorticoids,** the adrenal cortex has far-reaching and important effects on intermediary metabolism and electrolyte balance in the body. Glucocorticoids such as **cortisol** play a major role in the regulation of carbohydrate, protein, and lipid metabolism, and they also modulate the effects of other hormones on these same processes. **Aldosterone,** the most important mineralocorticoid produced by the adrenal cortex, participates in the regulation of renal sodium and potassium reabsorption and excretion, thereby affecting blood pressure homeostasis. The importance of mineralocorticoid secretion is illustrated by the life-threatening nature of various adrenal cortical diseases. Several **androgens and estrogens** are also produced by the adrenal cortex, but they are of relatively little biological significance under normal circumstances.

Cortisol and aldosterone are produced in anatomically distinct portions of the adrenal cortex, and the control of secretion of each is independent of the other. Thus, there is a functional zonation of the adrenal cortex that corresponds with the anatomical zonation of the gland. Aldosterone is produced exclusively in the zona glomerulosa, whereas cortisol production is limited to the two inner zones of the cortex, the zona fasciculata and the zona reticularis.

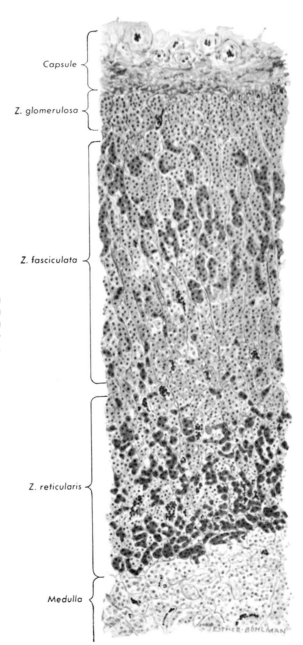

Capsule

Z. glomerulosa

Z. fasciculata

FIGURE 7–1. Histologic section through the adrenal gland of an adult human (x110). (From Bloom and Fawcett, A Textbook of Histology. W.B. Saunders Company, Philadelphia, p. 361, 1964.)

Z. reticularis

Medulla

Although the relative importance of the two inner zones in the production of cortisol has yet to be fully resolved, recent studies suggest that the zona fasciculata is the major source of cortisol. Adrenal androgens and estrogens are also produced by the inner cortical zones. The mechanisms responsible for the functional zonation of the adrenal cortex are described later in this chapter.

HORMONE BIOSYNTHESIS IN ADRENAL CORTEX

Sources of Adrenal Cholesterol

As noted in Chapter 1, cholesterol is the precursor to all steroid hormones. Adrenal cells are capable of synthesizing cholesterol *de novo*, but most of the adrenal cholesterol used for steroidogenesis is derived from circulating lipoproteins and in particular from low-density lipoproteins (LDL). The interaction of LDL with specific membrane receptors on adrenal cortical cells initiates their internalization, and subsequent lysosomal degradation of the LDL generates free cholesterol, which may be used for steroid hormone synthesis (see Fig. 1–4). The cholesterol that is not immediately used for hormone production is esterified and stored as cholesterol esters in lipid droplets within the cell. The cholesterol esters constitute the major storage form of steroids in adrenocortical cells and can be hydrolyzed to generate free cholesterol when the latter is needed for hormone production. As discussed later in this chapter, control of steroidogenesis is achieved primarily by the regulation of cholesterol metabolism.

Pathways of Hormone Production

The production of steroid hormones from cholesterol requires a series of enzymatic modifications of the cholesterol molecule (Fig. 7–2). In each steroid-producing cell, the relative abundance of the various steroidogenic enzymes determines the profile of secretory products for that cell. Although all of the compounds illustrated in Figure 7–2 can be synthesized by the adrenal cortex, the enzymes required for the production of testosterone and of estrogens are found in very low concentrations within adrenal cortical cells. Consequently, the latter compounds are normally produced only in very small quantities by the adrenal cortex. The steps involved in their synthesis are discussed in the chapters dealing with the testes and ovaries, the major sites of production of those hormones. The physiologically or quantitatively important secretory products of the adrenal cortex are shaded in Figure 7–2 and include the mineralocorticoid aldosterone, the glucocorticoid cortisol, and the androgen dehydroepiandrosterone.

Mineralocorticoid Synthesis (Fig. 7–2). The first step in the production of steroid hormones is the side-chain cleavage of cholesterol. This reaction ac-

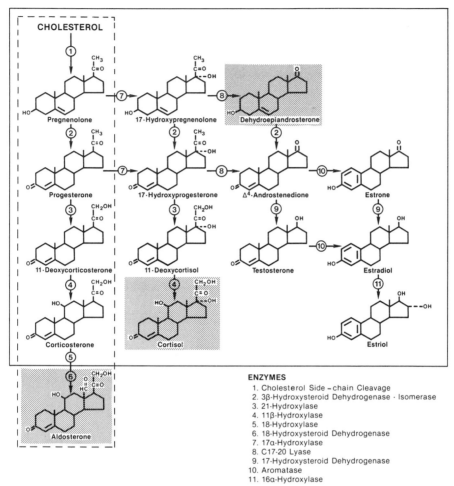

FIGURE 7–2. Steroidogenic pathways in the zona glomerulosa (within broken lines) and zona fasciculata–zona reticularis (within solid lines) of the human adrenal cortex. The major secretory products are shaded.

tually consists of two hydroxylations followed by cleavage of the cholesterol side chain, resulting in the production of pregnenolone. Pregnenolone has no known biological activity but is an intermediate in the production of all of the biologically active steroid hormones. For the production of aldosterone, pregnenolone must next be converted to progesterone.

That step occurs as a result of the coupled actions of two enzymes, 3β-hydroxysteroid dehydrogenase and Δ^5-3-ketosteroid isomerase. The former catalyzes the conversion of the 3-hydroxyl group of pregnenolone to a ketone, and the latter shifts the double bond between the fifth and sixth carbons of pregnenolone to between carbons 4 and 5. Although secreted in small quantities by the adrenal cortex, progesterone, like pregnenolone, serves principally as an intermediate in the synthesis of other adrenal steroids. Hydroxylation of progesterone at the 21-carbon position by the enzyme 21-hydroxylase results in the formation of 11-deoxycorticosterone (DOC). DOC is a fairly potent mineralocorticoid but is normally secreted in quite small quantities by the adrenal cortex (Table 7–1). However, in certain disease states, large amounts of DOC may be secreted, resulting in the symptoms associated with mineralocorticoid excess. Hydroxylation of DOC at the C-11 position, which is catalyzed by the enzyme 11β-hydroxylase, results in the formation of corticosterone, a steroid that has both glucocorticoid and mineralocorticoid activity. Corticosterone is the major glucocorticoid produced by many lower species but is a less potent glucocorticoid than cortisol and is secreted in far smaller quantities than cortisol by the human adrenal cortex (Table 7–1). Hydroxylation of corticosterone at the C-18 position by the 18-hydroxylase enzyme, followed by a dehydrogenase reaction at the same position, yields the potent mineralocorticoid aldosterone. Although produced in relatively small quantities, the potency of aldosterone makes it the physiologically most important mineralocorticoid produced by the adrenal cortex.

Glucocorticoid Synthesis (Fig. 7–2). The synthesis of cortisol involves some of the same enzymatic processes that are required for aldosterone production. However, since cortisol is a 17-hydroxycorticosteroid, the enzyme 17α-hydroxylase is also needed for its production. 17-Hydroxylation may occur either before or after pregnenolone is converted to progesterone, yielding 17-hydroxypregnenolone or 17-hydroxyprogesterone as the reaction product. 17-Hydroxypregnenolone is converted to 17-hydroxyprogesterone by the actions of the enzymes 3β-hydroxysteroid dehydrogenase and Δ^5-3-ketosteroid isomerase, the same enzymes that convert pregnenolone to progesterone. Hydroxylation of the 21 carbon results in the conversion of 17-hydroxyprogesterone to 11-deoxycortisol, and 11β-hydroxylation then converts 11-deoxycortisol to the potent glucocorticoid, cortisol. The 17-hydroxylated intermediates in cortisol synthesis—namely 17-hydroxypregnenolone, 17-hydroxyprogesterone,

TABLE 7–1. Steroids Secreted by the Human Adrenal Cortex

Steroid	Secretion Rate (mg/day)	Plasma Concentration (μg/100 ml)
Cortisol	12–30	10–25
Aldosterone	0.05–0.15	.002–.010
DHEA	7–15	0.2–1.0
DHEA-sulfate	10–25	80–250
Corticosterone	1–4	0.2–1.0
11-Deoxycorticosterone	0.05–0.2	.002–.012

and 11-deoxycortisol—have little biological activity and are normally secreted in small amounts by the adrenal cortex.

Androgen and Estrogen Synthesis (Fig. 7–2). Either 17-hydroxypregnenolone or 17-hydroxyprogesterone is required for androgen and estrogen biosynthesis. The enzyme C_{17-20} lyase cleaves the side chain of both compounds, yielding dehydroepiandrosterone (DHEA) or Δ^4-androstenedione, respectively. The latter may also be formed directly from DHEA by the dehydrogenase-isomerase reactions. Most of the DHEA that is produced is sulfated within the adrenal gland prior to secretion. DHEA, although secreted in large quantities by the adrenal cortex (Table 7–1), is a weakly androgenic compound when compared with testosterone, for example, and therefore is of little physiological significance in males. However, as discussed later, the adrenal androgens, DHEA and Δ^4-androstenedione, are of physiological significance in the female, in whom little testosterone is produced. Δ^4-Androstenedione may be converted to testosterone by reduction of the 17-ketone to a 17-hydroxyl group. Since little of this activity occurs in the adrenal cortex, the adrenal secretes only small amounts of testosterone. The androgens secreted by the adrenal cortex, DHEA and Δ^4-androstenedione, may be converted to testosterone at extra-adrenal sites. Similarly, although small amounts of estrogen are produced by the adrenal cortex, adrenal androgens may serve as precursors for estrogen synthesis in other tissues. The processes involved in estrogen biosynthesis are described in Chapter 9.

Functional Zonation of Steroidogenesis. The amount of hormone produced in any steroid-secreting cell is determined primarily by the amount of free cholesterol available for metabolism. However, it is the relative activities of the different steroidogenic enzymes within the cell that determine the identities of the secretory products, and the selective localization of key enzymes to certain cells limits the production of some steroid hormones to those cells. For example, only the adrenal cortex produces mineralocorticoids and glucocorticoids because the 11β-hydroxylase and 21-hydroxylase enzymes, which are required for their synthesis, are found only in adrenocortical cells. Similarly, within the adrenal gland, the functional zonation of the cortex is attributable to differences in the regional distribution of steroidogenic enzymes. The enzyme 18-hydroxysteroid dehydrogenase, which catalyzes the final step in the production of aldosterone, is found only in the zona glomerulosa of the gland. Accordingly, only the zona glomerulosa can synthesize aldosterone. On the other hand, the 17-hydroxylase, which is required for the synthesis of cortisol, androgens, and estrogens, is found in the inner zones of the cortex, the zona fasciculata and the zona reticularis, but not in the zona glomerulosa. Therefore, the latter compounds are produced in the inner zones of the adrenal cortex but not in the zona glomerulosa. The differences in the steroidogenic pathways between those zones are illustrated in Figure 7–2.

It is important to keep this functional zonation in mind especially when attempting to evaluate various adrenal cortical diseases. From a practical standpoint, it is useful to think of the zona glomerulosa and of the combined zona fasciculata–zona reticularis as distinct endocrine organs, since the secretory products of each are different, and the regulation of secretion in each is also different.

Inhibitors of Steroidogenesis. A number of the enzymatic reactions involved in the biosynthesis of adrenocortical steroids can be inhibited by various chemical agents. Some of those agents are highly specific for certain enzymatic steps. These inhibitors have been used primarily for experimental purposes, but some have also been used clinically to decrease adrenal steroid secretion in patients with adrenal cortical hyperfunction. In addition, metyrapone is an 11β-hydroxylase inhibitor that is widely used in the diagnosis of pituitary and adrenal diseases and is discussed later in this chapter.

SECRETION AND DISTRIBUTION OF ADRENAL HORMONES

As previously indicated in Chapter 1, steroid hormones are not stored in steroidogenic cells but are secreted immediately upon synthesis. Thus, the rate of steroid hormone secretion can be controlled only by regulation of biosynthesis. Once steroid hormones are produced, their lipid solubility allows them to diffuse across the cell membrane and into the circulation.

Lipophilic hormones such as the steroids are largely protein bound when they circulate in plasma. The extent of protein binding for the major adrenal corticosteroids is indicated in Table 7–2. It must always be borne in mind that only the free hormone is biologically active and able to exert the effects of the hormone. However, the free pool of hormone in blood is in equilibrium with the protein-bound fraction; therefore, the latter may provide free hormone as needed. Because of the limited water solubility of steroids, protein binding increases the amount of hormone that can circulate in the blood. In addition, since the protein-bound fraction of hormone is relatively resistant to metabolism, protein binding increases the plasma half-life of steroid hormones. Protein binding also limits the access of a hormone to its receptors in target cells.

The extent of protein binding and the proteins to which steroids are

TABLE 7–2. Amounts of Free vs. Protein-Bound Adrenocortical Hormones in Blood

Hormone	% Free	% Protein-Bound	
		CBG	Albumin
Cortisol	10	75	15
Aldosterone	40	10	50
DHEA-sulfate	2	–	98

bound vary from hormone to hormone (Table 7–2). Cortisol, for example, is approximately 90 per cent protein bound in plasma at physiological concentrations, and most of that binding is to a globulin that has a high affinity for cortisol and is known as **corticosteroid-binding globulin (CBG)**. The human CBG is also known as **transcortin**. Some cortisol in plasma is also bound to **albumin,** which has a far lower affinity for cortisol than CBG but which is present in large amounts. Aldosterone is protein bound to a far lesser extent than cortisol; most of this is low affinity binding to albumin. Only about 10 per cent of the aldosterone in plasma is associated with CBG. DHEA-sulfate is extensively protein bound in blood and virtually all of its binding is with albumin. The binding of other adrenal androgens and adrenal estrogens in the blood is the same as the sex hormones of gonadal origin (Chapters 8 and 9).

There are a number of physiological conditions as well as disease states in which the amount of binding protein in plasma is altered, resulting in a shift in the normal balance between free and protein-bound steroid hormones. Estrogens, for example, are known to stimulate hepatic synthesis of CBG. Therefore, during pregnancy when estrogen levels are high, or in women taking birth control pills, plasma CBG levels are elevated. As a result, protein-bound cortisol concentrations are abnormally high. However, since it is the free hormone that is biologically active and that is regulated, there should be no evidence of adrenal disease if everything else is normal. Under such conditions, total hormone levels in blood increase only because of the increase in the protein-bound fraction. On the other hand, if CBG production is abnormally low as may occur in some liver diseases, a decrease would occur in protein-bound cortisol levels, but again there should be no change in free cortisol and therefore no symptoms of adrenal dysfunction. Since it is total hormone levels in blood that are normally measured in the evaluation of adrenal cortical function, the clinician must be aware of the factors influencing the amount of protein-bound hormone in blood if an accurate diagnosis is to be made.

ACTIONS AND MECHANISM OF ACTION OF ADRENAL HORMONES

All of the adrenal cortical hormones exert their effects via the general mechanism described for lipophilic hormones in Chapter 1. That is, the hormone diffuses through the cell membrane in target cells and interacts with a cytosolic receptor specific for that hormone. As a result of the translocation of the hormone-receptor complex to the nucleus of the cell and subsequent effects on the transcription of specific genes, the synthesis of certain proteins is stimulated, resulting in the biologic action of the hormone.

As noted earlier, the adrenal cortical steroids can be subdivided into the glucocorticoids, typified by cortisol, and the mineralocorticoids, represented by aldosterone. However, it is important to recognize that for steroids in both categories there is some **overlap in biological activity.** That is, glucocorticoids exert some mineralocorticoid activity and mineralocorticoids have some glucocorticoid activity (Table 7–3). Thus, it should not be surprising that when large amounts of glucocorticoid are produced, as occurs in certain disease states, some mineralocorticoid effects are also manifested. It is the predominant biological activity that determines the classification of each steroid. For example, aldosterone exerts far greater mineralocorticoid than glucocorticoid activity and is therefore included in the former category, whereas cortisol is a potent glucocorticoid and has far less mineralocorticoid activity (Table 7–3). The relative glucocorticoid and mineralocorticoid potencies of other naturally occurring steroids tend to be intermediate between those of cortisol and aldosterone. With the objective of selectively enhancing either glucocorticoid or mineralocorticoid activity, a number of synthetic steroid analogs have been developed for clinical use. Some of those compounds are listed in Table 7–3.

Glucocorticoids

Glucocorticoids have a wide variety of effects in a large number of tissues. Some of the major effects and the corresponding sites of action are summarized in Table 7–4.

Physiological Effects. A number of the effects of glucocorticoids influence intermediary metabolism. One of the more prominent actions is **stimulation of hepatic gluconeogenesis,** the conversion of amino acids to carbohydrate. This effect results in part from induction of some of the enzymes involved in gluconeogenesis by glucocorticoids. Glucocorticoids also stimulate **protein degradation** in muscle, thereby increasing the mobilization of amino acids, which can serve as substrates for hepatic gluconeogenesis. As a result of the stimulation of gluconeogenesis, glucocorticoids **increase hepatic glycogen** content and also tend to raise blood glucose levels. The actions of glucocorticoids on gluconeogenesis and on muscle protein metabolism are catabolic in

TABLE 7–3. Relative Glucocorticoid and Mineralocorticoid Potencies of Various Steroids

Steroid	Glucocorticoid Potency	Mineralocorticoid Potency
	(Relative to Cortisol)	
Cortisol	1	1
Aldosterone	0.1	400
Corticosterone	0.2	2
11-Deoxycorticosterone	<0.1	20
Dexamethasone	30	2
Fludrocortisone	10	400
Prednisone	4	0.7
Triamcinolone	5	<0.1

TABLE 7–4.   **Glucocorticoid Effects and Target Tissues**

Effect	Site of Action
Stimulates gluconeogenesis	Liver
Increases hepatic glycogen	Liver
Increases blood glucose	Liver
Facilitates lipolysis	Adipose tissue
Catabolic (negative nitrogen balance)	Muscle, liver
Inhibits ACTH secretion	Hypothalamus, anterior pituitary
Facilitates water excretion	Kidney
Blocks inflammatory response	Multiple sites
Suppresses immune system	Macrophages, lymphocytes
Stimulates gastric acid secretion	Stomach

nature, increasing urinary nitrogen excretion and creating a **negative nitrogen balance.**

Glucocorticoids exert a number of effects on fat metabolism that are complex and not well understood. The stimulation of lipolysis by epinephrine is enhanced by cortisol. However, patients suffering from hypercortisolism often have an increase in fat deposition, and a decrease in fat synthesis is associated with adrenal insufficiency. The latter changes are difficult to interpret because of the possible compensatory effects of other hormones such as insulin. In addition, changes in food intake in patients with adrenal disease may further complicate interpretation of the actions of glucocorticoids on fat metabolism. The direct actions of glucocorticoids on adipose tissue seem to **facilitate lipolysis.**

Glucocorticoids exert effects on renal function that differ from those of mineralocorticoids. After adrenalectomy or in patients with adrenal insufficiency, there is a decrease in glomerular filtration rate and in renal blood flow. Such patients are also impaired in their ability to excrete a water load. These changes are corrected by administration of glucocorticoids such as cortisol but not by mineralocorticoids. The **negative feedback** effects of corticosteroids on pituitary secretion of adrenocorticotropic hormone (ACTH) are also directly related to glucocorticoid activity. That is, the greater the glucocorticoid potency of a steroid, the greater the inhibition of ACTH secretion. (The importance of this negative feedback activity in the regulation of cortisol secretion is discussed later in this chapter.) Effects of glucocorticoids on the gastrointestinal tract have also been observed. In particular, cortisol stimulates gastric acid secretion. Therefore, glucocorticoid treatment may be contraindicated in patients suffering from peptic ulcers.

A number of other effects of glucocorticoids have long been recognized but remain poorly understood. For example, glucocorticoids seem to have an important role in **adaptation to stress,** and indeed stress is one of the major stimuli for cortisol secretion. In adrenalectomized animals or in patients with adrenal insufficiency, severe stresses are poorly tolerated and may even be life-threatening. However, the precise role of glucocorticoids in the response to stress is not known. Glucocorticoids are also known to influence behavior and mood. Patients with adrenal hypofunction or hyperfunction often suffer from behavioral abnormalities that can be corrected by restoring normal hormone levels. The actions of glucocorticoids on behavior, like those on the response to stress, are not well understood.

Pharmacologic Effects. Supraphysiological concentrations of the naturally occurring glucocorticoids, such as cortisol, and the potent synthetic glucocorticoids exert important pharmacological actions, namely **anti-inflammatory and immunosuppressive effects.** Glucocorticoids have been widely used as anti-inflammatory agents in the treatment of diseases such as rheumatoid arthritis, disseminated lupus erythematosus, and rheumatic fever, in which the inflammatory response itself becomes a destructive process. Corticosteroids inhibit a number of the processes involved in inflammation, including capillary dilation, cellular exudation, and fibrin deposition. It should be emphasized that glucocorticoids modify these responses of the body to the disease but do not affect the underlying disease process.

One of the mechanisms of action of glucocorticoids on the inflammatory process is to inhibit the synthesis of prostaglandins, compounds that play a major role in initiating the inflammatory response. Glucocorticoids also decrease the release of biogenic amines by mast cells and leukocytes, thereby reducing the normal increase in capillary permeability that occurs during inflammation. Stabilization of lysosomal membranes, thereby decreasing the release of hydrolytic enzymes, and inhibition of the processes involved in mobilizing white blood cells to the inflamed area further contribute to inhibition of the inflammatory response by glucocorticoids.

The other major therapeutic use of glucocorticoids is as immunosuppressive agents. Glucocorticoids are used in the treatment of various allergic disorders, in some types of leukemia, in the prevention of organ transplant rejection, and for some autoimmune disorders. The immune response is complex, involving a number of different cell types, and glucocorticoids exert multiple effects on the overall process. For example, the proliferation of T lymphocytes (cells that play an important role in the immune response), is inhibited by corticosteroids. Glucocorticoids also inhibit immunoglobulin synthesis and kill B lymphocytes, the cells that are responsible for antibody production. As a result, antibody formation is inhibited. In addition, the production of complement, which is necessary for the killing actions of antibodies, is inhibited by glucocorticoids.

Mineralocorticoids

The major physiological effects of mineralocorticoids are on **electrolyte balance and blood pressure homeostasis.** Aldosterone is the most important of the naturally occurring mineralocorticoids and its principal site of action is

TABLE 7–5. Mineralocorticoid Effects and Target Tissues

Effect	Site of Action
Stimulates Na^+ reabsorption	Kidney, salivary glands, sweat glands
Stimulates K^+ excretion	Kidney, salivary glands, sweat glands
Stimulates H^+ excretion	Kidney

the distal tubule of the nephron in the kidney. The major effects of aldosterone are summarized in Table 7–5. Like other steroid hormones, mineralocorticoids interact with cytosolic receptors in their target cells, increasing RNA transcription and the synthesis of specific proteins. As a result of the production of these proteins by the renal tubular cell, aldosterone stimulates the **reabsorption of sodium ions** and enhances the **excretion of potassium and hydrogen ions.** The effects of aldosterone on sodium reabsorption promote expansion of the extracellular fluid volume. Therefore, the excessive production of mineralocorticoids often causes hypertension, whereas inadequate mineralocorticoid production is usually associated with low blood pressure.

The mechanism of action of aldosterone on sodium transport in the renal tubular cell is illustrated in Figure 7–3. The protein or proteins synthesized in response to aldosterone apparently stimulate sodium uptake by: (1) increasing the permeability of the luminal or apical membrane to sodium, (2) increasing mitochondrial ATP production, and (3) increasing Na^+/K^+-ATPase activity in the contraluminal or basal membrane. The latter effect may result in part from the increased ATP production. The net effect of these changes is to increase the renal reabsorption of sodium ions. The increase in sodium uptake in turn increases the negative potential in the lumen, which serves as a driving force for potassium ion excretion. This mechanism, therefore, tends to couple potassium excretion and sodium absorption, and this coupling is in fact normally observed. However, there are some exceptions. For example, it has long been recognized that the sodium-retaining effects of mineralocorticoids decline after several days, a process known as **renal escape.** Despite this decrease in sodium retention with time, the secretion of potassium ions continues to be stimulated by mineralocorticoids. Thus, mechanisms other than those involving sodium reabsorption may also contribute to the actions of mineralocorticoids on potassium excretion.

As noted earlier, mineralocorticoids stimulate renal excretion of hydrogen ions. Thus, hyperaldosteronism is often associated with metabolic alkalosis, and insufficient production of mineralocorticoids frequently causes acidosis. It is possible that hydrogen ions, like potassium ions, may be excreted by passive movement down the electrical gradient established by mineralocorticoid stimulation of sodium uptake. However, relatively little definitive information is available on the regulation of acid–base balance by mineralocorticoids.

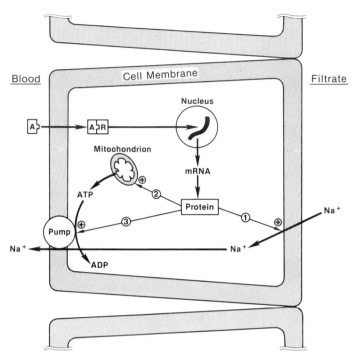

FIGURE 7–3. Mechanism(s) of action of aldosterone on sodium transport in the renal tubular cell. The numbered arrows indicate the three putative sites of action of aldosterone as described in the text. (A, aldosterone; R, receptor; +, stimulation.)

Androgens and Estrogens

The actions and mechanisms of action of adrenal androgens and estrogens are identical to those of the sex hormones of gonadal origin, and are discussed in Chapters 8 and 9. The estrogens of adrenal origin are produced in quite small quantities and have no known physiological significance. However, they may be important clinically in certain disease states characterized by feminization as a result of overproduction of adrenal estrogens. Large amounts of androgens are secreted by the adrenal cortex, but adrenal androgens are far less potent than the testicular androgen testosterone and are therefore of little physiological significance in the male. In females, on the other hand, the adrenal cortex is the major source of hormones having androgenic activity. Thus, androgen-dependent processes in the female such as development and maintenance of libido and growth of pubertal hair require adequate amounts of adrenal androgens. As discussed later in this chapter, the virilizing effects of adrenal androgens are quite prominent in a number of adrenocortical diseases.

METABOLISM OF ADRENAL HORMONES

Steroids are metabolized relatively slowly because of their extensive protein binding in plasma, which tends to protect them from degradation. In humans, cortisol has a plasma half-life of approximately 60 to 70 minutes. In contrast, the half-life of aldosterone, which is less extensively bound than cortisol in plasma, is only about 20 minutes. The metabolic clearance rate of aldosterone is far greater than that of cortisol, 2500 to 5000 liters/24 hours as opposed to 200 to 300 liters/24 hours. The rates and routes of metabolism of androgens and estrogens are discussed in Chapters 8 and 9, respectively.

The liver is the principal site of steroid metabolism, and for each steroid a large number of metabolites may be produced. Only the major pathways of metabolism are described in this text. In general, the enzymatic reactions involved in steroid metabolism tend to **decrease the biological activity of the hormones and increase their water solubility,** thereby facilitating their excretion in the urine. In humans, steroid hormones and their metabolites are excreted almost entirely in the urine. Consequently, estimates of steroid hormone secretion are often based on urinary metabolite levels.

The principal pathways of cortisol metabolism are illustrated in Figure 7–4. Other steroid hormones undergo similar types of structural changes in the course of hepatic metabolism. **Reduction of the double bonds and ketones** of the steroid molecule is a prominent feature of the metabolic pathway. Thus, saturation of the A ring of cortisol by hepatic enzymes results in the formation of the metabolite, tetrahydrocortisol. Further reduction at the C-20 position results in the formation of cortol (Fig. 7–4). Most of these reduced-steroid metabolites are conjugated at the 3-hydroxyl group before excretion. **Conjugation** greatly increases the water solubility of steroids, and glucuronides or sulfates are the most common conjugates produced; the former usually predominate for 21-carbon steroids. Thus, as shown in Figure 7–4, either tetrahydrocortisol or cortol may be converted to its glucuronide conjugate prior to excretion.

Other pathways of cortisol metabolism include oxidation of the C-11 hydroxyl group to a ketone, yielding the metabolite known as cortisone (Fig. 7–4). Cortisone may then undergo the same enzymatic modifications just described for cortisol. The corresponding metabolites would be tetrahydrocortisone, cortolone, and the glucuronide conjugate of each. Hydroxylation at the C-6 position of cortisol is a prominent reaction in infants but normally of little importance in adults. However, in certain disease states and in individuals treated with certain types of drugs, 6β-hydroxylation may become more important. Another minor metabolic pathway for glucocorticoids involves cleavage of the side chain of 21-carbon steroids, resulting in the production of 19-carbon metabolites having a ketone group at the 17-carbon position (17-ketosteroids).

A number of factors are known to influence the hepatic metabolism of steroids and consequently their rate of removal from the body. As examples,

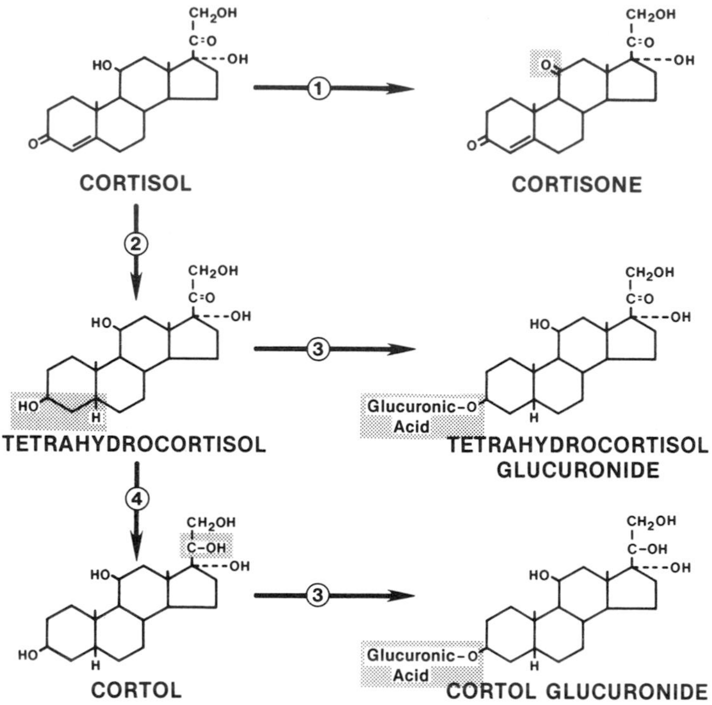

FIGURE 7–4. Principal pathways of hepatic cortisol metabolism. The numbers correspond to the following enzymes: (1) 11β-hydroxysteroid dehydrogenase; (2) Δ4–5 hydrogenase and 3-hydroxysteroid dehydrogenase; (3) glucuronyl transferase; (4) 20-hydroxysteroid dehydrogenase.

the rates of hepatic steroid metabolism are increased in patients with hyperthyroidism and decreased in hypothyroidism and in various types of liver disease. Although such diseases might produce transient changes in plasma steroid levels as a result of the changes in rate of hepatic steroid metabolism, adjustment in hormone secretion by the normal regulatory system tends to quickly return blood levels to normal. Age also seems to influence hepatic steroid metabolism; the plasma clearance of steroids is slower in infants and in very old persons than in normal adults.

REGULATION OF ADRENAL HORMONE SECRETION

Since there are different mechanisms involved in the regulation of cortisol, aldosterone, and androgen secretion by the adrenal cortex, each is described separately in this section.

Regulation of Glucocorticoid Secretion

Negative Feedback. Cortisol secretion by the adrenal cortex is regulated by a **negative feedback control** system involving the hypothalamus and anterior pituitary gland (Fig. 7–5). The hypothalamic and pituitary components of this regulatory system have been discussed to some extent in Chapters 4 and 5. The hypothalamus releases corticotropin-releasing hormone (CRH), which is transported to the corticotropin (ACTH)-producing cells of the anterior pituitary gland by the hypophyseal portal vessels. CRH, as a result of interactions with membrane receptors on the corticotropes, stimulates ACTH secretion. The mechanism of action of CRH has not been fully elucidated but seems to involve cyclic AMP (cAMP) as an intracellular mediator. The ACTH that is secreted in response to CRH is carried by the blood to the adrenal cortex, where it interacts with membrane-bound receptors on adrenocortical cells and stimulates cortisol secretion. The feedback control loop is completed by the inhibitory effects of plasma free cortisol on CRH and ACTH secretion by the hypothalamus and anterior pituitary, respectively (Fig. 7–5). The negative feedback effects of cortisol, like those of most other steroid hormones, are exerted primarily at the level of the hypothalamus. However, there is also some evidence for feedback effects by cortisol on the anterior pituitary gland to directly inhibit ACTH secretion.

The negative feedback system does not produce a uniform rate of cortisol release by the adrenal cortex. Instead, there are periods of secretory activity or "bursts" of secretion followed by periods of quiescence. The pattern of

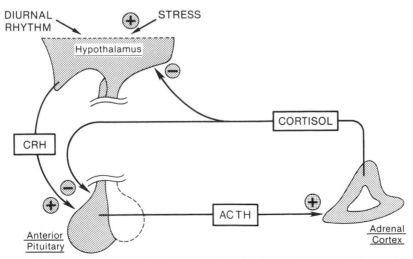

FIGURE 7–5. Regulation of cortisol secretion by the hypothalamo-pituitary axis. (+, stimulation; –, inhibition.)

adrenal cortisol secretion simply reflects the pattern of pituitary ACTH secretion that was discussed in Chapter 4. There tends to be relatively little variation in the rate of cortisol secretion from one secretory episode to the next. Therefore, the total amount of cortisol secreted during the course of a day is determined largely by the number of secretory periods.

Diurnal Rhythm and Stress. The negative feedback just described is the mechanism that is primarily responsible for regulation of cortisol secretion by the adrenal cortex. However, superimposed upon this basic control system are two additional factors that influence cortisol synthesis and release. One of those factors is a **diurnal rhythm.** In humans, the frequency of cortisol secretory bursts is greatest during the early morning hours and at a minimum late at night. As a result, there is a characteristic diurnal rhythm in plasma cortisol concentrations, with cortisol levels being far greater in the morning than at night (Fig. 7–6). It must be emphasized that the diurnal rhythm is in fact intrinsic to the hypothalamic-pituitary control system as described in Chapter 4. This diurnal pattern of secretion is related primarily to sleep and activity cycles and thus may be altered by changes in these habits. Those individuals who work nights and sleep days, for example, may have a diurnal pattern of cortisol secretion that is somewhat different from the majority of the population who work days and sleep at night. It is important for the clinician to be aware of the temporal pattern of cortisol secretion and of plasma cortisol levels when attempting to evaluate adrenocortical function. Thus, blood samples for

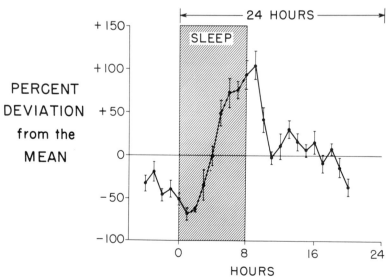

FIGURE 7–6. Diurnal rhythm in plasma cortisol concentrations. (From Orth, D.N., et al.: J. Clin. Endocrinol. 27:549, 1967.)

cortisol measurements must be drawn at standardized times of the day and the values interpreted in relation to what is appropriate for that time of day.

In addition to the diurnal rhythm, the other major factor that interacts with the negative feedback control system in the regulation of cortisol secretion is **stress.** It has long been recognized that all kinds of nonspecific stresses, both psychological and physical, can elicit dramatic increases in ACTH release and consequently in cortisol secretion. The effects of stress on cortisol secretion, like those of diurnal rhythm, are mediated through the central nervous system. Both are independent of, and in fact override, the negative feedback effects of cortisol on the hypothalamus and anterior pituitary. Therefore, acute stresses may produce dramatic increases in plasma cortisol levels. The magnitude of the cortisol secretory response is usually proportional to the intensity of the stimulus. Mild stresses may have relatively modest effects on cortisol secretion, whereas severe stresses will evoke major increases in cortisol output. The effects of acute stress tend to be greatest because adaptation occurs to certain types of chronic stress. As noted earlier in this chapter, the adrenal secretory response to stress seems to serve an important function because experimental animals as well as humans whose adrenal function is compromised are not able to tolerate stressful situations. For example, patients with adrenocortical insufficiency are very poor surgical risks because of the stress associated with surgery. Despite extensive investigation, the manner in which corticosteroids assist in the adaptation to stress is still not known.

Mechanism of Action of ACTH. Those factors described earlier that influence the rate of cortisol secretion do so by modifying the amount of ACTH that reaches the adrenal cortex. ACTH is the only known stimulus for cortisol secretion by the adrenal cortex, and cortisol secretion in general is directly controlled by plasma levels of ACTH. The actions of ACTH are primarily on the cells of the inner two zones of the adrenal cortex, the zona fasciculata and zona reticularis. As discussed more fully in the next section of this chapter, ACTH has relatively little effect on the function of the zona glomerulosa, namely aldosterone secretion. The actions of ACTH on the adrenal cortex include both **acute and chronic effects.** The long-term effects include stimulation of blood flow to the gland, a generalized stimulation of adrenal protein synthesis, and growth of the gland. As a result, under conditions of excessive ACTH secretion, the adrenal cortex becomes enlarged, and in the absence of adequate amounts of ACTH, the gland decreases in size or atrophies. Such changes in adrenal size are readily seen in various diseases associated with abnormally high or low ACTH secretion. Also included among the long-term effects of ACTH on the adrenal cortex is stimulation of the synthesis of the enzymes involved in steroidogenesis. Thus, the maintenance of the steroidogenic potential of the gland depends upon adequate amounts of ACTH. All of these long-term effects of ACTH appear to be **mediated by cAMP** since they are mimicked by administration of this second messenger.

The acute or short-term effects of ACTH on the adrenal cortex are con-

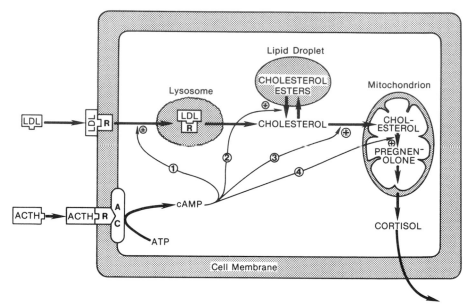

FIGURE 7–7. Mechanism of action of ACTH on adrenocortical steroidogenesis. The numbered arrows indicate the processes stimulated by ACTH as described in the text. (LDL, low density lipoprotein; R, receptor; +, stimulation.)

cerned primarily with the regulation of cortisol secretion. Administration of ACTH produces rapid changes in adrenocortical steroidogenesis. The acute actions of ACTH, like the chronic effects of the hormone on the gland, involve cAMP as the intracellular mediator. ACTH interacts with membrane-bound receptors on the cells of the inner two zones of the adrenal cortex and as a result activates adenylate cyclase, thereby increasing cAMP production (Fig. 7–7). cAMP then produces a number of effects that result in the **stimulation of cholesterol conversion to pregnenolone** (cholesterol side-chain cleavage), the rate-limiting step in cortisol production. ACTH promotes an increase in the amount of free cholesterol available for steroidogenesis by: (1) stimulating the uptake of low-density lipoproteins (Fig. 7–7), which are then further processed to generate free cholesterol as described in Chapter 1; (2) stimulating the hydrolysis of stored cholesterol esters within the adrenal cell, increasing the pool of free cholesterol, (3) stimulating the transport of cholesterol into mitochondria (Fig. 7–7), the location of the cholesterol side-chain cleavage enzyme; and (4) promoting the binding of cholesterol to the enzyme, an essential step for the initiation of enzyme activity. As a result of these effects of ACTH, cholesterol metabolism is accelerated, resulting in an increase in cortisol secretion. Conversely, in the absence of adequate amounts of ACTH, all of these processes decrease in activity, causing a decline in cortisol secretion.

There is evidence to indicate that in addition to cAMP, an intracellular protein mediator may be involved in the actions of ACTH on steroidogenesis. It has long been recognized that inhibitors of protein synthesis block the actions of ACTH on steroid secretion by the adrenal cortex. It appears that the requirement for protein synthesis resides at the level of the cholesterol side-chain cleavage enzyme. However, the identity of the protein factor and its specific function have not yet been determined.

Regulation of Mineralocorticoid Secretion

As noted earlier, the regulation of aldosterone secretion by the zona glomerulosa of the adrenal cortex is largely independent of cortisol secretion by the inner two zones of the gland. As might be predicted from the actions of mineralocorticoids, the regulation of aldosterone secretion is related principally to **electrolyte balance and blood pressure homeostasis.** Although several different factors interact in the overall regulation of aldosterone secretion, the renin-angiotensin system and plasma electrolyte concentrations are of the greatest physiological importance.

Renin-Angiotensin System. The renin-angiotensin system is a multicomponent system that plays an important role in the regulation of aldosterone secretion by the adrenal cortex (Fig. 7–8). Renin is an enzyme that is produced by the **juxtaglomerular apparatus** of the kidney and in response to appropriate stimuli is released into the blood. The renin then acts upon a circulating alpha-II globulin known as **angiotensinogen,** or renin substrate,

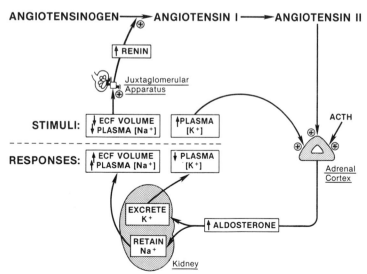

FIGURE 7–8. Regulation of aldosterone secretion by the zona glomerulosa of the adrenal cortex. (+, stimulation; −, inhibition; ECF, extracellular fluid.)

converting it to the decapeptide, **angiotensin I.** Angiotensin I is then converted to an octapeptide, **angiotensin II,** by an enzyme known as **converting enzyme.** The latter is found in particularly high concentrations in the pulmonary circulation. The angiotensin II may then be further processed to **angiotensin III** by removal of its amino terminal aspartic acid. However, the physiological significance of the latter conversion has not been fully resolved.

Angiotensin II as well as angiotensin III act directly on the cells of the zona glomerulosa to **stimulate aldosterone production** and secretion. The mechanism of action of the angiotensins on steroidogenesis in the zona glomerulosa has not been as clearly defined as that of ACTH in the other two zones of the adrenal cortex. The angiotensins interact with cell membrane receptors in the zona glomerulosa, and calcium, but not cAMP, is required for their actions on steroidogenesis. Recent studies indicate that an increase in phosphoinositol turnover may be involved in the actions of the angiotensins on aldosterone secretion. The angiotensins enhance aldosterone synthesis by stimulating cholesterol side-chain cleavage activity as well as by increasing the rate of conversion of corticosterone to aldosterone.

In addition to their effects on aldosterone secretion, the angiotensins also influence the size of the zona glomerulosa. Long-term effects of the angiotensins on the **growth of the zona glomerulosa** are analogous to those of ACTH on the zona fasciculata and zona reticularis of the adrenal cortex. Angiotensin II and angiotensin III also exert direct vasopressor effects on vascular smooth muscle; however, the physiological significance of these effects has not yet been determined. Angiotensin II and angiotensin III are approximately equipotent as stimulators of aldosterone secretion, but angiotensin II is a far more potent vasoconstrictor than angiotensin III.

The activity of the renin-angiotensin system is controlled primarily by blood pressure. The juxtaglomerular cells of the kidney are believed to act as baroreceptors, monitoring blood pressure in the afferent arterioles. A decrease in arterial pressure stimulates renin secretion by the juxtaglomerular cells, ultimately resulting in an increase in aldosterone secretion. Aldosterone, through its effects on renal sodium reabsorption, increases plasma volume and restores blood pressure to normal. Conversely, an increase in blood pressure in the afferent arterioles inhibits renin secretion, thereby decreasing aldosterone release by the adrenal cortex and ultimately producing a decline in blood pressure. Thus, the renin-angiotensin system and afferent arteriolar blood pressure tend to act as a negative feedback control system that serves to correct for any deviation from normal blood pressure (Fig. 7–8).

Blood pressure is not the only factor that controls the activity of the renin-angiotensin system. The sodium concentration of the renal tubular fluid may also play a role in the control of renin secretion. The **macula densa,** a group of specialized cells located at the origin of the distal tubule of the nephron, is believed to act as a chemoreceptor for sodium. According to this hypothesis, an increase in tubular fluid sodium concentration decreases renin release, and a decline in sodium levels stimulates renin secretion. In both cases, the corresponding change in aldosterone secretion would tend to restore sodium levels toward normal. Thus, a feedback control system involving renal tubular sodium concentrations may also participate in the regulation of aldosterone secretion.

Recent observations suggest that the sympathetic nerves innervating the kidney may also be involved in the regulation of the renin-angiotensin system. It has been demonstrated that the secretion of renin in response to various stimuli is blunted in the absence of those nerves. Prostaglandins may similarly influence the renin-angiotensin system since inhibition of prostaglandin synthesis decreases renin release. However, the importance of prostaglandins and of the renal sympathetic nerves in the overall regulation of the renin-angiotensin system is not known.

Estrogens, at least in large quantities, are known to influence the activity of the renin-angiotensin system. Women taking oral contraceptives and pregnant women have elevated plasma levels of both renin and aldosterone. The increased activity of the renin-angiotensin system probably accounts for the positive sodium balance and volume expansion that often accompany pregnancy or the use of oral contraceptives. Although it has been clearly established that large amounts of estrogens influence the renin-angiotensin system, it is not clear whether physiological amounts participate in the regulation of aldosterone secretion.

Plasma Potassium Concentrations. The second major regulatory factor involved in the control of aldosterone secretion is plasma potassium concentration. Changes in plasma potassium levels directly affect aldosterone secretion by the cells of the zona glomerulosa, independent of the renin-angiotensin system (Fig. 7–8). An increase in plasma potassium concentrations stimulates aldosterone secretion, whereas a decline in circulating potassium decreases aldosterone synthesis and release. Since one of the actions of aldosterone is to stimulate potassium excretion by the kidney, the secretory response in each case tends to restore plasma potassium levels to normal. Thus, plasma potassium and aldosterone comprise a feedback control loop that serves to regulate plasma potassium levels. Potassium appears to stimulate aldosterone secretion by stimulating an early step in the steroidogenic pathway, probably cholesterol side-chain cleavage. It is not clear whether plasma potassium levels *per se* or changes in the concentration of potassium within the cells of the zona glomerulosa mediate the effects of the ion on steroidogenesis.

ACTH. For many years it was believed that ACTH played no role in the regulation of aldosterone secretion since hypophysectomy has relatively little effect on the zona glomerulosa. However, in recent years, receptors for ACTH have been demonstrated on cells of the zona glomerulosa, and ACTH has been shown to stimulate aldosterone secretion in some circumstances. Nonetheless, any role for ACTH in the regulation of aldosterone secretion must be considered a minor one in relation to the renin-angiotensin system and plasma electrolytes. Various polypeptide fragments derived from the ACTH precursor pro-opiomelanocortin can also stimulate aldosterone secretion by zona glomerulosa cells. However, the physiological significance of these peptides in the regulation of aldosterone secretion is not yet known.

Regulation of Adrenal Androgen Secretion

In general, adrenal androgen and cortisol output parallel each other. Thus, under most circumstances, ACTH appears to be the major regulator of adrenal androgen secretion. However, there are times when androgen and cortisol output by the adrenal cortex diverge. For example, at about the time of puberty there is a dramatic increase in adrenal androgen secretion but little change in cortisol output. The change in adrenal function that occurs at this time is known as the **adrenarche;** it is this change that initiates the development of androgen-dependent processes in females. In addition to the divergence of androgen and cortisol secretion at adrenarche, with advancing age there is a decline in adrenal androgen secretion but no apparent change in cortisol output. Similarly, various disease states and other abnormal conditions have differing effects on androgen and cortisol secretion by the adrenal cortex. As a result of this occasional divergence the involvement of factors other than ACTH in the regulation of adrenal androgen secretion has been proposed for a number of years. Conflicting reports on the effects of prolactin on adrenal androgen secretion have appeared in the literature, but other known pituitary hormones appear to have little or no effect. Recent reports suggest that an as yet unidentified pituitary peptide may selectively stimulate androgen secretion by adrenocortical cells. However, at this time, the role of factors other than ACTH in the regulation of adrenal androgen secretion remains unresolved and further investigation is clearly needed.

CLINICAL APPLICATION

Although not common, a number of different disorders of adrenal cortical function may occur. Since an understanding of the procedures involved in the evaluation of adrenal cortical function is essential for the differential diagnosis of the various adrenal disorders, some of the more common diagnostic procedures are briefly described before diseases of the adrenal cortex are discussed.

Diagnostic Procedures

Some of the more common tests of adrenal cortical function are listed in Table 7–6 and are divided into those procedures used to evaluate glucocorticoid function and those used to evaluate mineralocorticoid function. In both cases, one of the simplest approaches is to measure **plasma steroid concentra-**

TABLE 7–6.   Diagnostic Tests for Evaluating Adrenocortical Function

Test	What Is Measured	Expected Result in Normal Person
Glucocorticoid		
Plasma steroids	Cortisol	9–24 μg/dl at 8–9 A.M.
Diurnal rhythm	Plasma cortisol	High in morning, low at night
ACTH stimulation	Plasma cortisol	Increases after ACTH
Insulin-induced hypoglycemia	Plasma cortisol and/or ACTH	Increases after insulin
Dexamethasone suppression	Plasma cortisol	Decreases after dexamethasone
Metyrapone test	Plasma 11-deoxycortisol or Urinary 17-OH-cortico-steroids	Increases after metyrapone
Mineralocorticoid		
Plasma steroids	Aldosterone	1–5 ng/dl (supine position)
Plasma renin activity	Conversion of renin sub-strate to angiotensin I (or II)	0.5–3.0 ng angiotensin I/ml plasma/hr (10–40 pg angiotensin II/ml/hr)
Sodium depletion (furose-mide)	Plasma renin activity and/or aldosterone	Increases after furosemide
Sodium loading	Plasma renin activity and/or aldosterone	Decreases

tions to determine if values are in the normal range. For plasma cortisol determinations, the time of drawing blood is important because of the **diurnal rhythm** in plasma cortisol levels. Since the absence of a diurnal rhythm may indicate adrenal cortical disease, plasma cortisol levels should be measured early in the morning and late at night to test for the presence of a diurnal rhythm. The ability of the adrenal cortex to respond to appropriate stimuli may be evaluated by measuring plasma cortisol concentrations before and after **ACTH administration** or **insulin-induced hypoglycemia.** In normal individuals, plasma cortisol levels should increase in response to both stimuli.

The normal functioning of the negative feedback control system that regulates cortisol secretion may be evaluated by the **dexamethasone suppression test** or the **metyrapone test** or both (Table 7–6). Dexamethasone is a very potent glucocorticoid; therefore, in normal individuals it should suppress ACTH secretion and decrease plasma cortisol levels. Metyrapone is an inhibitor of 11β-hydroxylation, the reaction that converts 11-deoxycortisol to cortisol. Thus, in a normal person, metyrapone administration blocks cortisol production, thereby bringing about a compensatory increase in ACTH secretion. ACTH in turn stimulates the steroidogenic pathway in the adrenal cortex. However, because 11β-hydroxylation is blocked, the immediate precursor to the reaction, 11-deoxycortisol, is secreted in very large quantities. Thus, after administration of metyrapone, plasma levels of 11-deoxycortisol and urinary excretion of its metabolites increase dramatically in normal individuals.

Tests of mineralocorticoid function include evaluation of the activity of the renin-angiotensin system, the major physiological regulator of aldosterone secretion. For example, **plasma renin activity** (the capacity of plasma samples to catalyze the conversion of angiotensinogen to angiotensin I or angiotensin II) is widely used as an index of the functional status of the renin-angiotensin system. In a normal individual, **sodium depletion,** induced by the diuretic furosemide, increases plasma renin activity as well as plasma aldosterone levels. Conversely **sodium loading** by intravenous administration of sodium chloride should suppress plasma renin activity and decrease plasma aldosterone concentrations if the renin-angiotensin system is functioning normally (Table 7–6).

Diseases of the Adrenal Cortex

Cushing's Syndrome. The disease characterized by **excessive cortisol secretion** is known as Cushing's syndrome. Some of the more common symptoms of Cushing's syndrome are summarized in Table 7–7. All of the symptoms are attributable to excessive cortisol or androgen secretion and the resulting actions of those hormones. The hypertension is a reflection of the mineralocorticoid activity that may be manifested by large amounts of glucocorticoids. Patients often show a typical central pattern of obesity known as **centripetal obesity,** as well as a rounding and fullness of the cheeks (moon facies). Many of the other symptoms of Cushing's syndrome represent an exaggeration of the physiological effects of cortisol, particularly of its catabolic actions (Table 7–7).

There are three major types of Cushing's syndrome based upon the causes of the disorder (Fig. 7–9). The type caused by excessive pituitary secretion of ACTH is also known as **Cushing's disease.** Cushing's syndrome may

TABLE 7–7. Symptoms of Cushing's Syndrome

Symptom	Frequency of Occurrence (%)
Centripetal obesity	95
Hypertension	82
Hyperglycemia	80
Amenorrhea or impotence	75
Hirsutism	75
Purple striae	65
"Moon" facies	60
Osteoporosis	60
Easy bruisability	60
Personality change	55

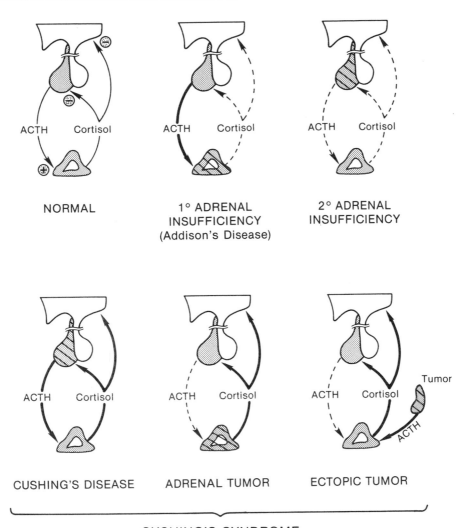

NORMAL

1° ADRENAL
INSUFFICIENCY
(Addison's Disease)

2° ADRENAL
INSUFFICIENCY

CUSHING'S DISEASE

ADRENAL TUMOR

ECTOPIC TUMOR

CUSHING'S SYNDROME

FIGURE 7–9. Pathophysiology of primary (1°) and secondary (2°) adrenocortical insufficiency and of the different types of Cushing's syndrome. The bold arrows indicate greater amounts than normal and the broken arrows less than normal. (+, stimulation; −, inhibition.)

also be caused by **autonomously functioning adrenal tumors** or by **ectopic ACTH-secreting tumors,** most commonly of the lung. It is important to be able to differentiate among the different types of Cushing's syndrome because the appropriate treatment depends upon its cause. In all forms of Cushing's syndrome, plasma cortisol levels are usually elevated and the diurnal rhythm

TABLE 7–8. Differential Diagnosis of Various Types of Cushing's Syndrome

	Cushing's Disease	Adrenal Tumor	Ectopic ACTH
Plasma cortisol	↑	↑	↑
Diurnal rhythm	Absent	Absent	Absent
Plasma ACTH	↑	↓	↑
Plasma cortisol after:			
Low-dose dexamethasone	No change	No change	No change
High-dose dexamethasone	↓	No change	No change
Response to metyrapone	↑	No change	No change
(cortisol + 11-deoxycortisol)			
ACTH stimulation	↑	Variable	Variable
(plasma cortisol)			

in plasma cortisol is absent (Table 7–8). Measurement of plasma ACTH concentrations, although not routinely done in most laboratories, may be helpful in making a differential diagnosis. Plasma ACTH concentrations are elevated in patients with Cushing's disease or with ectopic ACTH production but decreased in patients with functional adrenal tumors because of the negative feedback effects of cortisol on pituitary ACTH secretion. The dexamethasone suppression test is often useful in the diagnosis of Cushing's disease (Table 7–8). Although low doses of dexamethasone generally fail to suppress all types of Cushing's syndrome, higher doses will usually decrease plasma cortisol levels in patients whose disease is of pituitary origin. Apparently, in Cushing's disease the negative feedback control system is not completely lost but is far less sensitive to steroid feedback than normal. Patients with Cushing's disease will also usually respond to metyrapone (Table 7–8), whereas those with adrenal tumors or with ectopic tumors do not respond because of the autonomous nature of ACTH production by tumors. In patients with ectopic ACTH producing tumors, symptoms associated with the primary lesion—that is, the tumor itself—are often useful in determining the etiology of Cushing's syndrome.

Adrenal and ectopic tumors are treated by surgical removal of the tumors. In patients with Cushing's disease, if a pituitary tumor can be located, it too should be surgically removed. If a pituitary tumor cannot be identified, alternative approaches include radiation of the pituitary gland, bilateral adrenalectomy, and treatment with inhibitors of adrenal steroidogenesis such as aminoglutethimide or metyrapone.

Adrenocortical Insufficiency. The inadequate production of corticosteroids by the adrenal cortex may be caused by a pituitary abnormality resulting in insufficient secretion of ACTH or by a defect within the adrenal cortices rendering them unable to synthesize normal amounts of steroid hormones. The latter is known as **primary adrenocortical insufficiency, or Addison's disease,** and the former is known as **secondary adrenocortical insufficiency.** The pathophysiology of primary and of secondary adrenocortical insufficiency is illustrated in Figure 7–9. In Addison's disease, because the pituitary is normal, the decline in cortisol secretion brings about an increase in ACTH output by the pituitary. In secondary adrenocortical insufficiency, by contrast, both ACTH and cortisol secretion are below normal. In addition, in primary adrenocortical insufficiency, secretion of all adrenal steroids, including aldosterone, is below normal. However, since ACTH has little effect on mineralocorticoid production by the adrenal cortex, there is little or no change in aldosterone secretion in secondary adrenocortical insufficiency.

Some of the more common symptoms of primary adrenocortical insufficiency are listed in Table 7–9. Most of the symptoms are a direct result of inadequate cortisol or aldosterone secretion. The hyperpigmentation is caused by the excessive secretion of ACTH as well as of MSH. Hyperpigmentation is not seen in secondary adrenocortical insufficiency because ACTH levels are not elevated and are in fact below normal. Similarly, in secondary adrenocortical insufficiency there is usually no change in plasma potassium or sodium levels because the decline in ACTH secretion has little effect on the mineralocorticoid functions of the adrenal cortex.

Differentiation between primary and secondary adrenocortical insufficiency can be made by determination of plasma ACTH concentrations or more commonly with the ACTH stimulation test (Table 7–10). In the primary form of the disorder, plasma ACTH levels are above normal, whereas in secondary adrenocortical insufficiency, ACTH levels are subnormal. In Addison's disease, the adrenal cortex is unable to make adequate amounts of corticosteroids despite already high levels of ACTH. Therefore, stimulation with exogenous ACTH has no effect on plasma cortisol levels. In secondary adrenocortical insufficiency, by contrast, since an ACTH deficiency is the cause of the disorder, administration of exogenous ACTH will usually elicit an increase in cortisol secretion, although treatment for several days may be required to elicit the response.

Treatment of Addison's disease requires both glucocorticoid and mineralocorticoid replacement because secretion of both cortisol and aldosterone is

TABLE 7–9. Symptoms of Primary Adrenocortical Insufficiency

Symptom	Frequency of Occurrence (%)
Weakness and fatigability	100
Weight loss	100
Hyperpigmentation	92
Hypotension	88
Hyponatremia	88
Hyperkalemia	65
Gastrointestinal problems	55

**TABLE 7–10.   Differential Diagnosis of Primary vs. Secondary
Adrenocortical Insufficiency**

	Primary	Secondary
Plasma cortisol	↓	↓
Response to metyrapone	↓	↓
Response to insulin-induced hypoglycemia	↓	↓
Plasma ACTH	↑	↓
ACTH stimulation (plasma cortisol)	No change	↑

subnormal. In secondary adrenocortical insufficiency, however, treatment with glucocorticoid is sufficient. Although primary adrenocortical insufficiency may be caused by a number of different invasive processes such as infiltration of the adrenal cortex by carcinomas or by tuberculosis, the most common cause is idiopathic atrophy of the gland. An autoimmune etiology for idiopathic Addison's disease is highly probable.

Hyperaldosteronism. Excessive production of aldosterone by the adrenal cortex may be caused by a functional tumor of the gland or by inappropriately high activity of the renin-angiotensin system. The former condition is known as **primary hyperaldosteronism or Conn's syndrome,** and the latter is called **secondary hyperaldosteronism** (Table 7–11). The secondary form of the disease can be caused by any of a number of conditions, including liver and kidney (renovascular) disease, that cause edema and a decrease in effective arterial volume. As a result, the renin-angiotensin system is inappropriately activated, increasing renin and aldosterone secretion.

In both primary and secondary hyperaldosteronism, plasma aldosterone levels are elevated and the symptoms are those associated with mineralocorticoid excess—namely hypertension, hypokalemia, and metabolic alkalosis (Table 7–11). Patients with primary hyperaldosteronism usually do not have edema because after several days the sodium-retaining effects of aldosterone

TABLE 7–11.   Pathogenesis of Primary vs. Secondary Hyperaldosteronism

Primary Hyperaldosteronism

$$\uparrow \text{Aldosterone} \rightarrow \uparrow \text{Na}^+ \text{retention} \rightarrow \begin{bmatrix} \uparrow \text{ECF volume} \\ + \\ \uparrow \text{Renal perfusion pressure} \end{bmatrix} \rightarrow \downarrow \text{Renin}$$

Secondary Hyperaldosteronism

$$\downarrow \text{Renal perfusion pressure} \rightarrow \uparrow \text{Renin} \rightarrow \uparrow \text{Aldosterone} \rightarrow \begin{bmatrix} \uparrow \text{Na}^+ \text{retention} \\ + \\ \uparrow \text{ECF volume} \end{bmatrix}$$

are lost, although potassium continues to be excreted. Differentiation between primary and secondary hyperaldosteronism is important for determining the appropriate treatment and is normally quite straightforward. In the secondary form of the disease, high plasma aldosterone levels are accompanied by high plasma renin activity, whereas in the primary form of the disease the volume expansion caused by excessive aldosterone production decreases renin production by the juxtaglomerular cells (Table 7–11). Therefore, the differences in plasma renin activity readily indicate the distinction between the two types

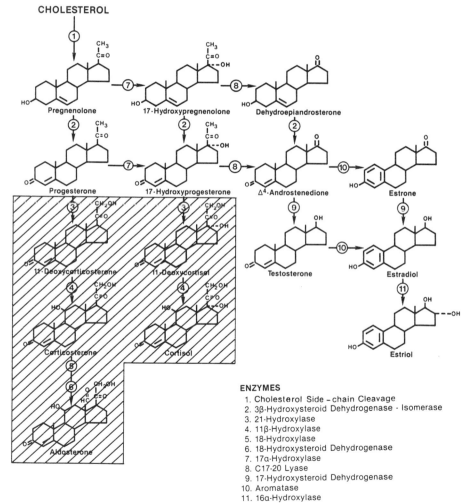

ENZYMES

1. Cholesterol Side–chain Cleavage
2. 3β-Hydroxysteroid Dehydrogenase · Isomerase
3. 21-Hydroxylase
4. 11β-Hydroxylase
5. 18-Hydroxylase
6. 18-Hydroxysteroid Dehydrogenase
7. 17α-Hydroxylase
8. C17-20 Lyase
9. 17-Hydroxysteroid Dehydrogenase
10. Aromatase
11. 16α-Hydroxylase

FIGURE 7–10. Consequences of a 21-hydroxylase (enzyme number 3) deficiency on adrenocortical steroidogenesis. The shaded area contains the hormones that cannot be synthesized as a result of the defect.

of hyperaldosteronism. Primary hyperaldosteronism is treated by removal of the tumor causing the disorder. With secondary hyperaldosteronism, the primary lesion that caused activation of the renin-angiotensin system must be treated. Drugs that block the effects of mineralocorticoids on the kidney are often useful in treating the edema accompanying secondary hyperaldosteronism.

Congenital Adrenal Hyperplasia. Congenital adrenal hyperplasia (CAH) encompasses a group of disorders characterized by an **inherited enzymatic defect in the steroidogenic pathway.** The defect may cause either a partial or complete block in one of the enzymatic steps required for cortisol synthesis. As a result of inadequate cortisol production, a compensatory increase in ACTH secretion results, causing the production of excessive amounts of those steroids in the pathway that precede the block. The specific symptoms vary with the site of the enzymatic defect because the pattern of steroid secretion is determined by the site of the block in the steroidogenic pathway. When the defective enzyme is one that is found in the testes or ovaries as well as in the adrenal cortex, the defect also occurs in the gonads, affecting synthesis of androgen or estrogen or both in those organs. It should be noted that many variants of CAH have been described and only a few of the simpler types are described in this chapter.

The consequences of a **21-hydroxylase deficiency,** the most common variant of CAH, are illustrated in Figure 7–10 and summarized in Table 7–12. As can be seen, the enzymatic deficiency blocks the production of cortisol and of aldosterone. The decline in cortisol production elicits an increase in ACTH secretion that stimulates the steroidogenic pathway, but because of the enzy-

TABLE 7–12.   Major Types of Congenital Adrenal Hyperplasia in Decreasing Order of Frequency and Their Symptoms

Enzyme Defect	Steroid Abnormality	Symptoms
21-Hydroxylase	↓ Cortisol ↓ Aldosterone ↑ Androgens	Masculinization Salt loss
11β-Hydroxylase	↓ Cortisol ↓ Aldosterone ↑ Androgens ↑ DOC	Masculinization (mild) Hypertension
3β-Hydroxysteroid dehydrogenase	↓ Cortisol ↓ Aldosterone ↑ DHEA	Salt loss Masculinization (mild) in ♀
17α-Hydroxylase	↓ Cortisol ↓ Androgens and estrogens ↑ DOC and corticosterone ↓ Aldosterone	Hypertension Hypokalemic alkalosis Sexual infantilism

matic defect, cortisol cannot be synthesized and large amounts of adrenal androgens are produced. The increase in androgen production accompanied by the decline in mineralocorticoid secretion results in virilization as well as in sodium loss and hypotension. The characteristic steroid abnormalities and symptoms of several other types of CAH are summarized in Table 7–12. In general, treatment of congenital adrenal hyperplasia requires administration of those hormones that cannot be synthesized because of the enzymatic defect in the steroidogenic pathway.

REFERENCES

Bondy, P.K.: Diseases of the adrenal cortex. *In* Williams' Textbook of Endocrinology, 7th ed. J.D. Wilson, and D.W. Foster, editors, W.B. Saunders Company, Philadelphia, p. 816, 1985.

Farese, R.V.: Phosphoinositide metabolism and hormone action. Endocrine Rev. 4:78, 1983.

James, V.H.T.: The Adrenal Gland. Raven Press, New York, 1979.

Makin, H.L.J.: Biochemistry of Steroid Hormones. Blackwell Scientific Publications, London, 1975.

Munck, A., Guyre, P.M., and Holbrook, N.J.: Physiological functions of glucocorticoids in stress and their relation to pharmacologic actions. Endocrine Rev. 5:25, 1984.

O'Dell, W., and Parker, L.: Control of adrenal androgen secretion. *In* Adrenal Androgens. A.R. Genazzani, et al. editors. Raven Press, New York, p. 27, 1980.

Simpson, E.R.: Cholesterol side-chain cleavage, cytochrome P-450, and the control of steroidogenesis. Mol. Cell Endocrinol. 13:213, 1979.

Strauss, J.F. and Menon, K.M.J.: Lipoprotein and Cholesterol Metabolism in Steroidogenic Tissues. George F. Stickley Co., Philadelphia, 1985.

8

REPRODUCTIVE FUNCTION IN THE MALE

INTRODUCTION

The function of the male reproductive system is to produce sperm and deliver them to the female. This function requires three distinct processes that involve separate anatomical compartments. One function obviously essential to male reproduction is the formation of sperm from germ cells. This process is called **spermatogenesis** and takes place in the seminiferous tubules, one of the major compartments of the testes. A second compartment within the testes, the Leydig cells, is responsible for the **endocrine** component of male reproduction. Leydig cells secrete the male sex steroid, testosterone, which plays a critical role in many aspects of reproductive function. The third component is a **delivery system** that consists of a series of ducts and associated secretory glands referred to as the male reproductive tract.

SPERMATOGENESIS

Gametogenesis in the male is a complex process by which relatively undifferentiated germ cells, containing a diploid complement of 46 chromosomes, are turned into extremely specialized sperm. During this process, the chromosome number is reduced by half, and the cytoplasm is extensively remodeled so all that remains in a mature sperm is a nucleus, a means of mobility (the tail and associated mitochondria), and an enzymatic drill (the acrosome) for entering the ovum. Spermatogenesis takes 64 days in men, but asynchrony among germ cells ensures a continuous production of sperm and the normal adult produces approximately 30 million sperm/day.

Stages of Spermatogenesis

Spermatogenesis can be divided into three major stages: mitotic proliferation, meiosis, and packaging. It begins with the **mitosis** of a germ cell, or spermatogonium, to form two daughter cells (Fig. 8–1). One of these cells then

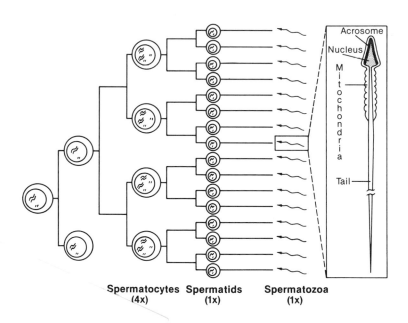

Spermatocytes   Spermatids   Spermatozoa
    (4x)   (1x)   (1x)

Meiosis —+— Packaging—|

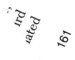

nesis in man. Two of the 23 pairs of chromosomes
ıber of chromosome sets at each stage is indicated

continues on to form sperm, while the other remains as a resting spermato-gonium, thus maintaining the germ cell line. The former cell undergoes a se-ries of mitotic divisions, the number of which is species-dependent. After the final division, the cells, now called spermatocytes, enter a resting phase dur-ing which chromosomes are duplicated in preparation for meiosis. In man, the daughter cell divides twice producing four spermatocytes, each containing double the normal number of chromosomes.

During **meiosis**, the spermatocyte divides twice without DNA replication so the resulting four spermatids each contain 23 unpaired chromosomes. This ensures that sperm carry half the normal amount of genetic information so that fertilization of the haploid ovum restores the normal complement of 46 chro-mosomes. In addition to this important reduction in chromosome number, the process of meiosis allows some chromosomes to exchange segments of DNA, thus mixing their genetic information.

Even after meiosis, spermatids in most respects resemble normal epithe-lial cells. Production of mature spermatozoa requires extensive remodeling of both nucleus and cytoplasm. This **packaging**, or spermiogenesis, includes con-densation of chromatin into a tight inert packet, formation of the acrosome by aggregation of Golgi-produced enzymatic vesicles, growth of the tail out of one centriole, and extrusion of most of the cytoplasm. In man, the spermatogenic sequence can theoretically produce a clone of 16 spermatozoa each time a spermatogonium initiates this process. However, this high efficiency is rare because some cells are usually lost in each stage of spermatogenesis.

Anatomical Aspects of Spermatogenesis

The location of the testes in the scrotum is essential for spermatogenesis because this process is **temperature-sensitive** and cannot occur at normal body temperature. In the scrotum, testicular temperature is lowered suffi-ciently to allow spermatogenesis. The temperature differential between testes and abdominal cavity is maintained, in part, by the close apposition of sper-matic artery and vein so the incoming arterial blood is cooled by the colder venous outflow. Contraction or relaxation of scrotal muscles on exposure to a cold or hot environment, respectively, also helps maintain the appropriate testicular temperature by altering the distance between the testes and ab-domen.

Approximately 80 per cent of testicular mass consists of numerous semi-niferous tubules that empty into the epididymis via the rete testes (Fig. 8–2). These tubules contain two functionally important cell types, germ cells (sper-matogonia and developing sperm) and Sertoli cells, which provide crucial sup-port for spermatogenesis. Examination of these tubules in cross-section re-veals an **anatomical progression** that parallels the temporal sequence of spermatogenesis. Sertoli cells and undifferentiated spermatogonia line the outer basement membrane while each clone of differentiating daughter cells

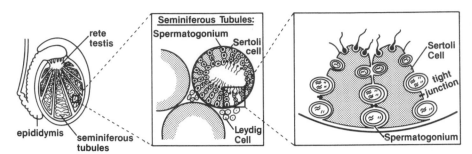

FIGURE 8–2. Components of testes at three magnifications.

migrates toward the tubule lumen as it moves progressively through the stages of spermatogenesis (Fig. 8–2). This histological picture, however, is complicated because the time between initiation of two successive spermatogenic generations is approximately a quarter of that required for completion of spermatogenesis (e.g., 16 days in men). Thus, when one clone of daughter cells is a quarter of the way through gametogenesis the next clone begins to form, and four successive clones, each further along in development and closer to the tubular lumen, are visible in a single histological specimen. This migration allows the completed spermatozoa to be released into the lumen of the seminiferous tubule, from which the sperm can be transported to the epididymis and then into the male reproductive tract.

Sertoli Cells

Sertoli cells perform several tasks essential for normal spermatogenesis. First, a **blood-testes barrier** is maintained by tight junctions between adjacent Sertoli cells (Fig. 8–2). This barrier prevents movement of proteins, charged organic molecules, and ions from interstitial fluid into the seminiferous tubules. Consequently, the composition of intratubular fluid differs markedly from interstitial fluid, and this composition may be critical for later stages of spermatogenesis that occur in the intratubular compartment. The blood-testes barrier also provides important immunological protection, preventing the formation of antibodies against the highly differentiated spermatozoa. Second, Sertoli cell cytoplasm completely surrounds the developing sperm providing important **nutrients** and perhaps helping to direct cytodifferentiation of spermatids. Third, these cells **secrete seminiferous tubule fluid**. This secretion literally washes the released sperm from the tubular lumen into the epididymis. It contains high concentrations of KCl, inositol, and glutamate but very little protein. It does, however, contain an androgen-binding protein, secreted by Sertoli cells, that maintains very high androgen levels within the male reproductive tract. Finally, Sertoli cells have an important **phagocytic function**, destroying cytoplasm extruded from the developing sperm as well as those sperm that fail to successfully complete all stages of spermatogenesis.

MALE REPRODUCTIVE TRACT

The male reproductive tract, which delivers sperm to the female in a vehicle (semen) conducive to sperm viability, can be divided into a sequence of ducts and three major secretory glands. Moving from testes to penis, sperm pass through the epididymis, ductus (or vas) deferens, ejaculatory duct, and urethra (Fig. 8–3). The major accessory sex glands, which provide most of the semen, are the seminal vesicles, prostate, and bulbourethral gland.

Ducts

In addition to transporting sperm, the ducts of the male reproductive tract have important functional roles. The **epididymis**, a convoluted tube of smooth muscle lined with secretory epithelium, is the site of final sperm maturation. Sperm leaving the seminiferous tubules are incapable of either movement or fertilization but in their passage through the epididymis gain both capabilities. The epididymis also absorbs most of the fluid entering from the seminiferous tubules, concentrating sperm 100-fold, and adds some enzymes and organic molecules to this fluid. Slow rhythmic contractions of the epididymal smooth muscle move the maturing sperm through the epididymis and into the **ductus deferens**, which carries the sperm back into the abdominal cavity through the inguinal canal. The ductus deferens has a thick muscular lining and at the urethral end enlarges considerably to form the ampulla, an important site of sperm storage. A short **ejaculatory duct** from each ampulla then converges to join the **urethra**, which carries the sperm on the final stages of their journey out of the male during ejaculation.

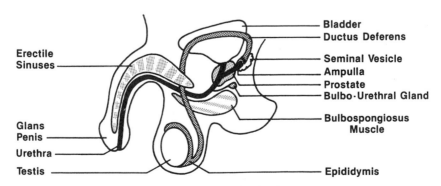

FIGURE 8–3. Male reproductive tract.

TABLE 8–1. Some Major Components of Semen

Constituent	Source	Probable Function
Sperm	Testis	Fertilization
Glycerophosphorylcholine	Epididymis	Secondary energy source
Carnitine	Epididymis	Unknown
Fructose	Seminal vesicles	Primary energy source
Prostaglandins	Seminal vesicles	Contractions of female reproductive tract
Fibrinogen	Seminal vesicles	Substrate for clotting enzymes
Ascorbic acid	Seminal vesicles	Unknown
Acid phosphatase	Prostate	Formation of glycerophosphate from glycerophosphorylcholine
Clotting enzymes	Prostate	Formation of coagulum
Fibrinolysin	Prostate	Breakdown of coagulum
Buffers	Prostate	Neutralize acid secretions of female reproductive tract
Citric acid	Prostate	Unknown

Accessory Sex Glands

Most constituents of semen (Table 8–1) are produced by two accessory sex glands, the seminal vesicles and prostate. The **seminal vesicles** are bilateral glands that empty into the ampulla of the ductus deferens (Fig. 8–3). Histologically, they consist of a convoluted network of ducts lined with secretory epithelia and surrounded by smooth muscle. These glands secrete a viscous fluid containing ascorbic acid, prostaglandins, a number of proteins including fibrinogen, and fructose, which is the primary source of energy for ejaculated sperm. This fluid, which makes up over half of the semen, is ejected shortly after the sperm leave the ampulla and helps wash them into the urethra.

The **prostate** is a large gland surrounding the ejaculatory duct and urethra and composed of several lobes inside a connective tissue capsule containing smooth muscle fibers. The prostatic secretion, which is released into the urethra, is a thin relatively alkaline fluid that contains phosphate and bicarbonate buffers, citric acid, and a number of enzymes including acid phosphatase, clotting enzymes, and fibrinolysin. The prostate gland contains a high zinc concentration and appears to need this element for normal function. The final major accessory sex gland is the **bulbourethral** (or Cowper's) gland that secretes a mucus-like substance prior to ejaculation.

Although seminal fluid is not absolutely essential for fertilization, it has several functions that greatly facilitate this process. First, it provides the bulk of the semen. This volume not only helps to wash the sperm into the urethra but also dilutes the thick mass of sperm, allowing the spermatozoa to develop motility. Second, sperm are highly sensitive to pH so the buffers and relative alkalinity of seminal fluid are probably important for neutralizing the acidic secretions of the female reproductive tract. Third, fructose and glycerophosphate (derived from glycerophosphorylcholine) provide energy necessary for sperm motility. Fourth, the clotting enzymes of the prostate act on fibrinogen from the seminal vesicles to form a coagulum that may help keep the sperm in the female reproductive tract during disengagement. This coagulum is broken down by fibrinolysin 15 to 20 minutes after coitus, releasing motile sperm. Finally, it has been suggested that prostaglandins in the seminal fluid stimulate muscular contractions in the female reproductive tract and that these contractions help transport the sperm to the ovum located in the oviduct.

MALE SEX ACT

Ultimately, delivery of semen into the female requires the male sex act, a complex reflex involving all parts of the male reproductive tract, the lumbar and sacral portion of the spinal cord, and the autonomic nervous system. The major source of tactile input to this reflex comes from sensory nerves in the genital region, and particularly those in the glans penis. In addition to these integral components, this reflex is usually influenced by descending input from the central nervous system so that psychic stimuli often play a critical role.

The first step in the male sex act is **erection** of the penis, initiated by tactile or psychic stimuli. Erection is caused by parasympathetic impulses that dilate the major penile arteries, increasing blood flow into the sinuses of the penis. The resulting increase in blood volume compresses the veins, decreasing venous return, and contributing to a further buildup of blood that eventually produces an erection. Parasympathetic impulses also cause secretion of mucus from the bulbourethral gland, which passes through the urethra to aid in lubrication. With sustained sexual stimulation, sympathetic impulses cause sequential contraction of smooth muscles in the prostate, epididymis, ductus deferens, and seminal vesicles. This causes **emission**, which is the sequential delivery of first prostatic fluid and sperm and then seminal vesicle fluid to the urethra. Finally, filling of the urethra with semen triggers nerve impulses that activate the bulbocavernosus muscles at the base of the penis, and the resulting rhythmic increases in pressure produce **ejaculation** of the semen. The male sex act is usually associated with a set of systemic changes including increases in respiration, heart rate, and blood pressure, that reach their peak during ejaculation. Afterward, during a **resolution phase**, the male becomes refractory to further sexual stimulation and detumescence occurs. Because of the complex nature of this reflex, it is particularly susceptible to disruption by both physical (e.g., circulatory or nervous damage) and psychological disturbances.

ENDOCRINE FUNCTION OF THE TESTES

The testes, in addition to producing sperm, secrete **testosterone**, the hormone primarily responsible for maintenance of the male reproductive system. Testosterone is produced by **Leydig** cells, which are located in the interstitial tissue connecting the seminiferous tubules (see Fig. 8–2) and are sometimes referred to as interstitial cells. They are closely associated with blood vessels and are histologically typical of steroid-producing cells, containing a large number of lipid droplets and extensive smooth endoplasmic reticulum.

Structure and Synthesis of Androgens

Testosterone is one of a group of steroids called **androgens**, all of which produce masculine characteristics. The major naturally occurring androgens are all C-19 steroids with a hydroxyl or ketone group on both the C-3 and C-17 positions (e.g., see testosterone in Fig. 8–4). By far the most potent androgens are testosterone and 5α-dihydrotestosterone (DHT); the latter is formed from testosterone by reduction of the double bond between the C-4 and C-5 positions. The testes secrete little or no DHT so that virtually all the DHT in the circulation is derived from the metabolism of testosterone in nonsteroid-producing tissues (Table 8–2). The testes secrete other androgens such as dehydroepiandrosterone (DHEA) and androstenedione, but because of their relatively low secretory rates and potencies, these compounds are not biologically important in the male. In fact, the adrenal cortex is the major source of DHEA and androstenedione in both men and women (Chapter 7). Consequently, in terms of testicular function, testosterone is the major steroid that needs to be considered.

The biosynthesis of testosterone begins with cholesterol and follows the common pathway already described for steroid biosynthesis (Fig. 8–4). In rodent testes, unlike other steroidogenic tissues, cholesterol is derived primarily from *de novo* synthesis rather than from serum lipoproteins; whether this is also true for men remains to be established. The rate-limiting step for testos-

TABLE 8–2. Major Androgens in Males

	Testosterone	DHT	Androstenedione	DHEA
Potency (Arbitrary units)	100	200	15	8
Testicular secretion rate (mg/day)	7	0	0.4	0.7
Circulating levels (ng/dl)	250–1000	10–45	40–110	200–1000

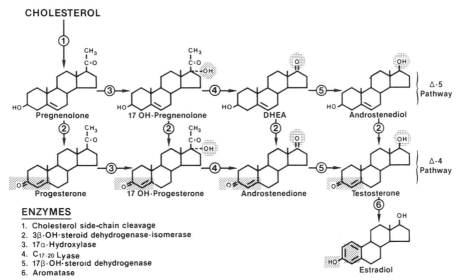

CHOLESTEROL

ENZYMES

1. **Cholesterol side-chain cleavage**
2. **3β-OH-steroid dehydrogenase-isomerase**
3. **17α-Hydroxylase**
4. **C₁₇₋₂₀ Lyase**
5. **17β-OH-steroid dehydrogenase**
6. **Aromatase**

FIGURE 8–4. Major pathways for testosterone biosynthesis. Circles depict changes occurring in the horizontal direction; rectangles, changes occurring in the vertical direction.

terone synthesis, as for all steroids, is the side-chain cleavage of cholesterol to form pregnenolone. This reaction occurs in the mitochondria, requires NADPH and O_2, and is under hormonal control. After this critical step, conversion of pregnenolone to testosterone can occur via either a Δ-5 pathway (intermediates contain a double bond between C-5 and C-6) or a Δ-4 pathway (intermediates with a C4-C5 double bond) as illustrated in Figure 8–4. The relative importance of these two pathways varies among species, but in men the Δ-5 pathway predominates. The reactions along either pathway are essentially identical and involve cleavage of carbons 20 and 21 and addition of a hydroxyl group at the C-17 position. The enzymes catalyzing these reactions—as well as 3β-hydroxysteroid dehydrogenase, which converts Δ-5 intermediates to analogous Δ-4 steroids (e.g., DHEA to androstenedione, Fig. 8–4)—are all located in the smooth endoplasmic reticulum.

In addition to androgens, the testes also secrete some estrogens, principally estradiol-17β (10 μg/day). Estradiol is formed from testosterone by an enzyme that aromatizes the A ring. In some species, this reaction occurs primarily in the Sertoli cell, but in humans the Leydig cell appears to be the main testicular site of estradiol production. Testosterone can also be aromatized in other tissues, and most of the circulating estrogens (60 to 75 per cent) are produced by peripheral metabolism of androgens. Estrogens have some effects on the reproductive tract and on gonadotropin secretion from the pituitary gland in males, but the physiological importance of these effects is not clear.

Circulating Form of Testosterone

Once released into the blood, testosterone circulates largely bound to proteins that are produced by the liver. Most of the testosterone binds with high affinity to a specific β-globulin, known as **sex steroid–binding globulin** (or testosterone-binding globulin). There is also a significant (about 40 per cent) low affinity binding to **albumin.** Only 1 to 3 per cent of the circulating testosterone is unbound, and this is the only active form of the hormone in the circulation. Changes in serum binding proteins are rare in healthy men but they can occur in some pathological situations, such as cirrhosis of the liver. Levels of sex steroid–binding globulin can also be modulated by steroids, with androgens inhibiting and estrogens stimulating production. Changes in binding protein levels will alter blood testosterone concentrations without necessarily affecting the amount of biologically active free hormone; such alterations must be taken into account clinically when total circulating testosterone is measured.

Actions of Testosterone

The overall function of androgens in the male is to ensure delivery of sperm to the female, and testosterone affects virtually all aspects of this process (Table 8–3).

Male Reproductive Tract. Testosterone has three major effects that are absolutely essential for the normal development and function of the male reproductive tract. First, testosterone causes differentiation of the reproductive tract *in utero*, an action that will be considered in Chapter 11. Second, rising

TABLE 8–3.   Actions of Testosterone

1. Reproductive tract and external genitalia
   a. Differentiation *in utero*
   b. Maturation at puberty
   c. Maintenance in adult (tract only)
2. Development of secondary sexual characteristics (at puberty)
   a. Male pattern of hair growth
   b. Deep voice
   c. Increased muscle growth
3. Other reproductive effects
   a. Development of libido at puberty
   b. Required for spermatogenesis
   c. Inhibition of gonadotropins
4. Nonreproductive effects
   a. Anabolic actions
   b. Pubertal growth spurt and then closure of epiphyses
   c. Increased secretion of sebaceous glands

testosterone concentrations at puberty are responsible for maturation of the external genitalia, causing an eightfold increase in the size of the scrotum and penis, and of the internal reproductive tract. Both the sizes and secretory activities of the epididymis, seminal vesicles, and prostate increase dramatically so that production of seminal fluid is initiated. Third, testosterone is required for maintenance of the internal reproductive tract, but not the external genitalia, in the adult. Castration results in involution and cessation of secretory activity of the accessory sex glands, and testosterone therapy restores normal function. The source of testosterone for maintenance of these glands can be the systemic circulation or the seminiferous tubular fluid; the latter seems to be particularly important for the epididymis.

Secondary Sexual Characteristics. Testosterone is also responsible for the development of several masculine traits that are only peripherally related to reproduction. These secondary sexual characteristics include a **deep voice** resulting from enlargement of the larynx and thickening of the vocal cords, **muscular development**, and the male pattern of **hair growth** (pubic hair that grows upward toward the umbilicus, beard and mustache, axillary and chest hair). Testosterone also suppresses hair growth on the skull, causing a receding hairline in most men and baldness in those individuals genetically disposed to this condition.

Other Reproduction-Related Actions. Testosterone also affects several other systems important for delivery of the sperm. This androgen is essential for development of **sexual libido** at puberty and helps to maintain the male sex drive in the adult. Once libido has developed, however, testosterone is no longer absolutely required; men often remain sexually active, albeit at a reduced level, for years after castration. In animals, androgens also increase aggressive behavior at puberty, but the importance of this action in humans is still being debated. Testosterone is also necessary for **spermatogenesis** and normal control of **gonadotropin secretion** from the pituitary gland, actions that are described in detail later in this chapter.

Nonreproductive Actions. Finally, testosterone has several important effects not related to reproductive function. First, this androgen has an **anabolic** effect, causing increased protein synthesis in many tissues throughout the body. The anabolic action accounts for the changes in muscle mass occurring at puberty. In bone, this anabolic effect is manifested as increased deposition of collagen, which eventually calcifies increasing bone thickness and strength. At puberty, testosterone acts on the **epiphyseal plates** of long bones, causing first a growth spurt, and then cessation of growth owing to fusion of the epiphyseal plates. These effects require the presence of growth hormone and are considered in more detail in Chapter 14. Testosterone also stimulates activity of the **sebaceous glands** in the skin. This action often results in acne in adolescents and thus may be considered (at least by teenagers) to indirectly alter some aspects of reproductive activity.

Mechanism of Action

The biochemical actions of testosterone in the accessory sex glands have been extensively studied and appear to follow the general model for lipophilic hormones (Fig. 1–8) with one major exception. In sex accessory tissues, testosterone diffuses into the cell and is **converted to DHT** by the enzyme 5α-reductase (Fig. 8–5). This is a membrane-bound (nuclear and endoplasmic reticulum) enzyme found primarily in the male reproductive tract and liver. Once formed, DHT binds to a cytosolic receptor, and the hormone-receptor complex then migrates to the nucleus and activates a number of genes. The resulting increase in enzymatic activity produces cellular hypertrophy and the onset of secretory activity. The DHT-receptor complex also activates the mitotic machinery of the cell, eventually producing hyperplasia. Together with hypertrophy of individual cells, hyperplasia accounts for the overall increase in target tissue mass. The role of DHT in the male reproductive tract accounts for the higher potency of DHT than testosterone and provides a straightforward explanation for the symptoms of a clinical syndrome in which growth of this tract is retarded due to a genetic deficiency in 5α-reductase.

While the conversion of testosterone to DHT is a critical step in the accessory sex glands, it does not appear to be obligatory for many of the other actions of androgens. In particular, the anabolic effects in muscle and bone

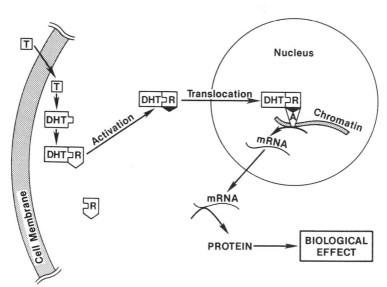

FIGURE 8–5. Mechanism of action of testosterone in the male reproductive tract. Testosterone (T) is converted to dihydrotestosterone (DHT) before binding to a cytosolic receptor (R). The hormone-receptor complex then binds to an acceptor site (A) on the chromatin.

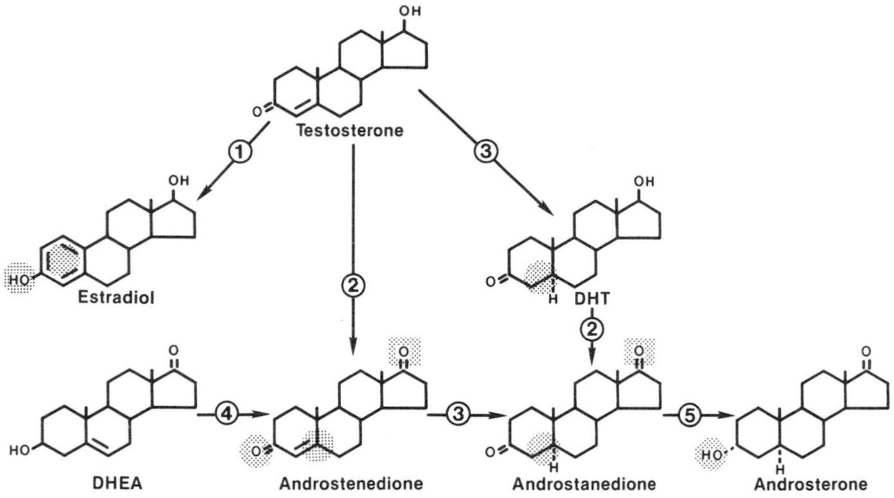

ENZYMES

1. Aromatase
2. 17β-OH-steroid dehydrogenase
3. 5α-reductase
4. 3β-OH-steroid dehydrogenase-isomerase
5. 3β-OH-steroid dehydrogenase

FIGURE 8–6. Major conversions of testosterone to either active metabolites or inactive 17-ketosteroids. Circles depict changes occurring in the horizontal (or diagonal) direction; squares, changes occurring in the vertical direction.

are probably due to a direct action of testosterone, as these tissues have little or no 5α-reductase activity. Finally, conversion of testosterone to another metabolite, estradiol (Fig. 8–6), may be important for some of its effects in the central nervous system. Some neural areas contain high levels of aromatase, the enzyme that converts testosterone to estradiol, and this estrogen appears to mediate some androgenic actions in rodents. However, the importance of aromatization to the actions of testosterone in the brain have not been clearly established in other species.

METABOLISM OF TESTICULAR HORMONES

Testosterone is metabolized rapidly and has a metabolic clearance rate of almost 1 liter/minute. Its major metabolites are 17-ketosteroids produced via either of the intermediates androstenedione or DHT (Fig. 8–6). The liver is the primary site of metabolism, although as already noted some production of DHT occurs in target tissues. The major end product of this pathway, androsterone, is conjugated with glucuronic or sulfuric acid and excreted in the urine. Because the hydroxyl on C-3 and the hydrogen on C-5 can be located above (β) or below (α) the steroid ring, a variety of stereoisomers of androsterone are excreted. Only small amounts of these metabolites are found in bile or feces.

As described in Chapter 7, the major adrenal androgen, DHEA, is also a source of urinary 17-ketosteroids. In fact, adrenal androgens account for approximately 70 per cent of the excreted 17-ketosteroids so that measurement of urinary 17-ketosteroids does not provide a reliable index of testicular androgen secretion. Two other testosterone metabolites appear in the urine in relatively small amounts: androstanediol, which is formed by reduction of the 3-keto group of DHT, and estrogen metabolites, which are formed after testosterone has been converted to estradiol.

REGULATION OF TESTICULAR FUNCTION

The testes, like the adrenals and thyroid, are controlled by hormones secreted from the anterior pituitary. Two pituitary hormones, however, are involved in regulation of testicular function, one for the endocrine component and the other for the gametogenic component. **Luteinizing hormone (LH)** acts on Leydig cells to stimulate testosterone secretion and **follicle-stimulating hormone (FSH)** acts on the seminiferous tubules to promote spermatogenesis. The names of these two gonadotropic hormones are derived from their actions in the female; LH has also been called interstitial cell–stimulating hormone (ICSH) for its actions in the male, but this terminology is no longer popular. As previously described (Chapter 4), secretion of both LH and FSH from the anterior pituitary requires the hypothalamic hormone, gonadotropin-releasing hormone (GnRH).

Release of LH and FSH from the pituitary forms one component of a **negative feedback loop** that regulates hormone levels throughout the hypothalamo-pituitary-testicular axis. The second component, closing the feedback loop, is the negative feedback action of testicular hormones that inhibits secretion of both LH and FSH (Fig. 8–7). As with other negative feedback loops (Chapter 1), this regulatory system functions to hold concentrations of LH, FSH, and testicular hormones within fairly narrow limits. In the rest of this section each of these components will be considered in detail.

Control of Gonadotropin Secretion

Before considering the negative feedback actions of testicular hormones, it may be useful to briefly review the role of GnRH in control of LH and FSH secretion. GnRH is released from hypothalamic neurons into capillaries of the hypophyseal portal circulation and carried by this system to the anterior pitu-

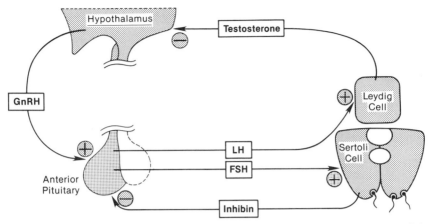

FIGURE 8–7. Negative feedback loops thought to control testicular function in adult males.

itary, where it stimulates release of LH and FSH. Under normal conditions GnRH release is episodic in that a burst of secretory activity is followed by relatively prolonged periods of quiescence. The resulting episodes of LH release produce abrupt increases in circulating LH concentrations, which then fall (as LH is metabolized) until the next secretory episode, a pattern often referred to as pulsatile. FSH is also secreted episodically. However, because of its slower metabolic clearance, levels of FSH fall only slightly between pulses, so that FSH concentrations remain relatively constant over time. The pattern of GnRH secretion is of some clinical significance because the pituitary cannot respond to GnRH if it is given continuously for a prolonged period. Thus, exogenous GnRH must be administered episodically to patients with deficiencies in endogenous GnRH release.

Control of LH Secretion. In men, testosterone is the primary negative feedback hormone controlling LH release. If plasma testosterone levels are decreased, LH secretion rises; androgen treatment prevents or reverses this increase, returning LH concentrations to normal. Testosterone produces some inhibitory effects directly at the pituitary, but most of its negative feedback action occurs in the central nervous system to decrease episodes of GnRH release. This, in turn, results in suppression of LH pulses, which are driven by GnRH. While testosterone is the most important inhibitor of LH release in men, recent evidence suggests that estradiol also produces some suppression of this gonadotropin. Since estradiol is derived mainly from peripheral aromatization of testosterone, this suppression can be considered an indirect androgen effect. Thus, testosterone released from Leydig cells acts both directly and indirectly, via its conversion to estradiol, to control LH secretion in men.

Superimposed on this negative feedback loop is a diurnal variation in testosterone secretion, with androgen levels somewhat elevated in the early morning. However, this variation is quite small in adults and probably of little physiological significance.

Control of FSH Secretion. Although FSH is also controlled by a negative feedback loop involving the testes, the nature of this inhibition is not as well understood as that of LH. Testosterone, by inhibiting GnRH release, is one important regulator of FSH secretion. However, androgen alone is not sufficient to account completely for the control of FSH secretion, indicating that some other hormone must be involved. Estradiol may be this second hormone, since a combination of androgen and estrogen is an effective inhibitor of FSH.

A more likely possibility is a putative hormone known as **inhibin.** Inhibin, which has recently been completely characterized, is a glycoprotein, consisting of an α and β chain. It is produced by the seminiferous tubules (and ovarian follicles) and acts on the pituitary to inhibit secretion of FSH but not LH. There is now strong circumstantial evidence that inhibin secretion by the seminiferous tubules participates in the control of FSH release; however, further work is needed to firmly establish the physiological role of this glycoprotein hormone.

Control of Testicular Function

The two gonadotropins, LH and FSH, control the endocrine and gametogenic components of the testes, respectively, by acting on different cell types (Fig. 8–8). LH acts on the Leydig cell to control testosterone secretion but has no direct effect on the seminiferous tubules. Although FSH has no effects on Leydig cell function, it is important for spermatogenesis, apparently by regulating the Sertoli cells. This specificity of gonadotropin action reflects a selective distribution of receptors. Leydig cells contain receptors for LH but not FSH, while Sertoli cells have receptors for FSH but not LH.

Control of Testosterone Secretion. LH has two important actions on Leydig cells. Acutely it acts to stimulate testosterone secretion and chronically it acts to maintain the structural and functional integrity of Leydig cells. The mechanism of the latter tropic effects remains a mystery, but the biochemical events leading to increased testosterone secretion are fairly well established.

LH acutely stimulates testosterone secretion by activating the rate-limiting step in testosterone biosynthesis, the side-chain cleavage of cholesterol to form pregnenolone. This increase in enzyme activity is the final step in a familiar sequence of events, namely those associated with the second messenger, cyclic AMP (cAMP) (Figs. 1–9 and 8–8). Thus LH binds to a high-affinity, low-capacity receptor located on the Leydig cell plasma membrane. This binding activates adenylate cyclase, increasing intracellular cAMP concentrations. The cAMP then binds to a protein kinase, freeing the catalytic subunit, which

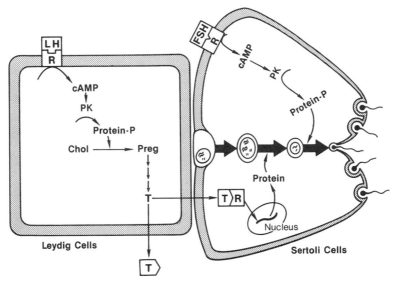

FIGURE 8–8. Hormonal control of testicular function. LH stimulates testosterone (T) release by binding to its receptor (R) and increasing the conversion of cholesterol (chol) to pregnenolone (preg) via a cAMP-protein kinase (PK) cascade. Spermatogenesis (bold arrows) is controlled by both FSH and T acting via the Sertoli cells. See text for further details.

phosphorylates a specific set of proteins. These phosphorylated proteins, in turn, increase the conversion of cholesterol to pregnenolone by two mechanisms: increased delivery of cholesterol to the mitochondria and increased activity of the enzyme that cleaves the side chain of cholesterol. The pregnenolone thus formed is rapidly converted to testosterone, which is released into the blood. After initiating this sequence of events, the LH-receptor complex is internalized by endocytosis and degraded, a process that may contribute to the loss of LH receptors produced by prolonged gonadotropin treatment.

This model of LH action implies that increases in LH will routinely produce increases in testosterone secretion, but this is not always the case. Leydig cells contain a large number of excess LH receptors so that occupancy of less than 5 per cent of the total produces a maximal increment in testosterone release. Thus, once LH concentrations reach a certain level, further increments will increase testicular binding but not testosterone secretion. However, the LH levels needed to produce a maximal response can be achieved only by exogenous LH administration. Another instance of dissociation between LH and testosterone secretion is of more physiological relevance. In normal men, endogenous pulses of LH often do not produce increments in testosterone secretion. The reasons for this lack of testicular response remain obscure; perhaps the tropic actions of LH to maintain Leydig cell structure and function are as important as its acute effects for the maintenance of normal testosterone levels. Regardless of which stimulatory action of LH is more important, the negative feedback loop between LH and testosterone will function to maintain relatively constant androgen levels in the adult.

Control of Spermatogenesis. Two hormones, **FSH and testosterone**, play direct, critical roles in spermatogenesis and each exerts its effect via the Sertoli cell (Fig. 8–8). Although both FSH and testosterone are required for the initiation of gametogenesis at puberty, there is still considerable controversy as to where in the spermatogenic process they act. In the rat, the mitotic phase of gametogenesis can occur without hormone stimulation, but testosterone is necessary for meiosis of spermatocytes to spermatids, and FSH is required for the later stages of spermatid maturation to spermatozoa. Although much less information is available in humans, it appears that testosterone is required for both mitosis and meiosis, while FSH is essential for spermatid maturation. It should be emphasized that the local production of testosterone is critical to spermatogenesis; only the extremely high androgen concentrations found in the testes will sustain sperm production.

One complicating factor in this story is that the hormonal requirements for maintenance of spermatogenesis in the adult may differ from those needed for its initiation at puberty. In the rat, once FSH and testosterone initiate spermatogenesis at puberty, testosterone alone is sufficient to maintain sperm production. The basis for the loss in the requirement for FSH and whether, in fact, the same phenomenon occurs in humans remain to be determined. This issue is of some practical importance since attempts to develop a male contraceptive by selectively inhibiting FSH are based on the assumption that this gonadotropin is required for sperm production in the adult.

While it is clear that FSH and testosterone affect spermatogenesis by altering Sertoli cell function, the exact mechanisms of these effects remain obscure. Testosterone acts via a cytosolic receptor to increase gene transcription (Fig. 8–8), but the specific proteins produced and their effects on germ cells are unknown. Similarly, the initial steps in FSH action (e.g., increased cAMP, activation of protein kinase) are much better established than its later effects. In addition to increasing protein phosphorylation, FSH stimulates production of several Sertoli cell proteins, including androgen-binding protein. This binding protein could be important for spermatogenesis by maintaining high intratubular testosterone concentrations.

It is important to realize that although FSH and testosterone are the only hormones directly controlling spermatogenesis, LH is also essential for this process. Without LH stimulation of the Leydig cells, intratesticular testosterone levels fall, which in turn disrupts sperm production. Thus, both gonadotropins are actually required for spermatogenesis, FSH acting directly and LH acting via its effects on testosterone production.

Other Factors Affecting Testicular Function

While LH and FSH are the principal extragonadal agents regulating the testes, other factors can influence reproductive function. In general, most of these agents alter spermatogenesis without greatly affecting testosterone secretion by the Leydig cells. As already mentioned, an **increase in temperature** can disrupt spermatogenesis. If the testes do not descend from the abdomen into the scrotum (a condition known as cryptorchidism), spermatogonia will not develop into sperm and will in fact eventually degenerate, producing permanent sterility. Therefore, it is important to move the testes surgically into the scrotum in cryptorchid boys before this degeneration occurs. Like most rapidly dividing cells, developing sperm are especially sensitive to **radiation**. Low doses of radiation can cause genetic damage resulting in embryonic abnormalities in any offspring, while high doses may cause sterility by destroying the spermatagonia. A variety of drugs, particularly **anticancer agents**, also affect mitotic cells and can disrupt spermatogenesis and produce temporary sterility. Finally, some of the **inhibitors of steroidogenesis** described in Chapter 7 may also inhibit testosterone biosynthesis, an effect that would disrupt normal function of both the Leydig cells and seminiferous tubules.

AGE-RELATED CHANGES IN THE MALE REPRODUCTIVE SYSTEM

In the adult, the negative feedback loop controlling the hypothalamo-pituitary-testicular axis ensures relatively constant testicular function. However, when examined throughout the life of an individual, four distinctly different reproductive periods can be described: prepuberty, puberty, adult, and senescence. The functioning of the male reproductive system in the adult has already been described; this section will briefly consider the other three periods.

Prepuberty

This period, which lasts from birth to approximately 10 years of age, is characterized by testicular quiescence. There is a burst of activity shortly after birth during which circulating concentrations of gonadotropins and testosterone increase substantially. Secretion of these hormones soon declines, however, with concentrations falling to very low levels within a year. The function of this transitory secretory activity is unknown. During the rest of the prepubertal period, secretion rates of LH and FSH are too low to stimulate any significant testicular activity. The testes and male reproductive tracts do grow in infants, but only in proportion to overall body growth. The prepubertal delay in the onset of reproductive function, which is observed in all animals, allows the body to develop so that it can more easily handle the stress of child-rearing. This is particularly important for the female, whose body must be able to support the developing embryo, but the male often participates in the feeding, care, and raising of the infant, activities that require physical and psychological maturity.

Puberty

This transitional period encompasses a complex sequence of endocrine, physical, and behavioral events leading to sexual maturity. The endocrine changes underlying this sequence of events have now been well characterized. Starting at some time between ages 8 and 12 years, an increase in the secretion of GnRH from the hypothalamus initiates the pubertal process. This GnRH release causes daily sleep-related increments in LH, which in turn produce brief nocturnal rises in testosterone secretion early in puberty. As puberty progresses, the duration of these secretory periods lengthens until only the slight diurnal variation evident in adults remains. These changes in GnRH output increase LH and FSH secretion, so that circulating concentrations of these gonadotropins gradually increase in parallel throughout puberty as illustrated for LH in Figure 8–9. Initially, the gonadotropins produce local changes in the testes; LH stimulates testosterone biosynthesis while FSH, together with the increasing intratesticular androgen concentrations, initiates spermatogenesis. It is the increase in volume of the seminiferous tubules that produces the first outward evidence of puberty, an increase in testicular size. Under continued LH stimulation, testosterone output from Leydig cells, and hence circulating androgen concentrations, rise progressively to induce the dramatic physical changes of puberty. Pubic hair appears first, followed shortly by growth of the penis and start of the adolescent growth spurt (Fig. 8–9). Other secondary sexual characteristics (beard growth, deepening of voice) and development of libido, as evidenced by interest in the opposite sex and nocturnal erections and ejaculations, begin later in puberty. Although the sequence of these changes is fairly constant, the time at which they start is quite variable so that some boys are just beginning puberty when others of their age are almost fully developed.

While the endocrine changes during puberty are well described, the fundamental mechanisms responsible for producing the initial changes in GnRH secretion are not. The low levels of gonadotropins during the prepubertal period appear to reflect an active neuroendocrine inhibition of GnRH release. This inhibition develops shortly after birth and suppresses the high levels of

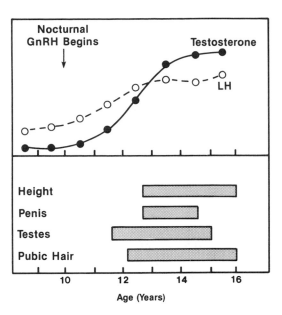

FIGURE 8–9. Time course of the major endocrine and physical changes occurring during puberty in adolescent males. (Bottom panel redrawn from Marshall, W.A. and Tanner, J.M.: Variations in the pattern of pubertal changes in boys. Arch. Dis. Child. 45:13, 1970.)

LH and FSH evident in the first few months of life. Both endocrine and neural components contribute to this prepubertal inhibition of GnRH. The endocrine inhibition is the result of a high sensitivity of the hypothalamus to the negative feedback actions of testosterone so that even the small amounts of testosterone produced by the prepubertal testes are able to inhibit GnRH release. At puberty the hypothalamus becomes less sensitive, the low testosterone levels no longer suppress GnRH, and hence GnRH and gonadotropin levels rise. This change in sensitivity to negative feedback is often referred to as the **gonadostat theory of puberty**. In addition to this testicular inhibition, a direct neural inhibition of GnRH occurs during the prepubertal period. In agonadal children, circulating LH and FSH levels are much lower than those in agonadal adults, but they rise to adult levels at the same age that puberty occurs in normal children. Since there is no testicular androgen production in these individuals, the rise in gonadotropin levels at "puberty" must reflect removal of a direct neural inhibition. It should be recognized that these endocrine and neural components could reflect different aspects of a single inhibitory system.

It is still not clear which event(s) is responsible for removing these inhibitory mechanisms at puberty. An age-related decrease in inhibitory activity within the central nervous system is one possibility that is supported by the ability of some neural lesions to produce precocious puberty. A second proposal suggests that achievement of a critical body weight or percentage of body fat (or both) induces a metabolic change responsible for increased GnRH release. While it is clear that nutritional levels—and hence body weight and composition—can profoundly alter reproductive function, direct evidence for their involvement at puberty is lacking. Finally, recent work has focused on a possible role for the pineal hormone melatonin at puberty. Melatonin secretory patterns change at puberty in humans and this hormone plays a critical role in the annual cessation and reinitiation of reproductive function in many seasonally breeding species. However, pinealectomy of subhuman primates has no effect on the pubertal initiation of reproductive function. Thus, the initial trigger for puberty in humans remains a mystery.

Senescence

News reports of paternity in aging politicians and movie stars clearly illustrate that reproductive fertility is often maintained into the seventh or eighth decade of life. Nevertheless, significant decreases in reproductive function do occur in older men, with many functions gradually declining after 45 to 50 years of age. These include a fall in the number of normal sperm produced and a gradual decline in circulating testosterone concentrations. The latter is accompanied by increasing levels of sex steroid–binding globulin so that free testosterone concentrations fall even more dramatically than total testosterone levels. This fall in free androgen partially removes the inhibitory control of gonadotropin secretion so that LH and FSH levels increase with age. Taken together, the rise in gonadotropins and fall in testosterone point to a primary deficit in testicular function in older men, which may be caused by degenerative changes in the microvasculature of the testes.

From a practical standpoint, changes in sexual behavior with aging are probably much more important than decreased testicular function. The decline in sexual activity actually precedes any endocrine changes, starting at about 35 to 40 years of age. These behavioral effects include decreased frequency of coitus, increased incidence of impotence, and a prolongation of the refractory period after orgasm. In most cases these changes will not greatly affect fertility but can have profound effects on the psychological well-being of the aging male.

PATHOLOGICAL CHANGES IN THE MALE REPRODUCTIVE SYSTEM

Hypogonadism

Decreased testicular function and hence infertility are much more common than hypergonadism. The causes of infertility can be divided into endo-

TABLE 8–4.   Clinical Features of Eunuchoidism*

Eunuchoidal skeleton
  Span more than 2 inches greater than height. Soles to symphysis more than 2 inches greater than symphysis to head. Delay in closure of epiphyses.
Lack of adult male hair distribution
  Sparse or absent facial and body hair. Scant pubic and axillary hair. Failure of hairline to recede.
High-pitched voice
Infantile genitalia
  Small penis, testes, and scrotum.
Poor muscular development
  Decreased muscle mass. Diminished endurance and strength.

*From Bardin, C.W. and Paulsen, C.A.: The testes. *In* Textbook of Endocrinology, 6th ed. R. Williams, editor. W.B. Saunders Company, Philadelphia, p. 313, 1983.

crine and nonendocrine factors. Nonendocrine causes are usually responsible for infertility that arises in adults, and the symptoms are generally limited to a decrease in the quality of semen (e.g., reduced quantity or motility of sperm). Endocrine causes often occur prepubertally and first become evident as a failure in sexual maturation. In the latter cases, referred to as **eunuchoidism**, the symptoms are much more severe, reflecting the lack of development of primary and secondary sexual characteristics (Table 8–4).

Endocrine hypogonadism is further divided into primary and secondary hypogonadism. In the former, the primary defect is at the gonadal level; because the resulting decrease in circulating testosterone concentrations causes LH and FSH levels to rise, this condition is often called *hyper*gonadotropic hypogonadism. In contrast, in secondary, or *hypo*gonadotropic hypogonadism, a deficit in pituitary LH or FSH secretion or in secretion of both is the cause of testicular dysfunction. This distinction is critical because the type of treatment will depend on the source of the problem. Several tests have been developed to distinguish between the two. In severe conditions, measurement of circulating LH and FSH is sufficient because they will be high in primary and low in secondary hypogonadism. LH is usually measured in samples taken at frequent intervals for several hours and then pooled to obtain an integrated value for LH; because of the episodic pattern of LH release, a single measurement does not provide an accurate index of secretion rate. When symptoms are less severe, hormone measurements alone may not be sufficient to locate the site of the deficit, and challenge tests are necessary. Testicular function is tested by examining the increment in testosterone resulting from an LH-like stimulus while pituitary function is usually tested by GnRH injection. The latter test is also helpful in determining whether a hypothalamic or hypophyseal problem is responsible for low gonadotropin levels.

The most common type of primary hypogonadism is **Klinefelter's syndrome**, a genetic abnormality occurring in 0.2 per cent of males. In the classical syndrome, there is essentially no gonadal function so that the symptoms of eunuchoidism develop at puberty. However, there can often be partial function, so that some development of the secondary sexual characteristics occurs. Other, much rarer, syndromes included within this classification are anorchia, in which no testicular tissue is present, and the Sertoli cell–only syndrome. In the latter, spermatagonia degenerate and FSH levels rise, but Leydig cell function is normal so that LH, testosterone, and masculine characteristics are normal. Since a testicular deficit is responsible for these syndromes, sperm production cannot be induced, but androgen treatment is given to ameliorate the other symptoms.

Hypogonadotropic syndromes can also vary in their intensity, with the worst being **panhypopituitarism**, in which deficits in GH, TSH, and ACTH as well as in the gonadotropins occur. Isolated gonadotropin deficiency, also called **hypogonadotropic eunuchoidism** or **Kallmann's syndrome**, is the second most common male endocrine disorder. It involves deficits in both LH and FSH and results in eunuchoid symptoms at puberty. Interestingly, this syndrome is associated with anosmia or hyposmia 80 per cent of the time. Instances of deficits in only one of the gonadotropins have also been reported. The only symptom of FSH deficiency is a decrease in mature sperm. Patients with low LH levels usually have normal spermatogenesis because there is sufficient LH to increase intratesticular androgen levels. However, testosterone secretion rates are low so that eunuchoidism, partial or complete, occurs. In all of these syndromes, the appropriate gonadotropin treatment restores spermatogenesis or testosterone production or both.

Finally, there are a few clinical situations in which a reproductive disorder results not from testicular problems but from abnormalities in androgen target cells. One such case is the deficiency in 5α-reductase already mentioned that delays development of the male reproductive tract. Another is **testicular feminization**, in which there is an absence of androgen receptors in target tissues. Individuals with this disorder develop a female physique despite the presence of abdominal testes secreting testosterone at a normal rate.

Adult Infertility

Infertility that arises in adult males is usually caused by a **primary deficiency in sperm production** without the major endocrine symptoms of eunuchoidism. It is important to realize that infertile males are not necessarily azoospermic (i.e., completely lacking in sperm). Sperm concentration averages 120 million/ml in normal adults and if this level falls below 20 million/ml, an individual is considered clinically infertile. Abnormal sperm motility and morphology also need to be taken into account in assessing the physiological status of a semen sample.

Seminiferous tubular failure is one obvious cause of infertility in the adult. This can result from exposure to a number of noxious agents (e.g., radiation) or contraction of mumps, which causes tubular damage in 15 to 25 per cent of the adult males who develop this disease. Infertility due to obstructions in the delivery system are less common and are fairly easily treated. However, most instances of infertility are the result of either a low sperm number (oligospermia) or low sperm motility of unknown etiology. In these cases, hormone treatments have not been particularly successful.

Impotence is another common cause of infertility in adults. Treatment for this disorder depends on whether it is psychological or physiological in origin. The latter can be subdivided into endocrine, vascular, or neural dysfunction. Androgen administration is sufficient treatment for the first type, and a variety of erectile-type penile implants have recently been developed for treatment of the latter two types.

Hypergonadism and Precocious Puberty

Hypersecretion from the testes is very rare in adults. Testicular neoplasms occur in only 0.002 per cent of the male population and 96 per cent of these involve the germinal epithelium. Hypersecretion is somewhat more common in the juvenile and the symptoms (premature sexual development and early cessation of growth) are much more dramatic. True precocious puberty can be either idiopathic or neurogenic in origin. The latter involves tumors in the brain that prematurely remove the systems that hold GnRH release in check. Treatment is focused on removal of the tumor using neurosurgery, radiotherapy, or chemotherapy. Treatment of iodiopathic precocious puberty has included the use of drugs, such as medroxyprogesterone or GnRH agonists, that inhibit gonadotropin secretion with some amelioration of symptoms.

Pseudoprecocious puberty results from increased circulating androgen levels because of ectopic LH or androgen production. Gonadotropin-secreting tumors are almost always malignant and hence need to be identified and treated as soon as possible. The most common cause of pseudoprecocious puberty is increased adrenal androgen secretion resulting from congenital adrenal hyperplasia (or adrenogenital syndrome). These individuals have a genetic enzyme deficiency (usually 21-hydroxylase) preventing or decreasing glucocorticoid production. This deficiency shunts adrenal steroid biosynthesis into the androgen pathway, and low cortisol levels cause ACTH concentrations to rise. ACTH stimulates adrenal cortical steroid biosynthesis and further increases androgen secretion. The net effect is precocious puberty in boys and virilization in girls. Adrenocorticoid treatment will not only alleviate the hypoadreno-cortical symptoms but also decrease androgen production by suppressing ACTH secretion.

Other Alterations in Reproductive Function

True delayed puberty, in which sexual development will eventually occur, needs to be distinguished from hypogonadism, which is often first evident as an absence of sexual development. This distinction is particularly difficult if the hypogonadism is caused by a secondary decrease in gonadotropin secretion. In these cases, physicians will often give intermittent gonadotropin therapy with hormone being administered for three months and withdrawn for three months. The boy can then be observed for spontaneous pubertal development during the latter three months, and treatment adjusted appropriately.

Hypertrophy of the prostate occurs in many older men. The prostatic lesion is usually benign, but the overgrowth will cause obstruction of the urethra. Benign prostatic hypertrophy does not result from the effects of androgens, so suppression of androgen secretion is not clinically useful. Prostatic cancer, on the other hand, is frequently exacerbated by testosterone so that inhibition of androgen production, either by suppression of gonadotropins or castration, can be beneficial. Cancer of the prostate is a common cause of death in older men.

Males wishing to voluntarily suppress fertility for contraceptive purposes still have only a limited number of options available. The only reliable, reversible male contraceptive now available is the condom. The other common method of male contraception is surgical disruption of the ductus (vas) deferens, a procedure known as **vasectomy**, but this usually produces permanent sterility. Even if the surgical disruption is repaired, fertility problems often persist, probably because antibodies to spermatozoa are produced when sperm leak into the body cavity after the vasectomy. A variety of drugs have been tested as male contraceptives, but no reliable compound that decreases sperm production without also suppressing libido is currently available.

REFERENCES

Barger, H. and de Kretser, D., editors: The Testis. Raven Press, New York, 1981.
Griffin, J.E. and Wilson, J.D.: Disorders of the testes and male reproductive tract. *In* Williams' Textbook of Endocrinology, 7th ed. J.D. Wilson and D.W. Foster, editors. W.B. Saunders Company, Philadelphia, p. 259, 1985.
Grumbach, M.M.: The neuroendocrinology of puberty. Hosp. Practice 15(3):51, 1980.

Harmon, S.M.: Clinical aspects of aging in the male reproductive system. *In* The Aging Reproductive System, E.L. Schneider, editor. Raven Press, New York, p. 29, 1978.

Johnson, M.H. and Everitt, B.J.: Essential Reproduction. Blackwell Scientific Publications, Oxford, 1980.

Plant, T.M.: Gonadal regulation of hypothalamic gonadotropin-releasing hormone release in primates. Endocrine Rev. 7:75, 1986.

Parvinen, M.: Regulation of the seminiferous epithelium. Endocrine Rev. 3:404, 1982.

Preslock, M.P. Steroidogenesis in the mammalian testis. Endocrine Rev. 1:132, 1980.

9

FEMALE REPRODUCTION

INTRODUCTION

Reproductive physiology in the female is more complex than that in the male because females perform two distinct reproductive functions: development of female gametes (ova) and maintenance of the fetus until it can survive in the outside world. To control these two functions, the ovary contains two related endocrine systems. The system that is responsible for gametogenesis (oogenesis) is analogous to the male reproductive system. It consists of an ovarian structure, the **follicle**, within which oogenesis occurs, and the hormone **estradiol**. Estradiol is produced by the follicle and performs functions in the female analogous to those of testosterone in the male. The other endocrine system is responsible for maintenance of the fetus and produces the hormone **progesterone**. This system becomes fully functional only during pregnancy (see Chapter 10), but it is partially active prior to pregnancy. In nonpregnant women, progesterone from the **corpus luteum** of the ovary prepares the reproductive system for gestation should conception occur.

In the normal adult, these two endocrine systems operate sequentially rather than simultaneously. It is this sequential activity of the follicular and luteal systems that produces the 28-day menstrual cycle. For approximately the first half of this cycle (the follicular phase), the first system operates to produce a mature ovum ready for fertilization. The second system then takes over during the next two weeks (the luteal phase) to prepare the female reproductive tract for pregnancy if fertilization occurs. If the ovum is not fertilized, this cycle begins again so that one mature ovum is produced each month.

FEMALE REPRODUCTIVE TRACT

Important functions of the female reproductive tract include reception of the ejaculated sperm, transport of the sperm to the ovum, maintenance of the developing fetus, and expulsion of the fetus at delivery. Since most of these functions relate directly to initiation and maintenance of pregnancy, they will be considered in detail in Chapter 10; this section will briefly describe the anatomy of the reproductive tract.

The female reproductive tract (Fig. 9–1) consists of two oviducts, the uterus and cervix, the vagina, and the external genitalia. The **oviducts** (or fallopian tubes), which connect the ovaries to the uterus, can be divided into three segments. The most lateral part is the fimbriated infundibulum, which picks up the mature ovum when it leaves the ovary. Next is the ampulla, which is the site of fertilization; it leads into the isthmus, a relatively short

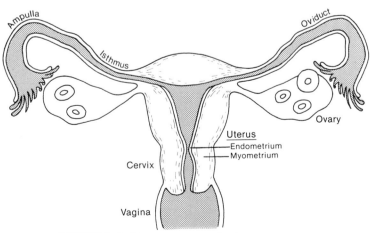

FIGURE 9–1. The female reproductive tract.

straight tube running into the uterus. In cross-section, the oviduct consists of an outer layer of smooth muscle and an inner mucosal lining. Two types of epithelial cells are evident on the inner surface of the oviduct: ciliated epithelia, which beat toward the uterus, and secretory epithelia. These cells are thought to aid in the transport and nourishment of the ovum and fertilized embryo.

The **uterus** is the organ primarily responsible for maintaining the fetus during its development and expelling it at the end of pregnancy. It consists of a well-developed muscular wall, the **myometrium**, and an inner mucosa or **endometrium** (Fig. 9–1). The endometrium contains an epithelial cell layer lining the uterine cavity and a deeper stromal layer that contains secretory glands. Blood is supplied to the endometrium by **spiral arteries**, which pass through the myometrium to the surface of the endometrium and give rise to extensive capillary networks within the stroma. The structure of both the endometrium and its spiral arteries changes dramatically throughout the menstrual cycle. These changes, which will be described in a later section, underlie the monthly bleeding (menses) that is the most obvious sign of cyclic reproductive function in women. The **cervix** is the lowest portion of the uterus and differs both anatomically and functionally from the rest of the uterus. The cervical canal connects the uterus and vagina and is lined with mucus-secreting epithelium. This mucus forms a barrier that helps prevent vaginal bacteria from entering the uterine cavity.

The **vagina** is essentially a muscular tube connecting the uterus to the outside environment. The walls of this tube are remarkably elastic. Under normal conditions the walls collapse so there is no vaginal lumen; during coitus the walls expand to receive the penis; during delivery they expand even further to form the birth canal. Squamous epithelial cells line the inner surface of the vagina. No secretory cells are evident, but the epithelial cells release glycogen into the lumen. Bacteria normally present in the vagina metabolize this glycogen to lactic acid, which accounts for the acidic nature of vaginal fluids.

The **external genitalia** include the vaginal orifice, clitoris, and the labia minora and labia majora. Functionally, the vaginal orifice (or introitus) includes the outer third of the vagina and plays a critical role in the physiological events leading to orgasm. The clitoris is a small erectile organ located anterior to the introitus. It is homologous to the glans penis of the male and is especially sensitive to tactile stimulation. The labia are folds of skin surrounding the other genitalia, with the labia minora being smaller and located inside the labia majora.

FEMALE SEX ACT

The physiological mechanisms responsible for orgasm are fundamentally the same in the two sexes. Thus, the female sexual response can be considered a complex neural reflex, initiated by stimulation of the external genitalia and integrated in the sacral and lumbar portion of the spinal cord. This reflex also receives input from and transmits signals to the brain, so that it is subject to psychic influences, and orgasm is accompanied by systemic sensations.

The first phase of the female sex act, **excitement**, can be initiated by either psychological or physical stimuli. Tactile stimulation of the clitoris and the surrounding perineal area usually produces a particularly strong sexual stimulus. These stimuli trigger, via spinal reflexes, parasympathetic impulses that dilate arterioles throughout the external genitalia and vagina. The increased blood flow causes vasocongestion, which is evident as swelling of the clitoris and labia. Vasocongestion causes the cervical end of the vagina to expand creating a space where the ejaculate is deposited. The increase in pressure within vaginal capillaries also produces a transudation of fluid into the lumen; this fluid is the main lubricant during coitus. Some additional lubrication is provided by mucus secreted by Bartholin's glands into the area surrounding the vaginal orifice. The second, or **plateau**, phase occurs during the few minutes just prior to orgasm. During this phase the uterus raises upward, lifting the cervix and enlarging the vaginal space created for the ejaculate. Further vasocongestion in the outer third of the vagina causes the introitus to decrease in diameter and tighten around the penis, thus increasing sexual stimuli to the male. If erotic stimulation is maintained, **orgasm** may be triggered by sympathetic impulses that cause contractions of the pelvic musculature. These include rhythmic contractions of the muscles surrounding the introitus and of the uterine myometrium. Orgasm usually lasts for only a minute or less and is followed by a **resolution** phase during which detumescence of the vagina and external genitalia occurs. Unlike the male, the female does not become refractory to sexual stimuli during the resolution phase so that multiple orgasms are possible. Systemic effects evident during the female sex act include nipple erection, flushing of the skin, and increased respiration, heart rate, and blood pressure.

ENDOCRINE TISSUES OF THE OVARY

Follicle and Gametogenesis

The ovary contains two endocrine glands: the follicle and the corpus luteum. However, these structures are coupled in that the corpus luteum is derived from follicular tissue. Thus, in a sense, the follicle can be considered the functional unit of the ovary. The mature follicle is a ball consisting of three cell types: thecal cells, granulosa cells, and the oocyte (Fig. 9–2). **Thecal cells** form the outer edge of the follicle and can be divided into two layers, a fibrous outer layer (theca externa) and a highly vascular internal layer (theca interna). **Granulosa cells** are the largest constituent of the follicle and have important

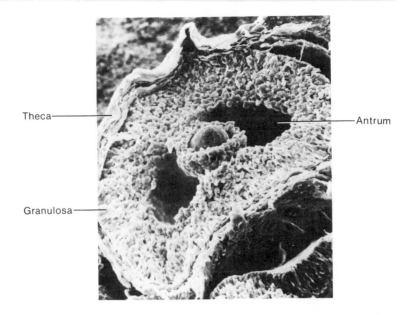

Theca

Antrum

Granulosa

FIGURE 9–2. The mature antral follicle. (Photograph by P. Bagavandoss taken from Richards, J.S.: Hormonal control of ovarian follicular development: A 1978 perspective. Rec. Prog. Horm. Res. 35:343, 1979.)

nutritive and endocrine functions. At the center of the follicle is the large **oocyte**, carrying the genetic contribution of the female. Finally, a fluid-filled cavity, the **antrum**, is evident in mature follicles.

Oogenesis, like spermatogenesis, requires mitosis, meiosis, and packaging to produce a mature ovum from the original germ cell. There are, however, major qualitative and quantitative sexual differences in gametogenesis. In addition to contributing half of the genes, the ovum provides almost all of the cytoplasmic components needed for early embryonic growth. Thus, in contrast to the highly differentiated spermatozoa, the ovum is a large, relatively undifferentiated cell containing numerous nutrients, organelles, and structural and enzymatic proteins. There are also striking quantitative differences between oogenesis and spermatogenesis; while the adult male produces 30 million sperm/day, the normal female produces at most 500 mature ova in her lifetime. Finally, gametogenesis in the female is tightly coupled to maturation of the ovarian follicle so that oogenesis is most conveniently divided into stages based on follicular events.

Folliculogenesis. The first stage of follicle formation (Fig. 9–3) is the mitotic proliferation of the primordial germ cells (oogonia), which begins shortly after these cells migrate to the fetal ovary. During this stage, the 1000 to 2000 germ cells that arrive in the ovary give rise to 6 to 7 million oogonia by the 20th week of gestation. However, mitotic proliferation ceases during the pre-

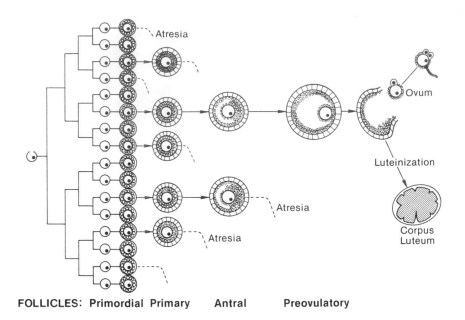

FOLLICLES: Primordial Primary   Antral   Preovulatory

├─Folliculogenesis─┼─────Follicular Development ────┼── Ovulation──┤
                                                      & Fertilization

FIGURE 9–3. Relationship between oogenesis and follicular function. Mitosis occurs only during folliculogenesis. One meiotic division occurs after ovulation and the other after fertilization, resulting in a mature ovum and two polar bodies.

natal period. All the oogonia begin the early steps of meiosis (the DNA replicates and homologous sets of chromosomes pair up to form tetrads) and become primary oocytes. These oocytes are quickly surrounded by a single layer of granulosa cells to form **primordial follicles**. Oocytes not incorporated into follicles degenerate so that at birth the ovary contains approximately 2 million primordial follicles. Since folliculogenesis and oogenesis do not occur postnatally, these follicles form the reservoir from which all ova in the adult must arise. In addition to protecting the germ cell, follicle formation inhibits any further development of the oocyte so that it becomes arrested in an early stage of meiosis. The oocyte will remain in this state of suspended animation until it is reactivated by follicular development, a period that can last up to 50 years for some oocytes.

    Follicular Development. For most of a woman's life, the pool of **primordial follicles** present at birth gives rise to a continuous trickle of developing follicles. Once a follicle begins to develop it is committed to one of two fates. If the hormonal milieu is appropriate, it will continue to develop and eventually release a mature ovum into the oviduct, by a process called **ovulation**. However, most (i.e., 99.9 per cent) follicles never ovulate; instead they degenerate by a process referred to as **atresia**. Atresia can occur at any stage of follicular development and eventually results in death of the oocyte. Thus, when a group of follicles begins to develop, almost all of them are destined to fall by the wayside, while normally one, or at most two, proceed all the way to ovulation (Fig. 9–3).

One of the first indications of follicular development is reactivation and growth of the oocyte. Meiosis does not resume at this time; instead this growth reflects the buildup of cytoplasmic materials that will be needed by the early embryo. The outer surface of the oocyte also becomes covered with a glycoprotein material that forms the zona pellucida. At the same time the granulosa cells proliferate so that several layers surround the oocyte, and stromal cells at the edge of the growing follicle differentiate to form a thin layer of thecal cells. The next stage of follicular development is the formation of the antrum, which is filled with follicular fluid originating partially from secretions of granulosa cells and partially from transudation of plasma. Coincident with antrum formation, the thecal cells differentiate into the theca interna and theca externa. This shift from a **preantral** (or primary) **follicle** to an **antral follicle** initiates a period of rapid growth during which the follicular diameter increases from less than 1 mm to 12 to 16 mm shortly before ovulation. During this time, granulosa and thecal cells continue to proliferate and the antrum increases dramatically to fill much of the **preovulatory** (or graafian) **follicle** (Fig. 9–3). The oocyte remains surrounded by a mass of granulosa cells and undergoes little further development during growth of the antral follicle.

Ovulation and Fertilization. The final stages of oocyte maturation, including both meiotic divisions, are coupled to ovulation and fertilization and thus occur in only a few ova. The maturing follicle is located in the cortical region of the ovary so that the dramatic increase in follicular diameter during follicular growth causes the preovulatory follicle to bulge on the ovarian surface. This creates a thin ischemic area (the stigma), which will rupture to release the ovum at ovulation.

One of the first indications of impending ovulation is resumption of meiosis by the oocyte. Meiosis progresses through the first division, producing two daughter cells each containing 46 chromosomes. However, the cytoplasm of the oocyte is not equally distributed between these two cells. Virtually all the cytoplasmic constituents remain with one cell, which is now called the **secondary oocyte**. The chromosomes of the second cell, together with a thin layer of cytoplasm, form the **first polar body**, which soon degenerates. This unequal distribution of cytoplasm preserves all the recently synthesized proteins and nutrients for the mature ovum. The first meiotic division is accompanied by synthesis of specific cytosolic proteins and organelles that prepare the oocyte for fertilization. Meiosis progresses to the beginning of the second division and then stops and the oocyte is ovulated in this condition.

While the oocyte is undergoing the first meiotic division, the follicle begins the process of ovulation. Intercellular connections between granulosa cells in the hillock containing the oocyte break down, allowing the oocyte and surrounding granulosa cells to float free in follicular fluid. An increase in blood flow to the follicle and in capillary permeability causes fluid movement into the follicle. Proteolytic enzymes released from follicular cells then begin to break down both the capillary endothelial cells and the follicular wall. The former action increases the rate of fluid movement into the follicle so that it rapidly swells. At the same time, digestion of the connective tissue in the follicular wall progressively decreases its ability to contain the swelling follicle. This weakening of the wall is particularly evident in the area of the stigma, which begins to balloon out and then ruptures, allowing follicular fluid to flow out of the ovary, carrying with it the secondary oocyte and attached granulosa cells.

When ovulation occurs, the oocyte is still arrested at the beginning of the second meiotic division. It does not develop further unless it is fertilized because entry of the sperm is needed to trigger the second meiotic division. If triggered, the second division follows the same pattern as the first, producing a second polar body and the **mature ovum**. This division completes oogenesis and sets the stage for formation of the embryo, which occurs a few hours later.

Corpus Luteum

Following ovulation, the granulosa and thecal cells remaining in the ruptured follicle undergo a dramatic structural transformation to form the corpus luteum, a process called **luteinization** (Fig. 9–3). These cells first collapse into the space left by the follicular fluid, which has been partially filled by clotted blood. Shortly thereafter, the granulosa cells begin to hypertrophy and take on the characteristics of a very active steroidogenic tissue, including extensive smooth endoplasmic reticulum, mitochondria, and lipid droplets. At the same time, blood vessels from the theca interna invade the luteinizing granulosa, and the corpus luteum becomes a highly vascularized tissue. Luteinization is directly coupled to ovulation so that the ruptured follicle always gives rise to the corpus luteum. Structurally, luteinization is complete within four days after ovulation, but the corpus luteum continues to increase in size for another four to five days. The bulk of the luteal tissue is derived from granulosa cells, but the outer layers of this gland are luteinized thecal cells that are sometimes called **paraluteal cells**.

Normally, the corpus luteum is a temporary tissue that regresses within 14 days of its formation. This process, termed **luteolysis**, involves degeneration and phagocytosis of luteal cells and proliferation of connective tissue within the corpus luteum. The vascular supply also regresses, producing an avascular fibrous tissue mass known as the **corpus albicans**.

Ovarian Hormone Production

The Follicle and Estrogen Synthesis. The major endocrine products of the follicle are **estrogens**, which are the steroids that produce female charac-

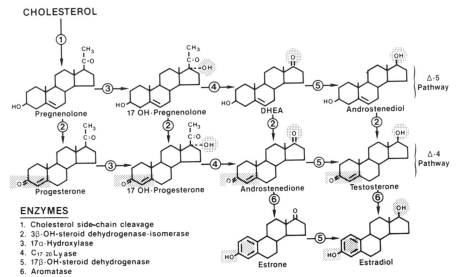

CHOLESTEROL

FIGURE 9–4. Biosynthesis of estrogens and progesterone. Circles depict changes occurring in the horizontal direction; rectangles, changes occurring vertically.

teristics. All naturally occurring estrogens are C-18 steroids with an aromatic A-ring and a hydroxyl group on the 3-carbon. There are three physiologically significant estrogens: **estrone**, which has a ketone group at the C-17 position (Fig. 9–4); **estradiol**, which has hydroxyl groups at both the C-3 and C-17 positions (Fig. 9–4); and **estriol**, which has hydroxyl groups at the C-3, C-16, and C-17 positions. These estrogens are often referred to as E_1, E_2, and E_3, respectively, with the subscripts indicating the number of hydroxyl groups attached to the steroid ring. In the nonpregnant adult woman, estradiol is the principal ovarian estrogen. The ovary secretes twice as much estradiol as estrone, and estrone has only 10 per cent of the estrogenic potency of estradiol. Estriol is the least potent of the three estrogens and in nonpregnant women is derived only from the metabolic degradation of estrone and estradiol. The placenta, however, produces large quantities of estriol, so this steroid is an important hormone of pregnancy.

The immediate precursors to estrone and estradiol are the androgens, androstenedione and testosterone (Fig. 9–4). Consequently, the pathway for estrogen synthesis is virtually identical to that for testicular androgen production. Synthesis begins with the side-chain cleavage of cholesterol to form pregnenolone in the mitochondria. The primary source of cholesterol for ovarian steroidogenesis appears to be circulating lipoproteins rather than *de novo* synthesis from acetate. As in all steroid-secreting tissues, the side-chain cleavage of cholesterol is a rate-limiting step in hormone production and is under hormonal control. The pregnenolone formed in the mitochondria moves into the smooth endoplasmic reticulum where it is converted to androgens via the Δ-4 or Δ-5 pathway. A critical step in estrogen synthesis is the aromatization of the A-ring and simultaneous removal of the C-19 methyl group. This conversion is catalyzed by the enzyme **aromatase**, requires NADPH and O_2, and occurs in the smooth endoplasmic reticulum. Aromatase activity is under hormonal control so that both the first and last steps in estrogen synthesis are regulated.

It now appears that both theca and granulosa cells participate in estrogen production. Granulosa cells can synthesize progesterone but are not able to convert progesterone to androgens. Thus, although granulosa cells contain high levels of aromatase activity, they cannot synthesize estrogens unless they are provided with androgens as substrates. In contrast, thecal cells readily produce androgens but have relatively low aromatase activity. Thecal cells can produce some estrogen, but most of the estrogen secreted by preovulatory follicles is probably synthesized in granulosa cells from androgens provided by thecal tissue. The participation of both theca and granulosa in estrogen synthesis has important implications for hormonal regulation of this process that will be considered later.

The ovary is the primary source of circulating estradiol, but plasma estrone is derived from a number of sources. In addition to the ovary, the adrenal cortex secretes some estrone and a significant amount of this estrogen is produced by the aromatization of androstenedione in other tissues. Adipose tissue is a major site of this conversion and can become a clinically important source of estrone in obese women. The ovarian follicle also secretes a number of other steroids including 17α-hydroxyprogesterone and several androgens. The major ovarian androgen is androstenedione, but the adrenal is a more important source of this androgen in women.

The Corpus Luteum and Progesterone Synthesis. Although progesterone is a precursor for most biologically active steroids, the only endocrine tissue that secretes large amounts of this steroid in nonpregnant women is the corpus luteum. This tissue also secretes two other steroids with progestational activity, 17α-hydroxyprogesterone and 20-dihydroprogesterone. These three steroids comprise the major naturally occurring "progestins," which are steroids that promote gestation. All three are C-21 steroids with a keto group at the C-3 position and a double bond between the 4- and 5-carbons (e.g., see Fig. 9–4). The latter two steroids are derived from progesterone, 17α-OH-progesterone by addition of a hydroxyl group at the C-17 position and 20-dihydroprogesterone by reduction of the C-20 ketone of progesterone to a hydroxyl group. Progesterone is much more potent than its derivatives and is the only important progestin produced by the corpus luteum.

Progesterone is synthesized in two steps starting with cholesterol derived from plasma lipoproteins. First, cholesterol is converted to pregnenolone by side-chain cleavage in the mitochondria. Pregnenolone then moves into the endoplasmic reticulum where it is converted to progesterone by the enzyme

3β-hydroxysteroid dehydrogenase-isomerase (Fig. 9–4). Cholesterol side-chain cleavage is the rate-limiting enzyme in this pathway and is the site of hormonal control of progesterone biosynthesis.

The corpus luteum also secretes estrogens, primarily estradiol. These estrogens are synthesized by the △-4 pathway (Fig. 9–4) and some evidence suggests that they are formed mainly by luteal cells originating from the theca interna. In contrast, granulosa-derived luteal cells are the primary source of progesterone.

ACTIONS OF OVARIAN STEROIDS

Circulating Form of Ovarian Steroids

As with other lipophilic hormones, most of the circulating estradiol and progesterone is bound to plasma proteins. Both steroids bind with a low affinity to albumin, but because of the high plasma albumin concentration, about half of the circulating estradiol and progesterone is bound to this protein. In addition, each steroid binds with a high affinity to a specific binding protein, **estradiol to sex steroid–binding globulin** (which also binds testosterone) and **progesterone to corticosteroid-binding globulin** (which also binds cortisol). Only 1 to 2 per cent of the circulating estradiol and progesterone are free and hence biologically active. Because estrogen stimulates the hepatic production of these steroid-binding proteins, concentrations in plasma may increase in women taking oral contraceptives or during pregnancy. Such changes will increase the percentage of bound steroid in the circulation, but compensatory endocrine mechanisms will ensure that these changes do not affect the concentration of free active steroid.

Actions of Estradiol

Estradiol and progesterone act in concert to promote conception and to prepare the reproductive system for pregnancy. In general, the actions of estrogens are important to preconception events; they are critical for follicular maturation and ovulation, development of physical characteristics that are sexually attractive to males, and transport of the sperm from the vagina to the oviduct where fertilization occurs (Table 9–1).

Female Reproductive Tract. Estradiol is responsible for **development** of the female reproductive tract **at puberty** and **maintenance** of the oviducts and uterus in the adult. At puberty, in response to increasing ovarian estradiol secretion, the oviducts enlarge and develop ciliated epithelia and the size of the uterus increases two- to threefold, primarily as a result of growth of the uterine myometrium. The vagina and external genitalia also enlarge in response to estrogens at this time, but in the adult the size of these tissues is no longer

TABLE 9–1. Actions and Sites of Action of Estradiol and Progesterone in Adults

Target Tissue	Estradiol	Progesterone
Oviducts	Maintenance ↑ Muscular contractions	↓ Muscular contractions
Uterus Endometrium Myometrium Cervical mucus	Maintenance Proliferation ↑ Blood supply ↑ Contractions ↓ Viscosity	Secretion ↑ Blood supply ↓ Contractions ↑ Viscosity
Mammary gland	Growth of ducts	Growth of alveoli
Other	Control of LH and FSH ↑ Follicular development	Control of LH and FSH ↑ Basal body temperature

estrogen-dependent. In contrast, the oviducts and uterus remain estrogen-dependent and thus will atrophy following ovariectomy of adult women. In addition to maintaining uterine and oviductal size, estrogens influence the histological and functional characteristics of these tissues. Specifically, estradiol causes **proliferation of the uterine endometrium**, increasing both its stromal and glandular components. Estrogens alter the composition of **cervical mucus**, dramatically increasing its water content. Finally, the **muscular activity** of both uterus and oviduct is stimulated by estrogen. The latter two effects play an important role in sperm transport, which is described in Chapter 10.

Secondary Sexual Characteristics. Estrogen secretion at puberty is responsible for development of many of the physical traits characteristic of the adult woman. These include the development of **breasts**, widening of the **pelvic girdle**, and deposition of **subcutaneous fat**, especially in the buttocks, thighs, and breasts. The increase in breast size that occurs at puberty is due primarily to fat deposition rather than development of the mammary gland. Estradiol does produce proliferation of the **mammary duct system**, but the ducts occupy little volume in the breasts of nonpregnant women. Two pubertal changes, growth of **axillary and pubic hair** and development of **libido**, are due to **adrenal androgens**, not estrogens. The action of these androgens on sebaceous glands also accounts for the occurrence of acne in adolescent females.

Other Actions. Estradiol has important effects on **follicular growth** and on **gonadotropin secretion**, which are described later in this chapter. Like testosterone in the male, estradiol acts on long bones to cause a pubertal **growth spurt** and then **fusion of the epiphyseal plates**, which terminates growth. Estrogens also increase plasma triglycerides and angiotensin levels, but these actions are probably not physiologically important.

Actions of Progesterone

Progesterone is primarily a hormone of pregnancy and most of its actions in nongravid women can be viewed as preparing the female reproductive system for gestation (Table 9–1).

Female Reproductive Tract. Progesterone **stimulates the secretory activity** of glands in the oviduct and uterus. This is particularly evident in the uterus where these glands increase dramatically in size as a result of the accumulation of glycogen and other nutrients, some of which are released into the uterine lumen for utilization by a developing embryo. Progesterone **suppresses muscular contractions** of the oviducts and uterus. As described in Chapter 10, this action of progesterone on the uterine myometrium is critical to the maintenance of pregnancy. Progesterone maintains the structure of the **spiral arteries** that provide blood to the secretory endometrium of the uterus. Finally, progesterone acts on the cervix to greatly increase the **viscosity of cervical mucus.** Thus, when progesterone levels are high, bacteria and other organisms, including spermatozoa, cannot pass through the cervix to the uterus. This action of progesterone may account for some of its effectiveness as a contraceptive.

Other Actions. Like estradiol, progesterone has important effects on **gonadotropin secretion**, which are described later. Progesterone acts on mammary tissue to promote development of the **alveoli and lobules** in which milk is synthesized and secreted. This action, however, requires relatively high progesterone concentrations, so that only limited development of these structures occurs before pregnancy. Finally, progesterone produces an increase in **basal body temperature.** The mechanism and physiological significance of this alteration in temperature are unknown, but it is of some clinical usefulness in monitoring events of the menstrual cycle.

Mechanism of Action

Both estradiol and progesterone exert their effects on target tissues via specific cytosolic receptors. The events initiated by receptor binding of these steroids follow the general model for the mechanism of action of lipophilic hormones (see Fig. 1–8). The hormone-receptor complex is first activated and then translocated to the nucleus, where it binds to acceptor sites on the chromosomes and initiates gene transcription. Finally, the mRNA resulting from gene transcription is used to synthesize specific proteins, which in turn produce the biological effect of the steroid.

One of the specific proteins induced by estradiol via this mechanism is the cytosolic receptor for progesterone. This observation provides a simple explanation for the well-established concept that progesterone requires estrogen priming to exert its biological effects. For example, estrogen pretreatment greatly increases the number of uterine progesterone receptors; consequently the uterus becomes extremely sensitive to the actions of progesterone.

METABOLISM OF OVARIAN STEROIDS

Estradiol

Estradiol is metabolized primarily by the liver via three pathways (Fig. 9–5). In one pathway, a hydroxyl group is added at the 16-carbon to produce **estriol**, which is then conjugated with glucuronic acid and excreted. In another pathway, estradiol is first converted to estrone by the enzyme 17-OH-steroid dehydrogenase. This is a reversible reaction and, in fact, the same enzyme catalyzes the conversion of estrone to estradiol in the ovary. Estrone can then be hydroxylated at either the 16- or the 2-carbon. 16-OH-estrone is then converted to estriol by 17-OH-steroid dehydrogenase, conjugated, and excreted. **2-OH-estrone** can be either conjugated directly or first converted to **2-methoxyestrone** before conjugation and excretion. Estradiol can also be hydroxylated at the 2-carbon, but very little 2-hydroxy- or 2-methoxy-estradiol appears in the urine. It is interesting to note that 2-hydroxylation of estrogens converts the A-ring of these steroids to a catechol, a structure also found in biologically active catecholamines (e.g., dopamine), and thus 2-OH-estrogens are often called **catechol estrogens**. Since neural tissue can convert estradiol to 2-OH-estradiol, it has been suggested that this catechol estrogen may medi-

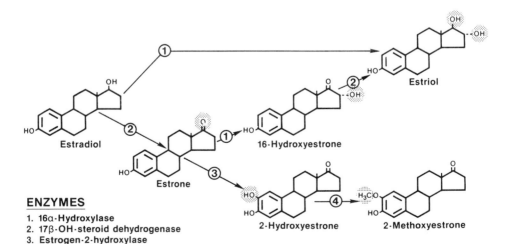

ENZYMES

1. 16α-Hydroxylase
2. 17β-OH-steroid dehydrogenase
3. Estrogen-2-hydroxylase
4. Catechol-O-Methyltransferase

FIGURE 9–5. Metabolism of estradiol to estriol and 2-methoxyestrone. Circles depict changes occurring at the previous step. Note that estriol contains two circles because two possible reactions lead to its formation.

ate some of the actions of estradiol in the brain. However, there is as yet no strong evidence for this hypothesis.

The metabolic clearance rate of estradiol is approximately 1.0 liter/min while the clearance rate of estrone is 1.5 liter/min. Since these estrogens are metabolized by the same pathways, this difference in clearance rate probably reflects the tighter binding of estradiol than estrone to serum-binding proteins. Estrogen metabolites are conjugated as sulfates or glucuronides, with the latter predominating. Most estrogen metabolites are excreted in the urine, but approximately 20 per cent appear in the bile.

Progesterone

The major metabolite of progesterone is **pregnanediol**, which is formed by reduction of the C-3 and C-20 keto groups and of the Δ-4 double bond of progesterone (Fig. 9–6). The specific intermediates between progesterone and pregnanediol depend on the order in which these reductions occur; if the C-20 keto group is reduced first, then 20-dihydroprogesterone is formed as an intermediate (Fig. 9–6). This means that hepatic metabolism of the 20-dihydroprogesterone secreted from the corpus luteum also contributes to the pregnanediol in the urine. Nevertheless, since the ovarian output of progesterone is five times that of 20-dihydroprogesterone, urinary pregnanediol measurements usually provide a reliable index of progesterone secretion. Progesterone is metabolized primarily in the liver, with a metabolic clearance rate of ap-

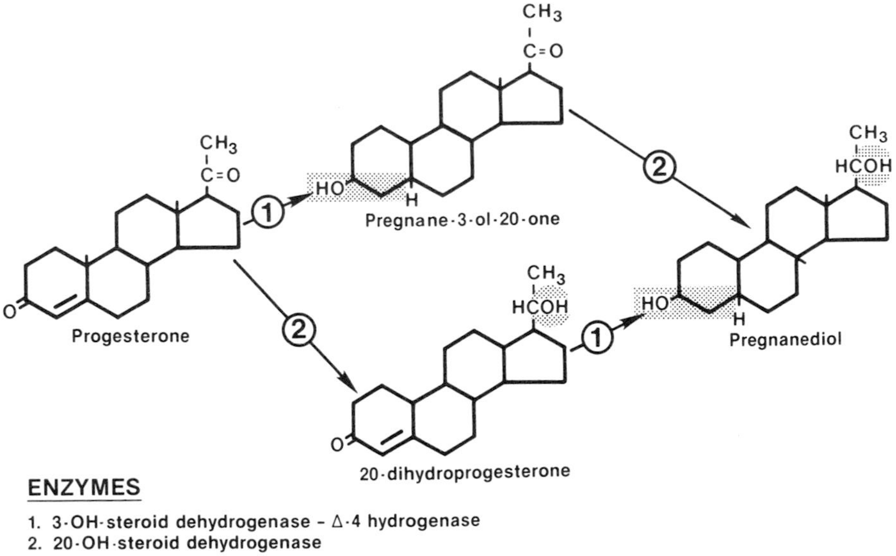

ENZYMES

1. 3-OH-steroid dehydrogenase – Δ-4 hydrogenase
2. 20-OH-steroid dehydrogenase

FIGURE 9–6. Hepatic metabolism of progesterone to pregnanediol. Rectangles indicate changes by enzyme 1; circles, changes by enzyme 2.

proximately 1.5 liters/min. The pregnanediol that is produced is conjugated to glucuronic acid and excreted in the urine.

REGULATION OF OVARIAN FUNCTION

As in the male, gonadal function in the female is controlled by the pituitary hormones, **luteinizing hormone (LH)** and **follicle-stimulating hormone (FSH)**; secretion of these gonadotropins is in turn regulated by the feedback actions of ovarian hormones and by the hypothalamic hormone, GnRH. However, this regulatory system in the female is complicated by the cyclic nature of ovarian function. For example, the ovarian effects of LH and FSH depend on the stage of the menstrual cycle because as the cycle progresses, the dominant endocrine tissue changes from a follicle to a corpus luteum. Futhermore, this endocrine system must be able to produce the cyclic fluctuations in steroid and gonadotropic hormones that occur throughout the menstrual cycle. This section will first describe the individual components of this control system and will then consider how these components interact to produce the menstrual cycle.

Hormonal Control of Follicular Function

As in the male, a major function of LH is control of steroidogenesis while FSH regulates gametogenesis or, more specifically, follicular development. However, this dichotomy of function is not as complete in the female; FSH has important effects on estrogen production and LH controls two aspects of follicular function, namely ovulation and luteinization.

Estrogen Secretion. Both LH and FSH are required for synthesis and secretion of estradiol by the follicle but these two hormones act on different cells and at different steps in the steroidogenic pathway. **LH acts on thecal cells** to stimulate androgen production while **FSH acts on granulosa cells** to ensure that thecal androgens are converted to estrogens (Fig. 9–7). The cellular specificity of the gonadotropins is due to the distribution of LH and FSH receptors. In antral follicles, LH receptors are found only on thecal cells and FSH receptors only on granulosa cells.

The actions of LH on thecal cells are virtually identical to its effects on Leydig cells in the testes. LH binds to its membrane receptor and stimulates production of cyclic AMP. The increased intracellular cAMP concentrations activate protein kinases, which ultimately increase the conversion of cholesterol to pregnenolone. Since side-chain cleavage of cholesterol is the rate-limiting step in ovarian androgen production, the overall effect of this sequence of events is to increase androgen synthesis. Some of this androgen diffuses into the blood, while the rest of it moves into the granulosa cell compartment to serve as a precursor for estrogen. A similar mechanism accounts for the ac-

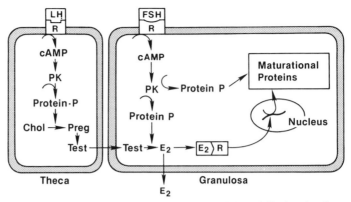

FIGURE 9–7. Actions of LH, FSH, and estradiol on follicular development. LH binds to thecal receptors and increases testosterone (test) production by increasing the conversion of cholesterol (chol) to pregnenolone (preg) via the cAMP–protein kinase (PK) second messenger system. FSH uses the same system to control the conversion of testosterone to estradiol (E_2) by granulosa cells.

tions of FSH on steroidogenesis in granulosa cells in that binding of FSH activates protein kinases by increasing cAMP concentrations. The ultimate effect of FSH on granulosa cells, however, is activation of aromatase. Thus, FSH is necessary for conversion of thecal androgens to estrogens (Fig. 9–7) within the granulosa cells.

Under physiological conditions, FSH plays largely a permissive role in estrogen production because basal FSH concentrations are sufficient to maintain high aromatase activity in the developing antral follicles. Consequently, changes in LH concentrations are primarily responsible for changes in ovarian estrogen secretion and there is a close correlation between LH and estradiol secretion. Finally, follicular estrogen secretion is also related to the total mass of thecal and granulosa cells. Thus, as the follicle grows, a given LH stimulus will result in more estradiol secretion simply because there are more cells present in the follicle.

Oogenesis and Follicular Maturation. FSH, LH, and estradiol are required for the complete development of the mature ovum, which involves both follicular and oocyte maturation. In describing the roles of these hormones it is useful to distinguish between the three stages of follicular maturation. Because folliculogenesis in the developing ovary *in utero* appears to occur independently of any hormonal regulation, this section will focus on the other two stages, follicular development and ovulation.

The factors initiating follicular development are not well understood. Exit of follicles from the resting pool of primordial follicles and the early stages of preantral development do not require gonadotropic stimulation. The number of follicles leaving the resting pool at any time is roughly proportional to the size of this pool, but the mechanisms that determine when a given follicle is activated are unknown. Once follicles reach the late preantral stage, they require hormonal support for further development, with FSH and estradiol being the most important hormones needed. FSH induces formation of the antrum and both hormones cause granulosa cell proliferation. Further, these hormones act synergistically in that estradiol increases the ovarian responsiveness to FSH. The molecular events underlying these actions are still being investigated, but one important effect of FSH is the induction of receptors for both FSH and LH on granulosa cells. The increase in FSH receptors further sensitizes the ovary to this gonadotropin, and the appearance of LH receptors on granulosa cells is a critical event in the development of the preovulatory follicle. It is important to realize that LH is also necessary for follicular development. Early in the life of antral follicles, LH is needed to maintain intrafollicular estradiol concentrations and may promote thecal cell proliferation. In addition, LH may act directly on granulosa cells to help maintain the preovulatory follicle, although such an effect has not been conclusively demonstrated.

Since a growing follicle either continues to develop or becomes atretic, the mechanisms controlling atresia are closely linked to those controlling follicular development. For example, it is not surprising that FSH and estradiol, which stimulate follicular development, also suppress atresia. Androgens, on the other hand, promote follicular atresia. How these factors interact to determine which follicles become atretic remains a mystery. However, given the antagonistic actions of androgens and estrogens, it is tempting to propose a critical role for granulosa cell aromatase activity. In those follicles with low aromatase activity, thecal androgens would not be rapidly converted to estrogens and would thus induce atresia. Conversely, high aromatase activity would result in high estrogen and low androgen levels in the follicle and thus promote follicular development.

Ovulation and Luteinization. Follicular development must precede ovulation because preantral and small antral follicles are incapable of ovulating. However, ovulation requires a specific endocrine signal that differs from those producing follicular growth. This endocrine signal is an abrupt, massive increment in LH secretion known as the **LH surge**. The induction of ovulation by the LH surge should not be confused with the steroidogenic action of LH required for estrogen production. The latter is seen only with low levels of LH; in fact, the LH surge has completely different effects on follicular steroidogenesis.

The LH surge induces ovulation and luteinization by binding to LH receptors on both granulosa and thecal cells. The former cells appear to be a critical site of action since granulosa cells within a follicle must develop LH receptors or the follicle will not ovulate in response to the LH surge. LH binding initiates the standard sequence of cyclic AMP-mediated events and

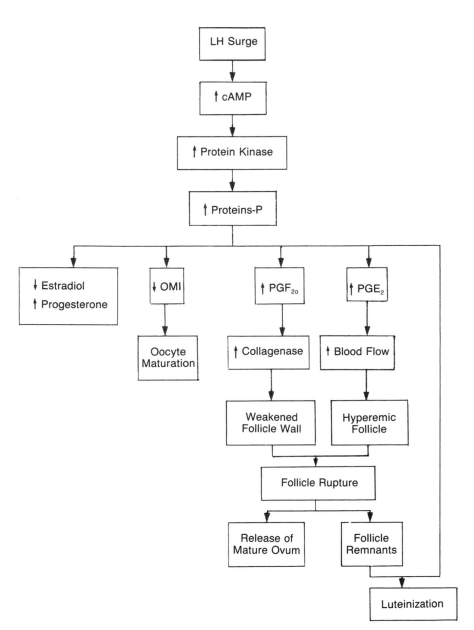

FIGURE 9–8. Effects of the LH surge on the preovulatory follicle.

results in the phosphorylation of specific proteins by protein kinases (Fig. 9–8). By initiating this sequence of events, the LH surge produces four major changes in the follicle. First, it **terminates estrogen** synthesis and **stimulates progesterone** production. Second, the LH surge **reinitiates meiosis in the oocyte**, apparently by suppressing release of an oocyte maturation–inhibiting (OMI) substance from granulosa cells. Third, it triggers a large **increase in PGE$_2$ and PGF$_{2\alpha}$** production. These prostaglandins induce follicular hyperemia and enzymatic digestion of the follicular wall, respectively, thus producing follicle rupture and ovulation. Fourth, the LH surge causes **differentiation of follicular cells to luteal cells** so that formation of the corpus luteum routinely follows ovulation.

Hormonal Control of Corpus Luteum

Control of luteal function can be divided into three distinct mechanisms: those responsible for corpus luteum formation, those controlling hormone secretion, and those determining when luteolysis occurs. Because the role of the LH surge in formation of the corpus luteum has already been described, this section will be limited to discussion of the latter two mechanisms.

Steroid Secretion. Only one hormone, **LH**, controls steroid secretion by the corpus luteum. The mechanism of LH action on steroidogenesis follows a familiar pattern: LH binds to its receptor on the cell membrane and increases cyclic AMP levels, which, acting via protein kinases, stimulate the side-chain cleavage of cholesterol. Since this reaction is the rate-limiting step in steroidogenesis, the net effect of LH is to increase the synthesis and secretion of progesterone and estradiol by the corpus luteum. Relatively low LH concentrations are sufficient for maintenance of progesterone and estradiol secretion, but in the absence of LH secretion, steroid output from the corpus luteum falls precipitously. The other major factor contributing to luteal steroid output is the **mass of luteal tissue.** For example, progesterone levels increase for several days after ovulation despite falling LH levels because the number of fully active luteal cells increases progessively as more and more granulosa cells complete their differentiation into luteal tissue. This illustrates the fact that, under most conditions, LH appears to play largely a permissive role in progesterone secretion so that increases in progesterone concentrations need not be preceded by increases in LH secretion.

Control of Luteal Life Span. In the nonpregnant woman, the corpus luteum functions for two weeks and then undergoes luteolysis. Although this 14-day life span is remarkably constant, the mechanisms responsible for it are not completely understood. In general, the demise of the corpus luteum is determined by the balance between **luteotropins**, which prolong luteal function, and **luteolysins**, which induce luteolysis. In nonpregnant women, **LH** is the primary luteotropin and **estradiol** the main luteolysin. Thus, either a fall in LH or a rise in estradiol could produce luteolysis; since both of these changes occur as the luteal phase progresses, both may contribute to the normal demise of the corpus luteum. Two other compounds may also play a role in determining luteal life span. $PGF_{2\alpha}$ is a potent luteolysin and there is some evidence that this prostaglandin mediates the actions of estradiol on the corpus luteum. Human chorionic gonadotropin (hCG) is an LH-like hormone that is produced during pregnancy. It has important luteotropic actions in pregnant women but plays no role during the normal menstrual cycle.

Control of Gonadotropin Secretion

Before describing the role of ovarian hormones in controlling LH and FSH secretion, it is necessary to understand two important aspects of gonadotropin secretion. First, as described in Chapter 5, release of LH and FSH from the anterior pituitary is driven by the hypothalamic hormone, **gonadotropin-releasing hormone (GnRH)**. GnRH is secreted by hypothalamic neurons in an episodic pattern and each bolus of GnRH travels down the hypophyseal portal vessels to produce a brief release of LH and FSH. This produces a pulsatile pattern in circulating LH levels, but similar short-term fluctuations in FSH concentrations do not occur because of the relatively slow metabolic clearance rate of FSH. Second, it is essential to understand the distinction between **basal (or tonic) LH secretion** and the **LH surge**. As previously discussed, tonic LH secretion controls ovarian steroidogenesis while the LH surge causes ovulation. In addition to producing different effects on the ovary, these two modes of LH secretion occur at different times during the menstrual cycle and are controlled by different neuroendocrine systems. It is thus necessary to consider the ovarian control of tonic and surge secretion of LH separately. The secretion of FSH can also be divided into tonic and surge components; however, since the FSH surge has no known physiological role in humans, only tonic FSH release will be considered.

Control of Tonic Gonadotropin Secretion. Tonic secretion of LH is controlled by the inhibitory actions of **estradiol** and **progesterone**. Since tonic LH stimulates secretion of these two steroids, this control system is a classic **negative feedback loop** (Fig. 9–9). Because both steroids participate in the inhibition of tonic LH, the absence of either estradiol or progesterone alone will allow basal LH levels to increase. Although the sites of action of progesterone and estradiol are still being debated, it appears that these steroids act at different loci. Estradiol acts primarily on the anterior pituitary to inhibit LH release by decreasing the response of the gonadotropes to GnRH. Progesterone acts mainly in the brain to decrease the episodes of GnRH release, thus indirectly suppressing tonic LH secretion. The inhibitory effects of progesterone, like most of its other actions, require either priming with, or the presence of, low levels of estradiol.

Tonic FSH secretion is also inhibited by estradiol and progesterone, but there is an important quantitative difference in the actions of these steroids.

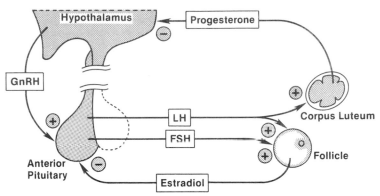

FIGURE 9-9. Feedback loops controlling tonic secretion of LH and FSH and steroidogenesis by the follicle and corpus luteum.

FSH release is more sensitive than LH to the negative feedback action of estradiol so that small amounts of estradiol can selectively inhibit FSH secretion. **Inhibin** may also contribute to the control of FSH secretion. This protein hormone that suppresses release of FSH, but not of LH, is produced by the follicle. There is as yet no strong evidence, however, that it plays an important role in the control of FSH during the normal menstrual cycle.

Control of the LH Surge. In contrast to tonic LH secretion, which is controlled by a negative feedback loop, the LH surge is produced by a **neuroendocrine reflex**. The reflex nature of this control system is clearly evident in some species, such as cats and rabbits, in which the LH surge is triggered by neural impulses initiated by coitus. In species such as humans, in which ovulation occurs spontaneously, the same basic neuroendocrine reflex is thought to be responsible for the LH surge, but in this case it is triggered by an endocrine signal rather than a neural one. In women, a sustained elevation in circulating concentrations of **estradiol initiates the LH surge** (Fig. 9–10). Since only mature, preovulatory follicles are capable of sustained estradiol secretion, this reflex ensures that the signal for ovulation (i.e., the LH surge) normally

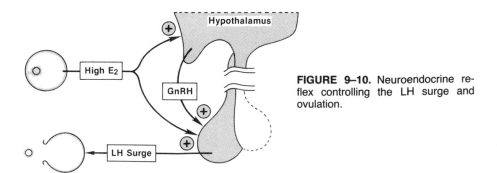

FIGURE 9-10. Neuroendocrine reflex controlling the LH surge and ovulation.

occurs only when the ovary contains a follicle ready for ovulation. Thus, in contrast to tonic LH secretion, which continues throughout the menstrual cycle, the LH surge occurs only for one to two days at midcycle, just before ovulation (Fig. 9–11). Induction of the LH surge by estradiol is often referred to as the "positive feedback" action of estradiol because in this case estradiol stimulates LH secretion rather than inhibits it; the negative feedback action

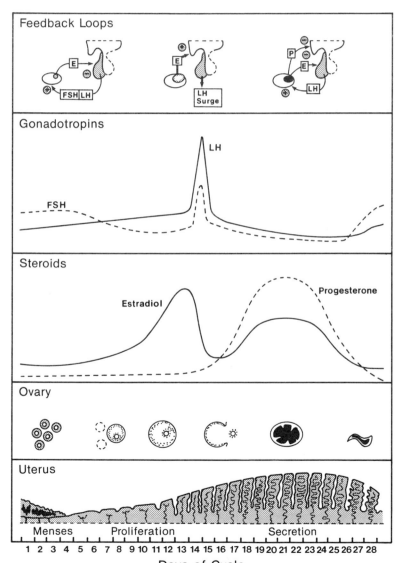

FIGURE 9–11. Events of the menstrual cycle.

of estradiol described earlier inhibits LH release but participates only in the regulation of tonic LH secretion.

In contrast to the effects of estradiol, progesterone inhibits the LH surge. This action of progesterone ensures that estrogen output from the corpus luteum does not induce an LH surge during the luteal phase and accounts for some of the contraceptive effects of progestin-containing oral contraceptives. Although there is considerable controversy as to the sites of action of estradiol and progesterone in controlling the LH surge, recent evidence suggests that these steroids exert their effects on both the hypothalamus and the pituitary. The major differences in control of tonic LH secretion and the LH surge are summarized in Table 9–2.

Control of the Menstrual Cycle

The average length of the menstrual cycle is 28 days, but there is considerable deviation from this mean value even in normal adults, and this variability is greatest in the years just after puberty and just before menopause. The most obvious sign of this cycle is the menstrual bleeding that occurs once per cycle. Underlying this outward manifestation is a complex sequence of events that produces the cyclic fluctuations in gonadotropic and ovarian hormones necessary for maturation and ovulation of a fertilizable ovum and preparation of the uterus for implantation (Fig. 9–11).

Events of the Follicular Phase. By convention, the first day of menstruation is considered the start of a new cycle and is designated day 1 of the follicular phase. Since the early stages of development of preantral follicles do not require hormonal support there is a constant supply of follicles reaching the late preantral stage throughout the cycle. However, only those follicles that reach this stage during the early follicular phase will continue to grow. At this time, circulating concentrations of estradiol and progesterone are low so that tonic FSH and LH secretion are elevated. The high FSH concentrations stimulate further follicular growth so a group of follicles develop antra and begin to secrete estradiol. Since estradiol alone does not completely suppress tonic LH secretion, basal levels of LH rise progressively throughout the follicular

TABLE 9–2. Comparison of the Characteristics of Tonic LH Secretion and of the LH Surge

Feature	Tonic LH	LH Surge
Function	Stimulates steroidogenesis	Induces ovulation
Occurrence	Throughout cycle	1–2 days at midcycle
Concentrations of LH	Low	High
Control system	Negative feedback loop	Neuroendocrine reflex
Actions of E_2	Inhibit	Trigger
Actions of progesterone	Inhibit	Inhibit

phase and provide a continuous stimulus for estradiol secretion. This stimulus, together with continued follicular growth, results in a progressive increase in plasma estradiol concentrations to a peak just prior to ovulation (Fig. 9–11).

The rising titers of estradiol during the follicular phase of the cycle produce three important effects. First, this steroid acts on the uterus to cause proliferation of the endometrium. Second, relatively early in the follicular phase estradiol (and possibly inhibin) begins to suppress FSH secretion. The resulting fall in FSH concentrations causes atresia of all but one (or two) follicle(s) so that usually only one ovum is released at ovulation. Third, estradiol concentrations eventually increase sufficiently to trigger the preovulatory LH surge (Fig. 9–11).

The estrogen-induced LH surge then initiates a sequence of ovarian changes that terminate the follicular phase and begin the luteal phase. The LH surge converts the follicle from an estrogen- to a progesterone-secreting tissue, and as a result plasma estradiol levels fall and progesterone concentrations begin to rise. This is followed by ovulation and luteinization of the granulosa and thecal cells remaining in the ruptured follicle.

Events of the Luteal Phase. As the remnants of the ruptured follicle develop into a fully active corpus luteum, they secrete increasing amounts of progesterone and estradiol (Fig. 9–11). The primary effect of the rise in circulating progesterone levels is production of a secretory endometrium capable of sustaining an embryo and allowing implantation. Progesterone also stimulates growth of the arterial supply to the endometrium and increases basal body temperature; the latter is often used as an indirect indication of normal ovulation and luteal function. The combination of progesterone and estradiol produces a strong inhibition of tonic gonadotropin secretion so that both LH and FSH reach a nadir toward the latter portion of the luteal phase.

On about day 10 or 11 after ovulation, either the low LH levels or the high estradiol levels or both induce luteolysis. As a result, steroid secretion declines over the last three days of the luteal phase (Fig. 9–11). Menstruation, which represents the involution and sloughing of the secretory endometrium, is a direct result of the fall in circulating progesterone and estradiol levels at the end of the luteal phase. Since these steroids are responsible for endometrial growth, their withdrawal at luteolysis produces the opposite effect (i.e., involution). At the same time, the fall in steroid levels stimulates release of uterine $PGF_{2\alpha}$; this prostaglandin causes vasospasms of the spiral arteries and thereby disrupts the blood supply to the endometrium. Hypoxia produces necrosis of the endometrium and its blood vessels and the resulting menstrual bleeding washes the dying endometrial tissues into the uterine lumen. The increase in $PGF_{2\alpha}$ often causes contractions of the uterine myometrium; these contractions help expel blood and endometrial tissue from the uterine cavity and can also produce the painful cramps that are frequently associated with menstruation.

Menstruation can be considered a cleansing process as it removes the secretory epithelium thus allowing the uterus to begin another wave of proliferation in response to the increasing estradiol concentrations during the follicular phase. In addition to preparing the uterus for the next ovarian cycle, the fall in progesterone and estradiol at luteolysis allows tonic secretion of FSH and LH to increase. This initiates the next follicular phase because the high FSH levels stimulate follicular growth. Thus, another cycle begins at the time of menstruation.

In some women, behavioral changes are associated with certain periods of the menstrual cycle. In general, there is a slight increase in libido at mid-cycle. Since androgens are the primary hormones maintaining libido in women, this is probably caused by the increase in ovarian androgen secretion that accompanies the rise in estradiol output late in the follicular phase. In a small percentage of women (5 to 10 per cent), the period of luteolysis is associated with increased irritability, depression, anxiety, or swelling of legs and breasts, a condition referred to as the **premenstrual tension syndrome**. The etiology of these symptoms is not understood, but they probably represent a response to the fall in progesterone and estradiol that occurs just before menstruation.

AGE-RELATED CHANGES IN FEMALE REPRODUCTIVE FUNCTION

The regular menstrual cycles characteristic of adult women are absent in young and aging females. However, the reasons for the anovulatory state in these two age groups are quite different.

Prepuberty

From birth until 8 to 10 years of age, ovulations and hence menstrual cycles do not occur because hypothalamic GnRH secretion is actively suppressed by mechanisms similar to those operative in prepubertal males; namely, a combination of direct neural inhibition and increased sensitivity to the negative feedback action of estradiol. These inhibitory mechanisms do not become fully functional until sometime after birth, so that during the first few months of life secretion of LH, FSH, and estradiol is relatively high. Thereafter, secretion of gonadotropins and estradiol declines and remains low until the onset of puberty. There is sufficient gonadotropin secretion throughout the prepubertal period to produce some antral follicles, but these follicles become atretic before reaching the preovulatory stage of development. This prolonged period of reproductive inactivity permits physical and psychological maturation so that the female is better able to handle the stresses of pregnancy and childrearing.

Puberty

The events initiating puberty are essentially identical in females and males (see Chapter 8 for a detailed discussion), but they begin one to two years earlier in females. Briefly, an as yet unknown maturational change removes the neuroendocrine inhibition of hypothalamic GnRH release. Consequently, GnRH output increases and stimulates gonadotropin secretion. This change is first limited to nocturnal bursts in LH and FSH secretion, but as the duration of these secretory episodes lengthens, there is a progressive rise in circulating FSH and LH levels. Since the gonadotropins stimulate follicular development, a parallel increase in circulating estradiol concentrations occurs that induces many of the female secondary sexual characteristics (e.g., breast development) and the adolescent growth spurt (Fig. 9–12). At the same time an increase in adrenal androgen secretion stimulates the growth of pubic hair and development of libido. This activation of adrenal steroidogenesis, which is called **adrenarche**, actually precedes activation of the ovaries and is thought to result from increased secretion of an unidentified hormone that specifically stimulates androgen production (Chapter 7). The activation of gonadal function eventually culminates in **menarche**, or the first menstruation, but this does not signal the beginning of regular ovulatory cycles. For the next few years, menstruation occurs at irregular intervals and most of these cycles are anovulatory. Even those cycles in which ovulation occurs are characterized by inadequate progesterone secretion during the luteal phase so that most women are infertile during this period. The reasons for this period of inadequate ovarian cycles remain obscure, but it does ensure full development of the female reproductive tract before any pregnancies occur.

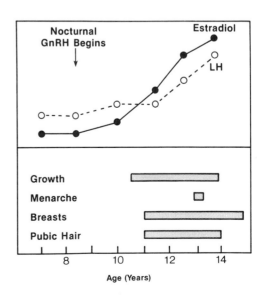

FIGURE 9–12. Events during puberty in the female. Bars indicate approximate ages during which the pubertal growth spurt occurs, breasts and pubic hair develop, and menses begins. (Bottom panel redrawn from Marshall, W.A. and Tanner, J.M.: Variations in the pattern of pubertal changes in boys. Arch. Dis. Child. 45:13, 1970.)

Menopause

The cessation of menstrual cycles in aging women (i.e., menopause) is a direct consequence of the termination of ovarian folliculogenesis *in utero*. At birth the ovaries contain all of the follicles available for development, and at sometime between 45 and 55 years of age, this reservoir is depleted so that ovarian cycles cease. The cessation of menstruation is preceded by a period of increasingly irregular cycles; some ovarian function persists for a few years into the postmenopausal period. This progressive failure in ovarian function, often referred to as the **climacteric**, is mirrored by a gradual decline in circulating estrogen concentrations. It is the absence of ovarian estrogen production that causes many of the clinical symptoms seen in postmenopausal women. Changes resulting directly from low estrogen levels include an increase in circulating gonadotropins, atrophy of the uterus, vaginal dryness that can cause discomfort during coitus, and a gradual decalcification of bone that can lead to osteoporosis in some women. Brief periods of increased body temperature (hot flashes or flushes) are one of the most common outward symptoms of menopause, but their etiology remains obscure. Menopause is also often associated with periods of depression, anxiety, and irritability, but whether these behavioral problems are caused by hormonal changes or reflect psychological adjustments to the implications of menopause is unknown.

CLINICAL CONSIDERATIONS

Abnormalities in ovarian secretory function fall into the same two broad categories as those for other endocrine tissues, namely hyposecretion and hypersecretion. However, because of the complex interactions required for the normal menstrual cycle, subtle changes in any component of the system are often sufficient to completely disrupt cyclic ovarian function. Thus, **amenorrhea** (the absence of menses) can occur without gross abnormalities in hormone output.

Hypogonadism

Inadequate ovarian function usually leads to amenorrhea, which can be classified as primary or secondary. This terminology should not be confused with primary and secondary **hypogonadism**, which refer to deficits at the ovary and pituitary, respectively. **Primary amenorrhea** is the absence of menses in females who have never menstruated, while **secondary amenorrhea** is the cessation of menses in patients who have menstruated previously. This is largely an artificial distinction, since the same pathology can cause either condition depending on whether it develops before or after menarche. Nevertheless, it remains a useful first step in diagnosis because most congenital disorders produce primary amenorrhea.

Primary Amenorrhea. It is important to distinguish between primary amenorrhea and delayed menarche. In the latter condition, menarche has not occurred by age 16, but normal cycles will eventually begin without treatment. Delayed menarche is diagnosed by the exclusion of other pathologies but may also be indicated by the appearance of secondary sexual characteristics (e.g., breast development), since these changes usually precede menarche (Fig. 9–12).

Primary amenorrhea is uncommon and is usually due to developmental anomalies in the ovaries or reproductive tract. The most common of these anomalies is **gonadal dysgenesis**, in which the ovaries fail to develop. Because of the absence of estrogen secretion, secondary sexual characteristics do not develop at puberty, but other symptoms depend on the type of gonadal dysgenesis. In its classic form (Turner's syndrome), there is a genetic defect that produces a combination of physical abnormalities including dwarfism and webbing of the neck. However, other forms of this syndrome are now recognized in which there is no major chromosomal abnormality and the only obvious symptom is sexual infantilism at puberty. Abnormalities in uterine development can also lead to primary amenorrhea, but in these cases, other aspects of sexual development at puberty will be normal.

A deficit in gonadotropin secretion is responsible for 20 to 30 per cent of the cases of primary amenorrhea. Such deficits can include all other pituitary hormones (panhypopituitarism) or be limited to LH and FSH release (Kallmann's syndrome). It is important to determine the genesis of amenorrhea, for if it is secondary to low gonadotropin secretion, appropriate treatment may restore fertility. If it is caused by a primary ovarian deficit, the patient will be infertile but hormone replacement is used to produce sexual development. Measurement of FSH (or LH) concentrations is the simplest method for distinguishing between these two conditions. Primary ovarian failure results in elevated gonadotropin levels because of the lack of steroid negative feedback, whereas gonadotropin levels are low if there is a secondary deficit in pituitary function.

Secondary Amenorrhea. The most common cause of secondary amenorrhea in premenopausal women is pregnancy. However, pregnancy is not considered a pathological condition and will be considered in detail in Chapter 10. By definition, secondary amenorrhea implies a previous history of ovarian function so that abnormalities in ovarian development can usually be ruled out as causative. However, ovarian failure (primary hypogonadism) may be caused in adults by autoimmune diseases or cancer therapy, both of which can produce depletion of ovarian follicles (Table 9–3). The most common pituitary cause of secondary amenorrhea is a prolactin-secreting adenoma; amenorrhea occurs in these individuals because **hyperprolactinemia** suppresses gonadotropin secretion (Chapter 10). At the hypothalamic level, psychological (or physical) **stress** will often suppress GnRH release and hence disrupt menstrual cycles. Extreme **weight loss** or **weight gain** can also cause amenorrhea (Table

TABLE 9–3. Some Common Causes of Secondary Amenorrhea

Site of Defect	Cause
Uterus	Adhesions after postpartum infection or surgery
Ovary	Autoimmune disease
	Radio- or chemotherapy
	Gonadotropin resistance
Pituitary	Hyperprolactinemia
	Postpartum panhypopituitarism
	Pituitary tumors
Hypothalamus	Psychogenic (stress)
	Starvation (anorexia nervosa)
	Hypothalamic tumors
Extrinsic to hypothalamo-hypophyseal-ovarian axis	Steroid ingestion
	Post-pill amenorrhea
	Extraovarian estrogen (obesity)
	Other endocrinopathies

9–3). The former appears to produce a hypoestrogenic prepubertal-like condition, whereas the increase in adipose tissue associated with the latter causes an increase in the conversion of adrenal androgens to estrogens. The excess estrogen disrupts the normal feedback relationship within the hypothalamo-hypophyseal-ovarian axis, producing secondary amenorrhea.

Hypergonadism

Excessive secretion of ovarian hormones can occur before or after menarche. If it occurs before puberty, early development of secondary sexual characteristics occurs, with or without normal menstrual cycles. Early maturation of the entire hypothalamo-hypophyseal-ovarian axis produces ovulatory cycles and is termed **true precocious puberty**. This can be caused by hypothalamic lesions that damage the neural systems suppressing GnRH release, but it is more often of unknown etiology. In contrast, **pseudoprecocious puberty** involves an increase in steroid hormone secretion in the absence of gonadotropic stimulation and ovulation. This is usually due to ovarian tumors, although adrenal tumors can also be responsible. The distinction between true and pseudoprecocious puberty is clinically important because the former is usually benign while the latter can be life-threatening.

Excessive secretion of ovarian hormones in the adult causes the same primary symptoms as hyposecretion, oligomenorrhea and amenorrhea. Estrogen- or androgen-producing ovarian tumors can cause secondary amenorrhea, but the most common cause of elevated ovarian steroid production is the **polycystic ovary syndrome** (PCO). In this syndrome, the ovary contains numerous atretic follicles and secretes excess androgen but little estradiol. Circulating estrone levels are elevated because of peripheral aromatization of androgen; LH concentrations are elevated but FSH levels are suppressed. The etiology of PCO is not completely understood, but it may be started by an abnormal elevation in ovarian androgen. The excess androgen promotes follicular atresia, which suppresses ovarian estradiol output. The resulting steroid secretory pattern results in an inappropriate feedback signal that elevates LH and inhibits FSH release. The increase in LH then stimulates androgen synthesis while the fall in FSH decreases aromatase activity so that the ratio of follicular androgen to estrogen increases, which exacerbates the initial condition. These hormonal changes establish a positive feedback loop that prevents follicular development and ovulation. Amenorrhea will thus continue until this loop is broken by treatment with FSH, with an antiestrogen (that elevates endogenous FSH), or by removal of ovarian tissue (ovarian wedge resection) to decrease androgen production.

Contraceptive Techniques

Women wishing to avoid pregnancy have a number of options available (Table 9–4) ranging from the noninvasive (e.g., rhythm method) to the surgical (e.g., tubal ligation). All available techniques involve some risks, including potentially lethal side effects (Table 9–4). A detailed consideration of these complications is beyond the scope of this text. Instead, this section will focus on the mechanisms of action of different contraceptive techniques.

Current Methods. All contraceptive methods now available act at one of three major steps in the reproductive process: ovulation, sperm transport to the ovum, or implantation (Fig. 9–13). **Oral contraceptives**, which usually

TABLE 9–4. Failure Rates and Mortality Associated with Contraceptive Techniques

Contraceptive Method	Average Failure Rate (Annual Pregnancies/100 Women)	Mortality Rate (Annual Deaths/100,000 Women)
None	90	8.3*
Tubal ligation	0.04	8†
Steroid pills	2–2.5	0.9 (5.2‡)
IUD	4	1.2
Barrier methods	10–15	1.2*
Coitus interruptus	23	2*
Natural methods	20–30	2*

*Birth related.
†Surgical complications.
‡Smokers.
Data for women 20–29 years old taken from Carr, B.R. and Griffin, J.E.: In Williams' Textbook of Endocrinology, 7th ed. J.D. Wilson and D.W. Foster, editors. W.B. Saunders Company, Philadelphia, 1985.

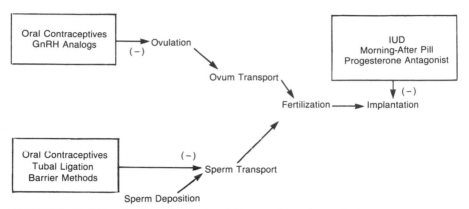

FIGURE 9–13. Sites of action of current and future contraceptive methods.

contain an estrogen-progestin combination, block ovulation by suppressing go-nadotropin secretion. The progestational activity of these pills also decreases sperm transport by decreasing muscular contractions in the female reproductive tract and increasing the viscosity of cervical mucus. Women who take oral contraceptives do have an increased risk of cardiovascular disease, especially if they also smoke tobacco. A different type of oral contraceptive sometimes used is the so-called morning-after pill. This high-estrogen content pill is taken during the early luteal phase and it prevents implantation by inducing premature luteolysis. The high dose of estrogen required for this effect often causes nausea and vomiting so that this contraceptive is not widely used.

Barrier methods of contraception (e.g., vaginal diaphragm) prevent sperm transport. These are most often used in conjunction with spermicidal agents and are quite effective if used conscientiously. The mechanism of action of the **intrauterine device** (IUD) is not completely understood. Most evidence suggests that the IUD induces a local inflammatory response that prevents implantation. Possible complications of the IUD include bleeding, uterine cramps, uterine perforation, and pelvic inflammatory disease following its insertion.

Future Trends. Several new approaches to contraception are now being clinically tested. **Long-acting injection** or subcutaneous **implantation** of steroids blocks ovulation and sperm transport (as do oral contraceptives) and is effective for three to six months. Oral administration of a **progesterone antagonist** during the luteal phase prevents implantation by antagonizing the actions of progesterone on the uterus. A variety of **GnRH analogues** have been tested for contraceptive activity. The most effective of these are long-acting GnRH agonists, which, paradoxically, suppress gonadotropin secretion. The inhibitory effects of these agonists reflect the inability of the pituitary to respond to a GnRH-like stimulus that is given continuously over a prolonged period.

REFERENCES

Carr, B.R. and Griffin, J.E.: Fertility control and its complications. *In* Williams' Textbook of Endocrinology, 7th ed. J.D. Wilson and D.W. Foster, editors. W.B. Saunders Company, Philadelphia, p. 452, 1985.

Grumbach, M.M.: The neuroendocrinology of puberty. Hosp. Practice 15 (3):51, 1980.

Johnson, M.H. and Everitt, B.J.: Essential Reproduction. Blackwell Scientific Publications, Oxford, 1980.

Knobil, E.: The neuroendocrine control of the menstrual cycle. Rec. Prog. Horm. Res. 36:53, 1980.

Ross, G.T.: Disorders of the ovary and female reproductive tract. *In* Williams' Textbook of Endocrinology, 7th ed. J.D. Wilson and D.W. Foster, editors. W.B. Saunders Company, Philadelphia, p. 206, 1985.

Serra, G.B.: The Ovary. Raven Press, New York, 1983.

Zeleznik, A.J. and Hillier, S.G.: The role of gonadotropins in the selection of the preovulatory follicle. Clin. Obstet. Gynecol. 27:927, 1984.

222

10

PREGNANCY AND LACTATION

INTRODUCTION

Male and female gonadal functions, described in the preceding chapters, are merely the initial steps in the overall process of reproduction. The remaining steps in the creation and nurturing of a new individual are extremely complex processes ranging from the molecular (e.g., fusion of male and female gametes) to the interpersonal (e.g., courtship). A detailed description of these events is beyond the scope of this text; rather, this chapter will focus on the contribution of the endocrine system to this process.

Several endocrine glands are essential for pregnancy and lactation. These include the **corpus luteum, anterior** and **posterior pituitaries,** and a temporary endocrine tissue, the **placenta.** The placenta, which develops at the interface between the uterus and embryo, has a remarkable capacity to secrete a

223

wide variety of protein, peptide, and steroid hormones. It is also unique among endocrine glands in that secretion of its hormones is subject to little or no extrinsic control. Instead, secretion rates depend primarily on the stage of pregnancy. Because of this feature of placental function, and because this chapter discusses a process rather than a system, the endocrinology of pregnancy and lactation is best described as a sequence of events with four major phases: initiation of pregnancy, maintenance of pregnancy, parturition, and lactation.

INITIATION OF PREGNANCY

The first phase of pregnancy begins with the infamous gleam in the parents' eyes and ends with union of sperm and ovum to form an embryo. The endocrine contributions to the initial steps in this process, sexual behavior and coitus, have already been described. Briefly, testicular androgens in men and adrenal androgens in women cause the development of the adult's sexual drive. Libido, however, is just one component of the complex interaction between a man and a woman that leads to sexual intercourse. Hormones can thus be viewed as building the foundation on which sexual behavior develops, while the specific expression of this behavior depends on a variety of other inputs, most of unknown origin.

Sperm Transport

Once sperm are deposited in the vagina, they must travel through the cervix, into the uterus, and then up the oviduct to its distal portion (the ampulla) where fertilization occurs. This is a formidable journey and sperm need the help of the female reproductive tract to complete it successfully. In addition, the endocrine environment, acting upon this tract, controls the transport of sperm from vagina to oviduct. To understand the involvement of hormones in sperm transport, it is important to realize that successful fertilization requires that coitus occur during the fertile period (usually from two days before to one day after ovulation). The ovum degenerates if not fertilized during the 24 hours postovulation, and sperm remain fertile for a maximum of 72 hours in the female reproductive tract. Because of this time restriction, sperm with a chance of fertilizing the ovum are transported in a reproductive tract that has been exposed to high estrogen concentrations (from the growing follicle destined to ovulate). In fact, this is the only endocrine condition in which sperm can successfully get to the oviduct.

The first, and most important, hurdle in this journey is the **cervical canal**. This passage into the uterus is filled with a viscous fluid, secreted by epithelial cells lining the cervix, the composition of which varies with the stage of the menstrual cycle. During most of the cycle, when progesterone concentrations are high or estrogen levels are low, cervical mucus is so viscous that sperm cannot penetrate the cervical canal. However, the high estrogen levels at the end of the follicular phase cause a large increase in the water content of cervical secretion, and the resulting decrease in viscosity allows sperm to traverse the cervical canal. The canal then remains open to sperm for two to three days, but even during this period only a small percentage of sperm in the ejaculate ever reach the uterus (Table 10–1). In addition to regulating sperm entry into the uterus, cervical mucus provides an environment much more conducive to sperm survival than does either the vagina or the uterus. The cervix thus serves as a site of temporary sperm storage and provides for a gradual release of sperm for one to two days after ejaculation.

Sperm migrate up the cervical canal under their own power in 10 to 15 minutes. Subsequent travel from the uterus to the ampulla of the oviduct, however, occurs much more rapidly than a sperm can swim (Table 10–1). Muscular contractions of the uterus and oviduct are thought to provide the primary propulsive force for this part of the journey to the ovum. In the **uterus,** myometrial contractions produce a churning action—much as in a washing machine—that quickly disperses the sperm throughout the uterine cavity. After traversing the uterotuberal junction, sperm must travel up the **oviduct** against the action of the cilia lining the tubule, most of which beat in the direction of the uterus. Antiperistaltic (i.e., upward) contractions of oviductal muscle propel sperm toward the ovum and may be aided by bands of cilia that beat toward the ovary in some portions of the oviduct. Uterine and oviductal sperm transport is facilitated by estrogens, which increase contractile activity in these tissues, and suppressed by progesterone, which inhibits contractions. Thus, this stage of sperm transport is also most efficient during the periovulatory period.

While sperm travel up the female reproductive tract they undergo a final maturation, referred to as **capacitation**. Prior to capacitation, sperm are incapable of fertilizing the ovum; after capacitation they are fertile, but the changes responsible for this maturation are unknown. During this same period, the ovum and attached granulosa cells are expelled from the ruptured follicle at ovulation. These cells are released into the peritoneal cavity but are

TABLE 10–1.   Transport of Sperm in the Female Reproductive Tract

Location	Time of Appearance (Minutes After Ejaculation)	Number* (% of Sperm Ejaculated)
Vagina	0	100
Cervical canal	1–3	3
Uterus	10–20	0.1
Oviduct	30–60	0.001

*Based on data from animals.

rapidly picked up by the fimbriated ostium of the oviduct. From there, they move quickly into the antrum, carried along by the downward beating cilia that line the oviduct. Because the ciliated epithelia of the oviduct are sensitive to estrogen, the cilia are most active at the time of ovulation.

Fertilization

The union of sperm and egg occurs in the ampulla. When a sperm encounters the granulosa cells surrounding the ovum, enzymes contained in the acrosome are released and break down the intercellular matrix holding the granulosa cells together. This enzymatic reaction creates a pathway for the sperm so it can reach the ovum and fuse with the surface membrane of the oocyte. Fusion of the first sperm with the ovum triggers an alteration in the zona pellucida surrounding the ovum that prevents entry of any additional sperm. Over the next two to three hours, the ovum completes meiosis, with one haploid set of chromosomes forming the female pronucleus and the other set being expelled as a polar body. During this period, the contents of the sperm diffuse into the ovum, which activates the chromatin to form the male pronucleus. As the two pronuclei move together, the chromosomes replicate. When they meet, the pronuclear membranes break down, allowing mixing of the genetic material and initiating the first mitotic division of a new embryo.

ROLES OF PROGESTERONE IN MAINTAINING PREGNANCY

While estradiol plays a critical role in the initiation of pregnancy, **progesterone** is the hormone responsible for its maintenance. Serum progesterone concentrations must remain elevated from the inception of pregnancy to its termination to avoid loss of the developing embryo. Progesterone has two major actions essential to pregnancy maintenance. Early in pregnancy, before the placenta develops, it **stimulates production of nutrients** needed for embryo survival. After the placenta develops and the fetus begins to grow, it inhibits **contractions of the uterine myometrium,** contractions that would expel the fetus if progesterone secretion fell. To ensure against premature onset of labor, circulating progesterone levels increase dramatically during pregnancy, reaching levels of close to 150 ng/ml during the third trimester (Fig. 10–1). The source of this progesterone and the mechanisms controlling its secretion vary with the stage of pregnancy.

Preimplantation

From fertilization to implantation, the progesterone needed for pregnancy maintenance is provided by the corpus luteum of the menstrual cycle. During this period, progesterone secretion from the corpus luteum is con-

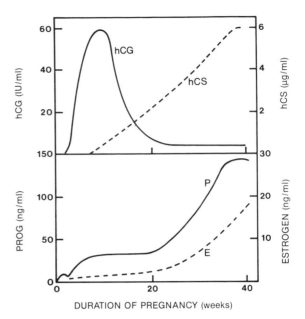

FIGURE 10–1. Plasma levels of the major maternal hormones in pregnancy: human chorionic gonadotropin (hCG), human chorionic somatomammotropin (hCS), progesterone (P), and estrogen (E).

trolled by mechanisms operable during the normal cycle (Chapter 9) so there is no endocrine indication that pregnancy has begun. Because of the absence of any overt signs of pregnancy during this period, clinicians often consider pregnancy to begin at implantation, not at fertilization.

Luteal phase progesterone has two important functions. First, it stimulates secretory cells lining the oviduct and the uterine endometrium to release nutrients (e.g., glycogen) used as energy by the developing embryo. Second, it induces structural changes in the endometrium that allow formation of a placenta upon implantation of the embryo. The significance of these progestational effects is illustrated by the observation that luteal phases with inadequate progesterone levels are almost always associated with infertility.

The embryo spends the first three or four days of the luteal phase in the oviduct, during which time several mitotic divisions occur to produce a ball of cells called the **morula**. Virtually all of this period is spent at the junction of the ampulla and isthmus, where a constriction prevents further movement toward the uterus. This temporal hiatus allows nutrients to accumulate in the uterine lumen; premature arrival in the uterus kills the morula. When this constriction relaxes in response to the increasing progesterone levels of the luteal phase, the embryo is rapidly moved into the uterus by peristaltic contractions of the isthmus. The embryo then floats freely in the uterus for three to four days, living on endometrial secretions and developing into a blastocyst. The blastocyst is a hollow ball of cells that contains two important cell types: **trophoblastic cells** on the outer surface and an **inner cell mass** (Fig. 10–2).

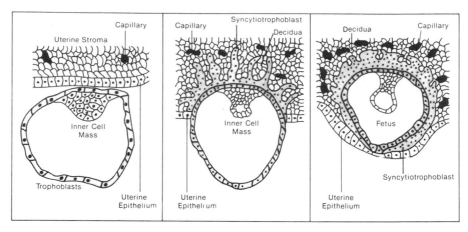

FIGURE 10–2. Implantation of the blastocyst. The panels depict the temporal progression from free-floating blastocyst to completely implanted embryo.

The inner cell mass develops into the fetus, whereas the trophoblastic cells initiate implantation and, together with endometrial tissue, develop into the placenta.

Implantation

Approximately six to eight days after fertilization, implantation begins when trophoblasts contact the endometrium and release proteolytic enzymes. These enzymes break down the adjacent endometrial cells and allow cords of trophoblastic cells to pass deeper into the endometrium where they continue to digest uterine cells (Fig. 10–2). At the same time, many of the invading trophoblastic cells fuse to form a syncytium (the **syncytiotrophoblast**). The initial attachment of the blastocyst to the uterus also triggers dramatic changes in the underlying uterine stroma. These changes include increased edema, vascularization, and storage of nutrients within stromal cells; the tissue so affected is called the **decidua**. The overall effect of these events is that the blastocyst literally creates a hole in the endometrium, enters this hole, and attaches to the decidual tissue. The syncytiotrophoblast continues to digest decidual cells and the nutrients released are passed on to the developing embryo. In this way, decidual tissue provides energy for the embryo until development of the placenta.

The **placenta,** which allows direct transfer of material between fetal and maternal circulatory systems, is derived from both trophoblastic and decidual tissue. As the syncytiotrophoblast, which has become part of the **chorion,** continues to grow, it develops an extensive network of lacunae. These lacunae soon fill with maternal blood as capillary walls within the decidua are digested by chorionic tissue. Simultaneously, embryonic capillaries grow into the tro-

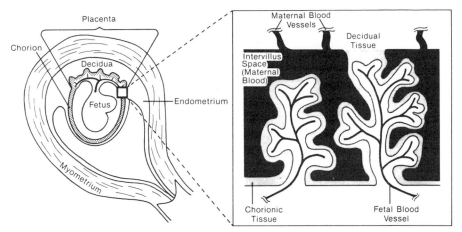

FIGURE 10–3. Structure of the placenta at the macroscopic (*left*) and microscopic (*right*) levels.

phoblastic chords to form placental villi (Fig. 10–3). Each villus contains fetal capillaries, which are separated from the maternal blood in the intervillus space by a thin layer of chorionic tissue. Some villi extend to the decidua and anchor the placenta to the uterus, but most simply project into the pool of maternal blood. This structure allows delivery of oxygen and nutrients to the fetus and removal of carbon dioxide and other waste products from it, without direct mixing of the fetal and maternal circulations. In addition to serving as an interface between mother and fetus, the placenta is the major endocrine organ of pregnancy and plays a critical role in its maintenance.

Early Postimplantation—Role of hCG

When implantation occurs (days 7 to 8 after ovulation), progesterone secretion from the corpus luteum of the menstrual cycle is maximal. However, in the absence of a signal from the embryo, luteolysis would soon occur, causing menstruation and loss of the implanted embryo. To prevent this, one of the first events following implantation is secretion of a hormone, **human chorionic gonadotropin (hCG),** that prolongs the life span of the corpus luteum. hCG is a glycoprotein, structurally similar to LH, that is produced by the syncytiotrophoblast. Like the other glycoprotein hormones (FSH, LH, TSH), hCG is composed of an α and β subunit; the α subunit is common to all four hormones. The β subunit is similar to that of LH except that it contains an additional 24 amino acids at the carboxyterminal end of the polypeptide chain. hCG binds to LH receptors and is capable of producing all the biological actions of LH. However, its primary, and perhaps only, function in the mother is to prevent luteolysis. Clinically, hCG is widely used as a substitute for LH because it is easily obtained from the urine of pregnant women, has no FSH activity, and has a long half-life in blood (30 to 40 hours) so that frequent injections are not required for sustained effects.

Circulating hCG concentrations begin to rise within one to two days of implantation and peak at approximately eight to ten weeks of gestation (see Fig. 10–1). This luteotropic stimulus maintains the structure and secretory activity of the corpus luteum (now referred to as the corpus luteum of pregnancy). The resulting elevated progesterone concentrations during this period prevent menstruation and maintain the decidual tissue necessary for early embryonic development. After about week 10 of pregnancy, hCG output declines to a relatively low secretion rate that is then maintained until parturition (Fig. 10–1). The fall in hCG occurs at a time when this hormone is no longer needed as a luteotropic stimulus because the placenta has begun to secrete significant amounts of progesterone. There is no known biological role for hCG during the second and third trimesters of pregnancy.

Second and Third Trimesters

Progesterone secretion from the placenta may begin shortly after implantation because the syncytiotrophoblast is capable of converting cholesterol to progesterone. However, this source of progesterone does not become important in pregnancy maintenance until the latter part of the first trimester. If the ovary is removed before approximately 10 weeks of pregnancy, abortion occurs due to insufficient progesterone secretion from the placenta. After 10 weeks, the ovary can be removed with no effect on the pregnancy because the placenta has taken over from the corpus luteum as the primary source of progesterone.

Because the placenta does not synthesize much cholesterol from acetate, progesterone synthesis and release depend on cholesterol obtained from the maternal circulation. Given an adequate supply of cholesterol, placental progesterone secretion appears to be independent of outside regulation and is largely proportional to placental weight. Therefore, the increase in circulating progesterone during the last two trimesters (Fig. 10–1) reflects placental growth during this period. The primary function of placental progesterone is to prevent abortion by suppressing contractions of the uterine myometrium. Progesterone produces this effect by inhibiting both spontaneous electrical activity and the ability of the myometrium to propagate an action potential. The very high local concentrations of progesterone may be particularly important in this regard.

The major roles of progesterone in pregnancy maintenance are summarized in Table 10–2. Other actions of progesterone are also important to pregnancy and lactation. The high progesterone levels of pregnancy cause cervical secretions to become so gelatinous that they form a "mucus plug," obstructing the cervical canal. This plug prevents bacteria and other pathogens from entering the uterus, protecting the embryo from infection. Second, progesterone

TABLE 10–2.   Maintenance of Pregnancy by Progesterone

Period	Source of Progesterone	Actions
Preimplantation	CL of menstrual cycle	Stimulates secretion of nutrients by oviduct and uterus Primes uterus so decidua forms at implantation
Early postimplantation	CL of pregnancy stimulated by hCG	Prevents menstruation; maintains decidual tissue
2nd–3rd trimester	Placenta	Prevents uterine contractions

may play a role in suppressing the mother's immune system so the fetus is not recognized as a foreign body and rejected. Finally, progesterone helps prepare the breasts for lactation, an action that will be considered later in this chapter.

ROLES OF OTHER PLACENTAL HORMONES

In addition to hCG and progesterone, the placenta produces a remarkable array of protein, peptide, and steroid hormones (Table 10–3). Of these hormones, the ones most important to pregnancy and lactation are estrogens and human chorionic somatomammotropin.

Estrogens

Like progesterone, circulating estrogen concentrations increase dramatically during pregnancy, reaching levels several hundred times higher than follicular phase estrogen concentrations (see Fig. 10–1). The circulating estrogens of pregnancy differ qualitatively from those during the menstrual cycle in that the major estrogen of pregnancy is **estriol**. Estriol is a weak estrogen that is produced in very small amounts in nonpregnant women by the addition of a hydroxyl group to the C-16 position of estradiol.

Estriol, like the other placental hormones, is secreted by the syncytiotrophoblast, but its synthesis requires a complex interaction between the pla-

TABLE 10–3.   Placental Hormones

Steroids:	Progesterone
	Estrogens (estriol, estradiol, estrone)
Proteins:	Human chorionic gonadotropin (hCG)
	Human chorionic somatomammotropin (placental lactogen)
	Human chorionic thyrotropin
	Human chorionic corticotropin
Peptides:	TRH
	GnRH

centa and fetus. The placenta does not contain the enzymes 17α-hydroxylase and C_{17-20} lyase, both of which are needed for the conversion of pregnenolone to dehydroepiandrosterone (DHEA). Thus, although it does have aromatase activity, the placenta cannot synthesize estrogens directly from pregnenolone. However, the fetal adrenal can convert cholesterol to DHEA, which is then sulfated and secreted. Most of the DHEA-sulfate is hydroxylated at the C-16 position by the fetal liver and the resulting 16α-OH-DHEA-sulfate is transported to the placenta. The placenta has an active sulfatase that removes the sulfate group and 16α-OH-DHEA is then converted to estriol by the same enzymes that normally convert DHEA to estradiol. Because of the multiple components of this biosynthetic pathway, estriol is often said to be produced by the fetoplacental unit. The role of the fetoplacental unit in steroidogenesis is described in more detail in Chapter 11.

Estrogen secretion during pregnancy is thought to stimulate the uterine myometrium, which increases in size throughout pregnancy. Estrogen, like progesterone, also stimulates mammary gland development in preparation for lactation. Estriol that is released into the maternal circulation is conjugated as a sulfate and/or glucuronide by the liver and excreted into the urine. Because of the fetal involvement in estriol production, urinary 16-OH-estrogens are often monitored as an index of fetal status in problem pregnancies.

Human Chorionic Somatomammotropin

Chorionic somatomammotropin (hCS), also called placental lactogen, is a placental protein hormone that has a structure very similar to growth hormone (GH). The concentration of hCS increases gradually throughout pregnancy and plateaus during the last month (Fig. 10–1). As its name implies, this hormone has both growth-promoting and lactogenic activities, but both are relatively weak. Two possible roles have been suggested for hCS during pregnancy. First, it may act on the mammary gland to induce the enzymes needed for milk synthesis. Second, it may produce important metabolic changes in the mother. During pregnancy, utilization of glucose by the mother decreases and she becomes relatively resistant to the hypoglycemic action of insulin. These metabolic changes may serve to shunt larger quantities of glucose to the fetus and, since similar effects can be produced by GH administration, they may be caused by increasing levels of hCS. Because pregnant women are insensitive to the actions of insulin, diabetes mellitus often first becomes evident during pregnancy. Consequently, urinary glucose levels are routinely determined during pregnancy to monitor the possible development of diabetes.

Other Placental Hormones

The placenta produces a number of other steroid and protein hormones. Interestingly, like hCG and hCS, most of the proteins are very similar or identical to pituitary or hypothalamic hormones (Table 10–3). However, the physiological importance of these hormones, if any, remains to be established.

PARTURITION

Preparation

Birth of an infant, or parturition, occurs approximately 38 weeks after conception. However, the timing of parturition is quite variable so that 37 to 43 weeks is considered a normal pregnancy length. Expulsion of the fetus requires both contractions of the uterine myometrium and opening of the cervix; as pregnancy progresses, the properties of these tissues change in preparation for parturition. As already mentioned, the uterine myometrium increases greatly in size throughout pregnancy in response to increasing estrogen levels. During the last month of pregnancy, this tissue becomes more and more sensitive to agents such as oxytocin that cause uterine contractions. Throughout most of pregnancy the cervix acts as a plug, keeping the fetus in and infectious agents out. At the end of pregnancy, the cervix begins to soften (or "ripen") as its collagen fibers dissociate and decrease in number. This softening of the cervix may be caused by **relaxin,** a polypeptide hormone produced by the corpus luteum of pregnancy and by the placenta. Relaxin also causes relaxation of the connective tissue between the pelvic bones and inhibits uterine contractions. Although the former action may aid passage of the fetus through the pelvis during delivery, the importance of relaxin for parturition in the human is still being evaluated.

Initiation

At the start of labor, the uterus changes from a relatively quiescent state to an active one in which rhythmic contractions become progressively stronger and more frequent. The agents responsible for triggering this change in uterine contractility in humans have not been established, but there are several possibilities. Since progesterone inhibits uterine contractility, a **fall in progesterone** could initiate uterine contractions; however, circulating concentrations of this steroid do not decrease prior to parturition. It is still possible that a local fall in uterine progesterone concentrations may be important. Alternatively, some workers have proposed that it is not the absolute progesterone levels that are important but the **ratio of estrogen to progesterone**. Since estrogens increase uterine contractility, an increase in this ratio might have the same effect as a fall in progesterone. This ratio does increase during the last month of pregnancy (see Fig. 10–1), but it does not change dramatically just before labor. $PGF_{2\alpha}$ is another possible candidate because this prostaglandin is a potent stimulator of uterine contractions and is necessary for parturition in a number of other species. However, most investigators have been unable to demonstrate an increase in $PGF_{2\alpha}$ release before labor in women, although it does increase dramatically during labor. A **fetal endocrine signal** may also play a role in initiating parturition. In a number of mammals increased output of glucocorticoids from the fetal adrenal appears to trigger labor and the human fetal adrenal secretes increasing amounts of cortisol during the last weeks of pregnancy. However, the absence of adrenal glucocorticoids in fetuses with congenital adrenal hyperplasia does not necessarily prolong pregnancy. Finally, **fetal size** may be an important trigger. Uterine myometrium, like other smooth muscle, contracts when stretched so that the growing fetus may initiate uterine contractions when it reaches a critical size. Proponents of this theory point out that twins are born one to two weeks earlier than a single fetus; its opponents note that, if size alone were important, twins would be born five to six weeks earlier. It may well be that in humans, there is no single signal triggering parturition. Instead, a number of these factors may act in concert, so that absence of any one of them does not greatly alter the initiation of labor.

Labor

Throughout most of pregnancy weak contractions (Braxton-Hicks contractions) occur, and these become much stronger and more frequent just before the onset of labor (false labor). True labor begins once these contractions become rhythmic and continue to increase in strength, duration, and frequency. At the beginning of labor, contractions occur only every 25 to 30 minutes and last 30 seconds or less; at the end they occur every 2 to 3 minutes and last 60 to 90 seconds.

The pattern of uterine contractions during labor is sustained by a **neuroendocrine reflex** involving **oxytocin,** the posterior pituitary hormone that causes uterine contractions (Fig. 10–4). Each uterine contraction begins at the top of the uterus (the fundus) and spreads toward the cervix but is much stronger in the fundus. Uterine contractions thus force the fetus toward the cervix and the pressure of the fetus on the cervix stretches it. Cervical stretch produces a neural signal that travels up the spinal cord to the anterior hypothalamus and triggers oxytocin release. Oxytocin then acts on the uterine myometrium to stimulate further uterine contractions. Note that each step in this pathway is stimulatory so that this circuit forms a **positive feedback loop**. This means that uterine contractions will continue, and indeed increase, until the pressure on the cervix is relieved by delivery.

Labor is divided into three stages. During the first stage, the positive feedback loop just described causes the cervix to dilate from 2 cm to 10 cm in diameter. This stage usually is the longest, lasting 8 to 24 hours in a first pregnancy. Stage 2, the actual delivery of the fetus, begins once the cervix is fully

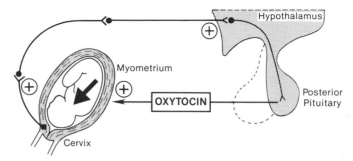

FIGURE 10–4. Positive feedback loop causing uterine contractions during labor. The initial uterine contractions force the fetus downward, stretching the cervix and triggering the neuroendocrine reflex.

dilated. Toward the end of stage 1, as the infant begins to move through the cervix, stretch receptors in the vagina activate a neural reflex that triggers contractions of the abdominal muscles. Once stage 2 has begun, these abdominal contractions, which occur simultaneously with uterine contractions, greatly increase the force pushing the infant through the vagina. Stage 2 ends with the delivery of the infant and usually lasts between 30 and 90 minutes. Stage 3 of labor, expulsion of the placenta, occurs 15 to 30 minutes after delivery. The uterus continues to contract for some time after delivery; this causes the placenta to first separate from the myometrium and then pass through the vagina. Separation of the placenta causes some uterine bleeding, but this is limited because continued muscular contractions of the myometrium constrict the maternal blood vessels supplying the damaged area. Oxytocin is often injected after delivery of the placenta to increase uterine contractions and help prevent hemorrhage.

Recovery

Shortly after delivery, the uterus begins to involute, a process that is usually complete in one to two months. This involution occurs largely because estrogen and progesterone concentrations fall precipitously when the placental source of these steroids is lost at delivery. Oxytocin that is released in response to suckling (see later discussion) may facilitate involution of the myometrium in nursing mothers by increasing uterine contractions and thereby maintaining its muscular tone. During involution, the tissue at the site of placental attachment dies. As the dying tissue is sloughed off it produces a vaginal discharge called "lochia" that continues for three to six weeks. After this period, the endometrium returns to its nongravid state, ready to support another pregnancy.

LACTATION

Milk is essential for survival of the neonate, although the origin of the milk can be either from the mother (nursing infants) or from an animal (bottle-fed infants). Milk contains **fat** (triglyceride), the carbohydrate **lactose,** a number of **proteins** including casein and α-lactalbumin, **vitamins,** and important **minerals,** particularly calcium and phosphate. The composition of milk changes during the early part of lactation. For the first five days postpartum it is called **colostrum;** it contains relatively low levels of lactose and fat but high concentrations of NaCl and proteins. The major proteins are lactoferrin, which has bacteriocidal activities, and immunoglobulins, which provide some protection against infection while the newborn's own immune system develops. From days 5 to 10 postpartum the milk is referred to as **transitional milk,** and after day 10 **mature milk** is produced, which contains high concentrations of lactose, fat, and CaPO₄, and low concentrations of protein.

Milk Production

The structure of the mammary gland resembles that of the lung. Branching out from the nipple is a network of progressively smaller **ducts** that terminate in **lobules** (Fig. 10–5). These lobules are made up of clusters of milk-containing **alveoli** that open into the lobular ends of the milk-collecting ducts. The constituents of milk are synthesized in epithelial cells lining each alveolus and then secreted into the lumen. Production of milk proteins follows the same intracellular pathway as that for protein hormones described in Chapter 1. The proteins are synthesized in the rough endoplasmic reticulum, packaged

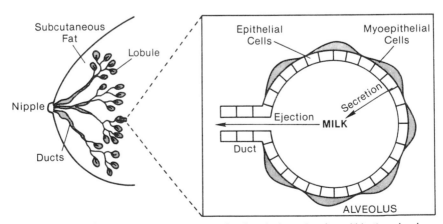

FIGURE 10–5. Structure of the mammary gland and of an alveolus within the gland.

into secretory vesicles in the Golgi apparatus, and released from the cell by exocytosis. Lactose and $CaPO_4$ are also secreted via Golgi-derived secretory vesicles. $CaPO_4$ binds to the casein within these vesicles and lactose is synthesized in the Golgi apparatus by the condensation of glucose and galactose. The enzyme catalyzing this reaction is located in the Golgi membrane but must be activated by α-lactalbumin. Lactose is produced only by the mammary gland because only this tissue makes α-lactalbumin. The fatty acids and glycerols that are required for the synthesis of triglycerides can either be synthesized *de novo* or obtained from the maternal circulation, and the relative importance of each source depends on the amount of fat in the mother's diet. Triglycerides, synthesized in the cytoplasm and smooth endoplasmic reticulum, coalesce to form lipid droplets and then move toward the apical plasma membrane. This movement continues after the droplets reach the plasma membrane so that they bulge out, become surrounded by the membrane, and eventually pinch off to form membrane-bounded fat globules in the milk. These lipid droplets also contain cholesterol and vitamins A, D, and E.

After the milk is secreted into the alveolar lumen, it is moved toward the nipple by a process called **milk ejection**. Each alveolus is surrounded by a network of myoepithelial cells (Fig. 10–5). When these smooth muscle cells contract, they decrease the volume of each alveolus, thereby forcing the milk into the ducts and hence toward the nipple. This milk ejection produced by positive pressure at the alveolar end of the mammary gland is required to get milk to the nipple because the infant, sucking on one end of an extensive network of ducts, cannot possibly create sufficient negative pressure to suck the milk out of the alveoli.

Hormonal Control

The development and function of the mammary gland requires at least eight hormones: estrogen, progesterone, prolactin and/or hCS, oxytocin, cortisol, insulin, parathyroid hormone, and growth hormone. Because the latter four hormones play largely a permissive role, this section will focus on the first four hormones. In general, the sex steroids cause development of the glandular tissue while prolactin and oxytocin are essential for milk production and delivery, respectively.

Development of the Mammary Gland. From birth to puberty, the mammary gland consists of just a rudimentary duct system. At puberty, the increased secretion of **estradiol acts on the ducts** to produce growth and branching, while **progesterone stimulates alveolar-lobular formation**. However, development of the mammary gland is very limited in nonpregnant women and the increase in breast size at puberty is due mainly to an increase in stromal and adipose tissue. During pregnancy, the extremely high concentrations of estrogen and progesterone promote extensive branching of the terminal ducts and hypertrophy and hyperplasia of the alveoli. Concentrations of both prolactin and hCS (placental lactogen) also increase throughout pregnancy, and these hormones contribute to alveolar development. These lactogenic hormones also induce the enzymes needed for the synthesis of milk, causing the alveolar epithelia to differentiate into secretory cells. Most of these changes occur during the first trimester and by the fourth month of pregnancy the mammary gland is fully developed.

Initiation and Maintenance of Lactation. Although the mammary gland is fully capable of producing milk by the middle of pregnancy, little or no secretion occurs until parturition. This delay occurs because the high estrogen and progesterone concentrations during pregnancy inhibit milk secretion. The **decreases in these steroids at parturition initiate lactation**.

Once milk production begins, two hormones are critical for its maintenance: prolactin, acting on the epithelial cells to stimulate milk secretion, and oxytocin, acting on the myoepithelial cells to produce milk ejection. Release of these hormones represents the efferent limb of a **neuroendocrine reflex,** which has already been described for oxytocin. Briefly, the suckling stimulus activates sensory nerves in the nipple and the resulting action potentials travel up the spinal cord to the oxytocin-producing cell bodies in the hypothalamus (Fig. 10–6). This afferent signal triggers a bolus of oxytocin release from the posterior pituitary, which travels to the breasts and stimulates contraction of the myoepithelial cells, causing milk ejection. This **milk ejection reflex** is an ideal system for the control of milk movement to the nipple since it ensures that milk ejection occurs when the infant needs milk but not at other times.

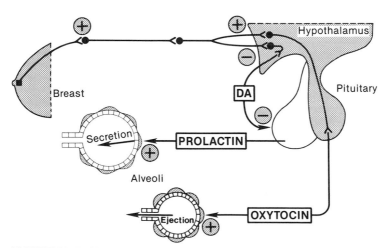

FIGURE 10–6. Neuroendocrine reflex controlling milk secretion and ejection. Note that the reflex stimulates prolactin release by either suppressing the prolactin-inhibiting hormone dopamine (DA), as illustrated here, or increasing release of an unknown prolactin-releasing factor.

This reflex is easily inhibited by psychological stress so a relaxed environment and positive attitude toward nursing are important for successful lactation. Lactation can become conditioned to stimuli other than suckling, so that handling the infant or the sound of its cry can trigger milk ejection.

An analogous neuroendocrine reflex stimulates prolactin release from the anterior pituitary in response to suckling. Recall that prolactin secretion is controlled by two hypothalamic substances: dopamine, which inhibits prolactin release, and an as yet unidentified prolactin-releasing factor (PRF). The afferent impulses initiated by suckling are carried by the spinal cord to the hypothalamus. There they inhibit dopamine or stimulate PRF secretion (or do both) (Fig. 10–6), stimulating prolactin release from the anterior pituitary. The prolactin then acts on the alveolar epithelium to promote secretion of the components of milk. The milk secretion produced by this reflex replenishes the milk lost from the alveolus by milk ejection. At the same time, prolactin promotes synthesis of milk proteins, including α-lactalbumin, which stimulates lactose formation and the enzymes needed for production of triglycerides. This ensures that synthesis of milk keeps pace with milk secretion. These effects of prolactin are not mediated by cyclic AMP; the actual second messenger for this hormone has not been determined. By coupling prolactin release to the suckling stimulus, this control system provides a simple mechanism for matching the rate of milk production to the needs of the infant for milk.

Cessation of Lactation. Two mechanisms contribute to the cessation of milk production when the infant is weaned. First, because there is no suckling stimulus, prolactin concentrations remain low so that there is no longer any stimulus for milk synthesis and secretion. However, even with abrupt weaning, this mechanism does not immediately terminate milk production. The prolactin-induced enzymes in the alveolar epithelial cells remain active for some time after the cessation of prolactin secretion, and consequently secretion of milk into the alveoli continues. The second mechanism inhibiting milk production results from the absence of oxytocin secretion. Because there is no milk ejection reflex after weaning, the milk secreted during this period accumulates in the alveoli, causing engorgement of the breast. The consequent buildup of pressure within the alveoli acts directly on the epithelial cells to suppress secretion and synthesis of milk. Thus, the absence of suckling-induced increases in both prolactin and oxytocin contribute to the cessation of lactation at weaning.

Effects of Lactation on Other Maternal Endocrine Systems

Lactation produces a tremendous metabolic drain on the mother. At its peak, a lactating woman produces over a liter of milk/day, which contains 40 to 50 gm fat, 9 to 10 gm protein, 70 to 100 gm lactose, and 0.3 gm calcium. Under normal conditions these substances are derived from the diet, but if nutrition is inadequate they are derived from maternal stores. Under the latter circumstances, lactation will cause an increase in the concentrations of parathyroid hormone to mobilize bone calcium and may shift the endocrine control of metabolism toward a "fasting-like" condition (see Chapter 15) to ensure delivery of calcium, glucose, and fatty acids to the breast.

Lactation also suppresses ovarian function, although the duration of this effect is quite variable. In those societies in which infants depend on breast feeding as a primary energy source for an extended period (two to three years), postpartum amenorrhea lasts for as long as three years and is an important means of contraception. In other societies breast feeding is usually not so intense or prolonged, and fertile cycles can return within two to three months postpartum. Lactation causes amenorrhea by inhibiting LH and FSH secretion. The suckling stimulus itself and the hyperprolactinemia of lactation probably both act to suppress GnRH release from the hypothalamus, thus inducing a hypogonadotropic state. Because this effect of lactation is weak and of variable duration in our society, it is not recommended that postpartum women rely on it as a means of contraception.

CLINICAL ASPECTS OF PREGNANCY AND LACTATION

In Vitro Fertilization

One of the most exciting recent developments in obstetrics is the perfection of *in vitro* fertilization techniques for couples who are infertile because of mechanical barriers between sperm and egg (usually blockage of the oviduct). In this procedure, growth of a crop of preovulatory follicles is stimulated, usually by the sequential injection of human menopausal gonadotropin and hCG, and the oocytes are collected with a laparoscope shortly before ovulation. The oocytes are fertilized *in vitro* and the embryos cultured for three to five days, during which time development up to the blastocyst stage occurs. An embryo is then placed into the uterus via the cervix, and pregnancy results approximately 20 per cent of the time.

Hormonal Measurements During Pregnancy

One of the earliest hormone assays developed for routine clinical use was the measurement of urinary hCG to determine if conception has occurred. Initially, a bioassay (induction of ovulation in rabbits) was used, but now more sophisticated immunological procedures are available. Although hCG can be measured by radioimmunoassay, an assay based on the ability of antibodies to cause hemolysis of red blood cells (RBCs) in the presence of complement is the most common procedure. hCG-coated RBCs are usually mixed with urine from the woman, antibodies against hCG, and complement. If hCG is present in the urine, it saturates the antibody present and prevents it from binding to the hCG on the RBC. Thus hemolysis does not occur and the RBCs form a ring as they settle to the bottom of the tube. If hCG is not present in the urine, the antibodies are free to bind to the hCG-coated RBCs. This causes hemolysis, and no ring is formed. This procedure is inexpensive, rapid (one to two hours), and so easy to do that kits are now available in drug stores and supermarkets.

Another hormone that is often monitored during pregnancy is estriol. Since the fetal adrenal and liver play essential roles in the synthesis of this steroid, measurement of circulating or urinary estriol is used as one index of fetal viability. In high-risk pregnancies (e.g., maternal hypertension), a marked fall in estriol concentrations often provides an early warning of impending fetal death.

Endocrine Abnormalities of Pregnancy

In the past, steroid treatments were sometimes used in an attempt to prolong difficult pregnancies. However, it is now recognized that malfunction of the endocrine system needed for the maintenance of pregnancy is uncommon, so steroid treatments are rarely used for this purpose. However, progesterone is sometimes administered early in pregnancy, if infertility is known to be caused by deficient progesterone secretion during the luteal phase. A number of cases of placental sulfatase deficiency have been reported. Since this enzyme is involved in estrogen synthesis by the fetoplacental unit, estriol concentrations remain quite low throughout pregnancy. The only obvious effects of this estrogen deficiency are a delay in parturition and uterine insensitivity to oxytocin. Interestingly, the offspring of these pregnancies have all been male.

One of the first clinical signs of pregnancy is the daily nausea and vomiting known as "morning sickness," although it can occur at any time of the day. This condition usually appears shortly after implantation and subsides by the end of the first trimester. Because the incidence of morning sickness coincides with the peak in hCG production, it has been suggested that hCG may be responsible for the nausea. However, there is no strong evidence supporting this proposal. Alternatively, the estrogen levels that begin increasing during this period could be responsible, since administration of estrogen often causes nausea and vomiting.

Prolactin and Abnormalities of the Mammary Gland

In considering abnormalities in prolactin secretion, it is important to distinguish between nursing and non-nursing conditions. During nursing only *hypo*prolactinemia is clinically significant, whereas if the patient is not nursing, *hyper*prolactinemia is the only condition that will cause clinical symptoms.

Lactation. The only clinically relevant disorder causing a deficiency in prolactin secretion is known as **Sheehan's syndrome**. This condition results from vascular damage to the pituitary caused by hemorrhage during delivery and is first apparent as a failure in lactation. Other pituitary deficiencies (e.g., hypothyroidism) become evident later and must be treated. In other instances of insufficient milk production, it is easier to supplement with bottle feeding than to determine the etiology and treat the problem.

If a woman chooses not to breast feed an infant, lactation usually stops within one to two weeks postpartum due to the absence of suckling-induced increases in oxytocin and prolactin. This process is accompanied by some discomfort due to breast engorgement, and non-nursing women formerly were given a combination of long-acting estrogen and androgen at delivery to inhibit milk secretion postpartum. Because of the potential side effects of estrogen administration, the preferred treatment is now either binding of the breasts and analgesics, or bromocriptine, a dopamine agonist that suppresses prolactin secretion.

Nonlactating Women. Galactorrhea is the persistent production of milk in the non-nursing individual; it usually results from excess prolactin secretion by pituitary adenomas. These tumors may be readily evident as an enlarged pituitary or may be microadenomas detectable only with sophisticated radiological scanning techniques. Hyperprolactinemia often, but not always, produces amenorrhea. If microadenomas are responsible for galactorrhea and fertility is not desired, treatment may not be necessary since a gradual reduction in serum prolactin levels and spontaneous remission will often occur. Large pituitary tumors usually require either surgical or radiological treatment. Infertile women with galactorrhea who wish to become pregnant are given bromocriptine to suppress prolactin secretion. This treatment routinely results in restoration of normal menstrual cycles and fertility. Bromocriptine is also often effective in shrinking prolactin-secreting tumors. However, tumor recurrence or return of hyperprolactinemia (or both) almost always occurs shortly after cessation of treatment with this drug.

Gynecomastia. Breast development in men results from either a deficiency in testosterone or an excess of estrogen. Hyperprolactinemia, by itself, does not produce breast enlargement in men. However, high prolactin levels can suppress LH and FSH release, and the resulting decrease in testosterone secretion can produce gynecomastia. Treatment with bromocriptine ameliorates these symptoms if they are caused by hyperprolactinemia.

REFERENCES

Buster, J.E.: Fetal, placental, and maternal hormones. *In* Fetal Physiology and Medicine, 2nd ed. R.W. Beard and P.W. Nathanielsz, editors. Marcel Dekker, Inc., New York, p. 559, 1984.

Casey, M.L., MacDonald, P.C., and Simpson, E.R.: Endocrinological changes of pregnancy. *In* Williams' Textbook of Endocrinology, 7th ed. J.D. Wilson and D.W. Foster, editors. W.B. Saunders Company, Philadelphia, p. 422, 1985.

Edwards, R.G.: Conception in the Human Female. Academic Press, New York, 1980.

Frantz, A.G. and Wilson, J.D.: Endocrine disorders of the breast. *In* Williams' Textbook of Endocrinology, 7th ed. J.D. Wilson and D.W. Foster, editors. W.B. Saunders Company, Philadelphia, p. 402, 1985.

Neville, M.C. and Neifert, M.R.: Lactation: Physiology, Nutrition, and Breastfeeding. Plenum Press, New York, 1983.

11

FETAL ENDOCRINOLOGY

INTRODUCTION

The study of endocrine function in the fetus is a relatively young branch of endocrinology. Because the technical difficulties involved in analyzing endocrine systems in the fetus have only recently been overcome, much of our current knowledge in this area derives from work in the last two decades. In its broadest sense, fetal endocrinology includes the origin and development of all endocrine glands, the factors controlling this development, the functioning of each endocrine system *in utero,* and the adaptations of each system to extrauterine life. This chapter will focus on the latter two aspects of fetal endocrinology and will consider in detail only those endocrine systems that appear to play important roles in fetal and neonatal development.

Although all endocrine systems show some activity in the fetus, many of them do not play essential roles in fetal homeostasis because the corresponding maternal system dominates. The ability of a maternal endocrine system to influence fetal homeostasis, however, depends to a large extent on the permeability properties of the placenta. If a hormone or hormonally controlled substance can cross the placenta, then a maternal endocrine system usually controls the circulating levels of that substance in the fetus. For example, glucose is readily transferred from mother to fetus, and because maternal insulin and glucagon maintain a constant glucose supply for the fetus, the fetal pancreas is not necessary for glucose homeostasis *in utero*. In contrast, the large peptide and protein hormones of the pituitary do not cross the placenta; therefore, the fetal pituitary must play a role in fetal endocrine function.

In addition to functioning as a passive "barrier" to transfer of some hormones between mother and infant, the placenta is an active participant in fetal endocrinology. As described in Chapter 10, the placenta produces a number of steroid and protein hormones that are released into both the maternal and fetal circulations. Some of these hormones play critical roles in the development and secretory activities of the fetal adrenals and gonads (to be described below). The placenta can also influence fetal endocrine systems by nonhormonal mechanisms. For example, it actively pumps calcium from mother to fetus. The resulting fetal hypercalcemia stimulates calcitonin secretion and inhibits parathyroid hormone release from fetal endocrine tissues, as it would in the adult (Chapter 16).

Of the classical endocrine glands, the three with clearly defined roles in fetal or neonatal development are the **thyroid, adrenal cortices,** and **gonads.** In turn, the development of these tissues is dependent to some extent on secretion of tropic hormones from the fetal **pituitary.** The rest of this chapter will focus on these four endocrine tissues. Factors influencing fetal growth are considered in Chapter 14.

HYPOTHALAMO-HYPOPHYSEAL UNIT

Development

The anterior pituitary develops from a dorsal outcropping of the buccal cavity known as **Rathke's pouch.** This tissue grows dorsally, contacting the ventral **infundibular process** of the hypothalamus by the fifth week of gestation. The infundibulum gives rise to the posterior lobe of the pituitary while the intermediate lobe is derived from the wall of Rathke's pouch, which directly contacts neuroectoderm. At eight to ten weeks all the major pituitary cell types are evident, and concentrations of all the pituitary hormones in the fetal circulation are low but detectable. By this time, the buccal connection has been broken and the pituitary is already partially surrounded by the sella turcica. Thereafter, pituitary weight and hormone content increase progressively to term.

Hypothalamic releasing factors are also detectable in neural tissue by eight to ten weeks, and the first hypothalamic nuclei and tracts can be identified in another week or two. The hypophyseal portal circulation develops somewhat later. The primary capillary plexus in the median eminence develops at 14 to 15 weeks, and the connection to the anterior pituitary is completed at about 19 to 20 weeks of gestation.

Hormone Secretion

Secretion of anterior pituitary hormones during fetal and neonatal development can be divided into four general stages. These stages are illustrated in Figure 11–1, using circulating GH levels as an example. The first, or **hyposecretory,** stage occurs during the early developmental period (5 to 13 weeks). As its name implies, this stage is characterized by relatively low secretion rates. This hyposecretion is due in part to the small size of the pituitary and in part to the absence of hypothalamic stimulation. Starting sometime between 13 and 16 weeks of gestation, there is a dramatic increase in the release of almost all anterior pituitary hormones. The onset of this **hypersecretory** stage correlates with the development of the hypophyseal portal vessels and is thought to be caused by unrestrained hypothalamic stimulation. Circulating levels of the anterior pituitary hormones peak at around 20 weeks and then decline throughout the rest of gestation. The decline can be fairly rapid as

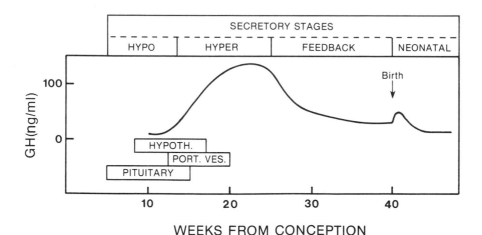

FIGURE 11–1. Development of the hypothalamo-hypophyseal axis. Horizontal bars depict the development of the hypothalamus (HYPOTH), hypophyseal portal vessels (PORT VES), and pituitary gland. The four stages of anterior pituitary hormone secretion indicated at the top of the figure are illustrated using circulating growth hormone (GH) levels as an example. (GH data drawn from Kaplan et al.: Rec. Prog. Horm. Res. 32:161, 1976.)

occurs for GH (Fig. 11–1), or gradual (TSH), or be delayed until the last few weeks of gestation (ACTH). This period of falling anterior pituitary hormone levels is referred to as the **negative feedback** stage because the pattern is thought to result from the maturation of the feedback control systems that are operational in the adult. The final, or **neonatal,** stage occurs during the early postpartum period. During this time, in general, a transitory hypersecretory period exists, after which hormone concentrations decline to the levels seen until adolescence.

Within this overall pattern, there is considerable variation in the exact time course of secretion for individual pituitary hormones. The maturation of the various feedback control systems occurs at different stages of development, ranging from midgestation (GH) to postpartum (LH and FSH), so that there is considerable variability in hormonal patterns during the third trimester. Similarly, the transitory postpartum increase can last for hours (TSH, ACTH), days (GH), or months (LH, FSH).

Secretion of one anterior pituitary hormone does not conform to the general pattern already described. Fetal prolactin concentrations remain quite low throughout most of gestation and then increase dramatically during the last two months. This distinct pattern of prolactin release is due in part to a basic difference in the hypothalamic control of this hormone. In contrast to the other anterior pituitary hormones, prolactin is controlled primarily by inhibitory hypothalamic input. Thus, during the hypersecretory stage for other pituitary hormones, prolactin is subjected to an unrestrained inhibition from the hypothalamus. The increase in circulating prolactin during the last stages of gestation is thought to be caused by the increasing placental estrogen secretion, because estrogens can act directly at the pituitary to stimulate prolactin release.

THYROID GLAND

Fetal hypothalamo-pituitary-thyroid axis function is largely independent of the mother because neither TSH nor thyroid hormones can cross the placenta. Although TRH can cross the placenta, the concentrations of this hypophysiotropic peptide in the maternal circulation are low. The placenta does produce a TSH-like hormone, but its role in fetal thyroid development is unknown.

Development

The thyroid develops from the floor of the buccal cavity and grows downward to reach the lower neck by six to seven weeks of gestation. Follicles become histologically evident at 10 to 11 weeks of age and are capable of thyroid hormone synthesis at this time. Although growth and development of the thyroid gland appear to occur independently of fetal TSH, this anterior pituitary hormone is required for the synthesis and secretion of thyroid hormones.

Hormone Secretion and Metabolism

Throughout most of gestation, the fetal thyroid secretes only **thyroxine** (T_4), although small amounts of triiodothyronine (T_3) are released during the last few weeks before parturition (Fig. 11–2). The secretory activity of the thyroid gland is dependent on fetal TSH, so that there is little secretion during the first trimester when TSH release is in its hyposecretory stage. Circulating T_4 concentrations increase rapidly between 20 and 30 weeks in response to the antecedent rise in TSH (Fig. 11–2). This increase in T_4 levels continues at a reduced rate after 30 weeks of gestation because TSH concentrations gradually decline in response to the negative feedback actions of T_4 (Fig. 11–2).

In contrast to metabolism in the adult, fetal monodeiodination of T_4 occurs exclusively on the inner ring, producing biologically inactive **reverse T_3** (**rT_3**), rather than biologically active T_3. Thus, the concentration of rT_3 in the fetal circulation increases in parallel with that of T_4 throughout gestation (Fig. 11–2). The thyroid begins to secrete T_3 during the last trimester, but even at term T_3 concentrations in the fetal circulation are much lower than those in the adult.

At birth there is a brief, but massive, outpouring of TSH; concentrations of this hormone peak within 30 to 60 minutes of delivery and then fall gradually to normal levels over the next day (Fig. 11–2). This neonatal TSH surge occurs, at least in part, in response to the rapid drop in ambient temperature

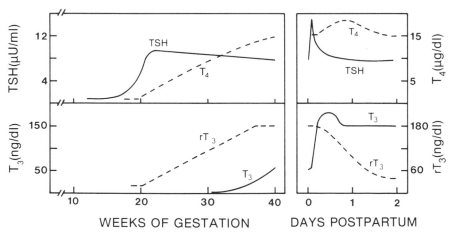

FIGURE 11–2. Circulating concentrations of TSH, T_4, rT_3, and T_3 in the fetal (*left*) and early neonatal (*right*) periods. Note the difference in time scales between the two panels. (Data replotted from Fisher, et al.: Rec. Prog. Horm. Res. 33:59, 1977.)

that the fetus experiences at birth. The rise in TSH stimulates T_4 and T_3 release from the thyroid so that the plasma levels of both hormones increase in the neonate. Concentrations of T_4 then return to the levels seen in the fetus but T_3 concentrations do not (Fig. 11–2). This maintenance of circulating T_3 levels is due in large part to a shift in the metabolism of T_4. During the first few weeks postpartum there is a gradual increase in monodeiodination of the outer ring of T_4. Consequently, rT_3 levels fall and T_3 levels remain elevated relative to their concentrations in the fetus. By one month postpartum, the activities of these two enzymes are similar to those in adults, as are circulating concentrations of T_4, T_3, and rT_3. The mechanisms responsible for these developmental changes in T_4 metabolism are not well understood, but there is some evidence that the increase in fetal adrenal cortisol secretion just prior to delivery may induce the enzymes that convert T_4 to T_3.

Actions and Significance of Thyroid Hormones to Development

Thyroid hormones are essential for normal **development of the central nervous system**. Untreated hypothyroidism leads to a permanent impairment in the functioning of the neocortex, cerebellum, and hippocampus, which is manifested as mental retardation. The mechanisms of thyroid hormone action on neural tissue remain largely unknown, although stimulation of neuronal DNA, RNA, and protein synthesis have been demonstrated. Fortunately, the phase of brain development during which thyroid hormone is essential occurs largely postnatally. Thus, early detection and treatment of neonatal hypothyroidism will prevent permanent mental retardation. The advent of radioimmunoassays for hormones of the thyroid axis has led to the routine screening of neonates for hypothyroidism so that replacement therapy can be started as soon as possible.

In addition to their essential role in neural development, thyroid hormones contribute to **neonatal thermogenesis**. Specifically, the cold-induced postpartum increase in T_4 and T_3 (Fig. 11–2) is thought to produce a transient hyperthyroid state that contributes to the maintenance of body temperature by newborn infants in the face of an abrupt drop in ambient temperature at birth.

THE ADRENAL CORTEX

Development and Morphology

In the fetus, the adrenal cortex consists of two distinct zones. The inner **fetal zone** is composed of large, lightly staining cells and comprises 80 per cent of the gland at term. The outer **definitive zone** contains smaller, darkly staining cells. After birth the fetal zone regresses and the definitive zone develops into the adult adrenal cortex.

The fetal zone of the adrenal appears at six weeks of gestation on the cranial end of each kidney. Two weeks later, the definitive zone begins to develop around the fetal zone. After its formation, the fetal adrenal dramatically increases in size throughout gestation. The weight of each gland increases from 50 mg to 1 gm between 10 and 20 weeks of gestation, doubles in weight between 20 and 30 weeks, and then doubles again to about 4 gm at term. After birth there is a decrease in weight of approximately 50 per cent as the fetal zone regresses and the definitive zone continues to develop.

Hormone Synthesis

The fetal adrenal cortex, like the adult gland, secretes principally cortisol, aldosterone, and dehydroepiandrosterone-sulfate (DHEA-sulfate). However, in the context of pregnancy, **DHEA-sulfate** and **cortisol** are its most important products. Cortisol induces a number of critical maturational events in the fetus, whereas DHEA-sulfate is important primarily as a precursor for estrogen synthesis by the placenta.

DHEA-sulfate is synthesized from cholesterol (via pregnenolone and 17-OH-pregnenolone) primarily in the fetal zone (Fig. 11–3). The sulfate group can be added at any step in this sequence and its addition decreases the androgenic potency of DHEA. Conjugation of DHEA thus protects the female fetus from the possible virilizing effects of adrenal androgens. After release from the fetal adrenal, most of the DHEA-sulfate is hydroxylated at the C-16 position by the fetal liver and the resulting 16-OH-DHEA-sulfate is the major precursor for **estriol** synthesis by the placenta (Fig. 11–3). As described in Chapter 10, since the placenta cannot synthesize androgens from cholesterol, the production of DHEA-sulfate by the fetal adrenal provides an essential substrate for placental estrogen production during pregnancy. Because of this interaction, estrogen is often said to be produced by the "**fetoplacental unit**," and maternal estriol levels can be used as an index of fetal viability.

The fetoplacental unit is also essential for fetal cortisol production. Throughout much of gestation, the fetal adrenal cortex has a deficiency in 3β-hydroxysteroid dehydrogenase-isomerase activity and therefore cannot convert pregnenolone to progesterone. Consequently, the fetal adrenal must use **placental progesterone** as a precursor for the synthesis of cortisol (Fig. 11–3). The synthesis of cortisol (and aldosterone) from progesterone occurs primarily in the definitive zone of the adrenal. Thus, both estrogen synthesis by the placenta and cortisol production by the fetal adrenal result from a synergistic interaction between these two tissues.

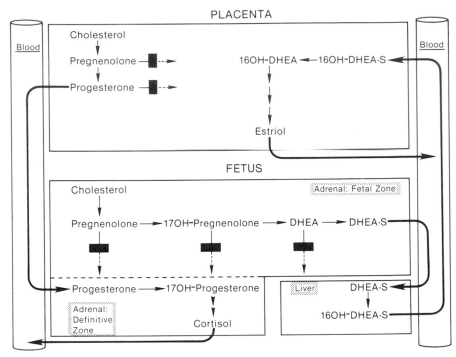

FIGURE 11–3. Biosynthesis of estriol and cortisol by the fetoplacental unit. Enzyme deficiencies in placenta and fetal adrenal are indicated by solid bars.

Hormone Secretion and Metabolism

Fetal cortisol concentrations increase slowly from the beginning of the second trimester to week 30 and then rise dramatically during the last 10 weeks of gestation (Fig. 11–4). Despite intensive investigation, the factors responsible for this pattern of cortisol secretion remain obscure. Fetal **ACTH** is clearly essential for the function of the adrenal cortex after week 20 of gestation. However, ACTH appears to play largely a permissive role. ACTH levels are relatively constant during the second trimester and decline during the period when cortisol increases at the end of pregnancy (Fig. 11–4). Recent evidence suggests that these ACTH levels are sufficient to stimulate maximal cortisol production by the adrenal. Other hormones, including prolactin and MSH, have been proposed as stimulators of cortisol secretion, but there is little support for these possibilities. Placental **hCG** is thought to help maintain the fetal zone during the first 20 weeks of gestation but is probably not important thereafter. In the absence of any clear hormonal stimulus, the rapid cortisol rise late in gestation may be largely caused by the **increase in adrenal size** occurring during this period, since as the adrenal mass increases the gland would be expected to secrete more cortisol. Another possible contributing fac-

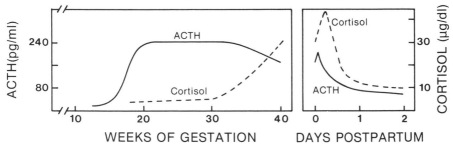

FIGURE 11–4. Temporal changes in ACTH and cortisol concentrations in fetal (*left*) and neonatal (*right*) circulation. Note differences in time scale between the two panels. (Data drawn from Winter et al.: J. Clin. Endocr. Metabol. 39:269, 1974 and Seron-Ferre and Jaffe: Ann. Rev. Physiol. 43:141, 1981.)

tor is a **decrease in the metabolism** of cortisol that occurs in a number of fetal tissues toward the end of pregnancy.

In response to the "stress" of exposure to the extrauterine environment there is a transient increase in ACTH secretion that peaks within two to three hours after delivery and falls slowly over the next 24 hours (Fig. 11–4). The changes in ACTH output cause a similar rise and fall in circulating cortisol concentrations. This transitory increase in cortisol is thought to aid in the physiological adjustments to life outside the uterus.

In the fetus, cortisol is metabolized primarily to **cortisone** by a variety of fetal organs and by the placenta. Since cortisol readily crosses the placenta, the latter is a particularly important site of metabolism. As a result of placental metabolism, most of the maternal cortisol is converted to cortisone before entering the fetal circulation so that the cortisol found in fetal plasma originates largely from the fetal adrenal. As already described, DHEA-sulfate is metabolized primarily to estriol by the placenta.

Importance of Cortisol to Fetal Maturation

Cortisol from the fetal adrenal is one of the most important hormonal factors controlling fetal development. Specifically, the increase in plasma cortisol levels that starts at about 30 weeks of gestation (Fig. 11–4) induces several functional changes that are critical for the survival of the infant after delivery. **Maturation of the lung** is perhaps the most important action of cortisol in the fetus. Cortisol increases the synthesis of pulmonary surfactant by inducing one or more of the enzymes involved in its synthesis. Surfactant is essential for alveolar stability, and together with cortisol-induced anatomical development of the lung, it ensures an adequate alveolar surface for gas exchange. Prematurely delivered infants, in whom this lung maturation has not occurred, are particularly susceptible to pulmonary failure, a condition known as the **respiratory distress syndrome** (**RDS**). Recognition of the role of cortisol in lung maturation has led to the development of a successful treatment for RDS. Glucocorticoid treatment, if given at least 48 hours before delivery (to allow time for enzyme induction) decreases the incidence of RDS by 55 to 65 per cent.

The prepartum rise in cortisol secretion induces a number of hepatic enzymes and stimulates the **deposition of liver glycogen**. This glycogen is the primary source of blood glucose during the first 24 hours of extrauterine life. Cortisol induces the enzymes that convert norepinephrine to **epinephrine** in the adrenal medulla and that convert T_4 to T_3 in nonthyroidal tissues, thus shifting these systems to their adult patterns. Cortisol also has important maturational effects on neural tissue. In several mammals, but apparently not humans, increased cortisol secretion from the fetal adrenal is the trigger for parturition (Chapter 10). Finally, it is important to realize that these maturational effects of cortisol are not limited to the prepartum periods; the postpartum surge in cortisol (Fig. 11–4) accelerates these maturational events in the newborn infant.

Thus, the fetal adrenal cortex plays a critical role in normal fetal development, and dysfunctions of this gland can also be the cause of abnormalities in development. The most common of these is **congenital adrenal hyperplasia**. As discussed in Chapter 7, the excess adrenal androgen secretion associated with some types of this disease produces virilization of the reproductive tract and of the genitalia in the female fetus.

THE GONADS AND REPRODUCTIVE TRACTS

Overview of Sexual Differentiation

The gonads and reproductive tracts are unique among fetal tissues in that completely different anatomical structures develop in males and females, a process called **sexual differentiation**. Sexual dimorphism occurs at three levels: **genetic, gonadal,** and **phenotypic**. Further, these three levels represent a hierarchy that directs sexual differentiation. Genetic sex, established at fertilization, determines gonadal sex (i.e., ovary or testes), and the gonadal sex then determines the phenotypic sex.

Before the factors controlling sexual differentiation are considered, there are two general features of this process worth emphasizing. First, each sexually dimorphic structure develops from an anlage with the **potential to be either male or female**. This is illustrated in Figure 11–5, which depicts the sexual differentiation of external genitalia in males and females from a common precursor. In both sexes, the undifferentiated genitals consist of a genital tubercle, urethral folds, and, more laterally, genital (or labioscrotal) swellings. In males, the urethral folds fuse to form the penis and the genital swellings fuse to form the scrotum. In females, these two structures do not fuse at mid-

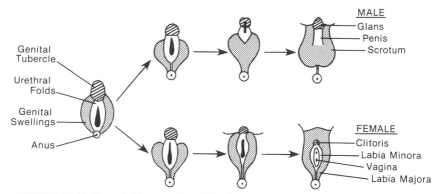

FIGURE 11–5. Sexual differentiation of the female and male genitalia from a common anlage. (Redrawn from Wilson et al.: Recent Prog. Horm. Res. 37:1, 1981.)

line but instead develop into the labia minora and majora, respectively. The tubercle gives rise to either the glans penis or clitoris, the major distinctions between the two being their size and the presence of the urethral opening in the former. The gonads and reproductive tracts also develop from sexually indifferent structures.

The second important feature of sexual differentiation is that the sexually indifferent anlage will develop into a female structure unless acted upon by masculinizing factors. Thus, **development of male structures requires an active stimulus, whereas female structures develop passively owing to the lack of male determinants**.

Factors Determining Sexual Differentiation

The mechanisms responsible for sexual differentiation vary depending on the level of sexual dimorphism (genetic sex, gonadal sex, and phenotypic sex).

Determination of Genetic Sex. The genetic sex of an individual is determined by two of the 46 chromosomes present in all human cells. If these two sex chromosomes are homologous (XX) the individual is genetically female; if they are heterologous (XY) the individual is male. Since the germ cells of females contain only X chromosomes, the ovum must also contain an X chromosome. Thus, the genetic sex of the fetus is determined by the genetic material of the **sperm**: Y-containing sperm will produce a male fetus at fertilization, whereas X-containing sperm produce a female fetus. Studies of chromosomal anomalies indicate that the presence or absence of the Y chromosome, not the number of X chromosomes, determines the gonadal sex; XO individuals have ovaries, XXY (or XXXY) individuals have testes. This does not imply that the X chromosome plays no role in sexual development. The X chromosome contains a number of genes essential to development of both females and males.

For example, the gene coding for androgen receptors is located on this chromosome. Similarly, genes located on some of the autosomal chromosomes are also necessary for normal sexual development. Thus, although the Y chromosome is the determinant of whether an individual is genetically male or female, it is not the only controller of sexual development.

Determination of Gonadal Sex. The indifferent gonadal anlage forms between weeks 5 and 6 of gestation with the arrival of the primordial germ cells, which migrate from their site of origin near the yolk sac. Differentiation of the testes is first evident around week 7 with the appearance of seminiferous cords in the **medullary** region of the gonad. As development of the testes continues, the medullary region expands while the cortex degenerates to form a fibrous layer. During this period, the medullary cords of the developing ovary begin to degenerate, but not until four months later do follicles begin to appear in the **cortical** region of this tissue. Consequently, during the first six months of gestation, the ovary continues to appear histologically indifferent, although it can be distinguished from the testes by the absence of medullary cords.

As just discussed, the Y chromosome is the genetic determinant of gonadal differentiation; in the presence of the Y chromosome testes develop, in its absence ovaries develop. The Y chromosome appears to exert this effect by controlling production of a specific protein, called the **H-Y antigen** (histocompatibility Y antigen). The H-Y antigen is a cell membrane protein found only in males. It is secreted by Sertoli cell precursors early in gestation; it binds to receptors on adjacent gonadal cells and causes testicular differentiation (Fig. 11–6). Gonadal cells in the ovaries also contain receptors for H-Y antigen, but since this protein is not produced in females, these cells never receive the signal for testicular formation. Consequently, they develop into ovaries.

Determination of Phenotypic Sex. Phenotypic sex refers to the structure of the reproductive tracts and external genitalia. As previously stated, male or female genitalia develop from the same common anlage, but this is not true for the reproductive tracts. The male reproductive tract is derived from embryonic structures known as the **wolffian ducts,** while the female tract develops from the **müllerian ducts.** The early embryo has the potential to develop either male or female reproductive tracts because both duct systems are present before sexual differentiation occurs.

Development of phenotypic sex is determined by two hormones secreted by the fetal testes, **testosterone** and **müllerian-inhibiting factor** (or antimüllerian hormone). Testosterone, released from the Leydig cells, stimulates development of the wolffian ducts and differentiation of the male genitalia; müllerian-inhibiting factor is produced by Sertoli cells and causes regression of the müllerian ducts (Fig. 11–6). Shortly after the fetal testes begin to form, both of these hormones are secreted. Consequently, the müllerian ducts regress and the wolffian ducts and genitalia develop into the male reproductive tract, penis, and scrotum. In the female, since there is no testosterone released by the ovary, the wolffian ducts regress and the external genitalia de-

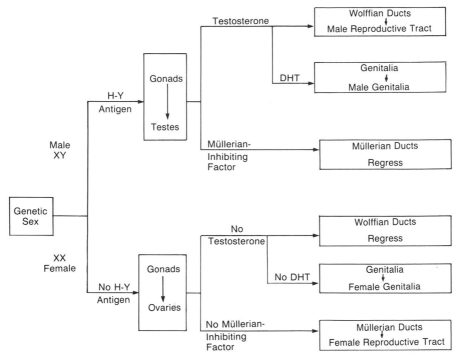

FIGURE 11–6. Factors controlling sexual differentiation.

velop into the clitoris, labia minora, and labia majora. At the same time, in the absence of müllerian-inhibiting factor, the müllerian ducts develop into the oviducts, uterus, and vagina (Fig. 11–6).

There are two important characteristics of the masculinizing actions of testosterone. First, most of these actions can occur only during a limited period of development. In the absence of testosterone, the wolffian ducts have regressed by week 14 of gestation, so that testosterone secretion after this time cannot stimulate development of the male reproductive tract. Similarly, androgens cannot produce fusion of the urethral or labioscrotal folds after 12 weeks of gestation, although testosterone can cause clitorial hypertrophy even after birth. Second, the mechanism of testosterone action differs, depending on the target tissue. Although testosterone must be converted to dihydrotestosterone (DHT) to cause virilization of the external genitalia, this conversion is not necessary for the effects of testosterone on the wolffian ducts (Fig. 11–6). Thus, individuals with a genetic deficiency of 5α-reductase (which converts testosterone to DHT) have female external genitalia but a male reproductive tract at birth.

Differentiation of phenotypic sex occurs fairly early in development. It starts shortly after the testes begin to form (week 9) and is essentially complete by week 14. During most of this period, there is little or no secretion of LH by the fetal pituitary, so LH cannot be responsible for the critical increase in testosterone production from the fetal testes. Instead, hCG from the placenta appears to be the stimulus for this early rise in testosterone secretion. In contrast, the testosterone stimulus needed for descent of the testes into the scrotum may be partially dependent on fetal LH, since this descent occurs much later in gestation.

Differentiation in the Central Nervous System. In most animals there are clear sexual differences in certain aspects of brain function. A variety of behaviors show some degree of sexual dimorphism, including **sexual behavior** and **aggression**. In addition, in many subprimate species the neural mechanisms responsible for the LH surge are absent in males so that the same estrogen treatment that induces an LH surge in females is ineffective in males. These differences in neural function are due to sexual differentiation in the central nervous system that is analogous to differentiation of the genitals. If **testosterone** is present during a critical period of development, male-type behaviors occur in the adult; if testosterone is absent during this period, female-type behaviors develop.

The importance of sexual differentiation of the central nervous system in humans is still being evaluated. An LH surge can be induced with the appropriate hormonal treatment in male primates, indicating that this system is not masculinized *in utero*. Sexual differences in four types of human behavior have been described (Table 11–1). However, because most of these behaviors occur only in humans, information on the genesis of this sexual dimorphism is limited to studies of pathological conditions, such as genetic females exposed to high androgen concentrations *in utero*. **Gender identity** appears to be determined during the first three to four years of life by the **sex of rearing** (i.e., whether the infant is reared as a male or female). For example, if an infant is raised as a female during this early postnatal period, she will consider herself a female, regardless of the secondary sexual characteristics that develop at puberty. Some recent evidence suggests that prenatal androgen exposure may influence the development of gender identity, but the sex of rearing is still

TABLE 11-1. Sexually Dimorphic Behavior in Humans

Behavior	Male Pattern	Female Pattern
Gender identity (self-image)	Male	Female
Childhood sexually dimorphic behaviors		
Energy expenditure (athletic play)	High	Low
Aggression (fighting)	High	Low
Preference for playmates	Male	Female
Parenting rehearsal (types of play)	Father	Mother
Sexual orientation	Female	Male
Cognition	Spatial perceptions	Verbal abilities

thought to be the primary determinant of this behavior. In contrast, a number of behaviors that show a sexual **dimorphism during childhood** (Table 11–1) are the result of **sexual differentiation**. Exposure to high androgen levels *in utero* results in a male-type pattern of behavior regardless of the genetic sex or the sex of rearing.

The role of early androgen exposure in the genesis of **sexual orientation** remains extremely controversial. There is some indirect evidence that male homosexuality may be due in part to low androgen production prenatally, but most data suggest that sexual orientation depends primarily on sex of rearing and other environmental influences. There is no apparent sexual dimorphism in general intelligence, but there are clear sex differences in **specific cognitive abilities** (Table 11–1). The limited information available suggests that the sex-related differences in these skills are not caused by hormonal exposure *in utero*. Thus, there appears to be some sexual differentiation within the human central nervous system, but the sex of rearing and other postnatal environmental factors are the primary determinants of human psychosexual development.

Clinical Abnormalities in Sexual Differentiation

Chromosomal anomalies usually result in inadequate gonadal development rather than affecting gonadal differentiation. For example, XXY patients (Klinefelter's syndrome) have nonfunctional testes (Chapter 9) while XO patients (Turner's syndrome) have ovaries that begin to develop and then regress *in utero* (Chapter 10). Some chromosomal abnormalities (XXX or XYY) are not associated with any clear pathological symptoms, but genetic counseling for these individuals should be considered because of the remote possibility of their producing XXY progeny.

Abnormalities in sexual differentiation are divided into three major categories: (1) **true hermaphrodism,** individuals with both ovarian and testicular tissue; (2) **female pseudohermaphrodism,** individuals with normal ovaries but masculinized genitalia; and (3) **male pseudohermaphrodism,** individuals with testes but incompletely masculinized genitalia (Table 11–2). True hermaphrodites are rare and are usually the result of abnormal production of the H-Y antigen in XX individuals or genetic mosaicism (presence of both XX and XY containing cells). In patients with a testis on one side and an ovary on the other, the ipsilateral tract is usually the same sex as the gonad. The genitalia can be either male or female but are most often ambiguous.

Pseudohermaphrodism occurs when the factors controlling phenotypic sex (Fig. 11–6) are inappropriate for the type of gonad present. In females, this condition is almost always the result of exposure to excess androgen *in utero* (Table 11–2); the most common cause is **congenital adrenal hyperplasia** (see Chapter 7 for the etiology of this syndrome). The degree of virilization depends on the time of initial exposure to androgen. After the 12th week of

TABLE 11–2.   Abnormalities in Sexual Differentiation

Classification	Most Common Causes
True hermaphrodism	XX with H-Y antigen XX/XY mosaicism
Female pseudohermaphrodism	Excess adrenal androgen Excess maternal androgen
Male pseudohermaphrodism	Low androgen production: LH/hCG unresponsiveness Steroidogenic enzyme defect
	Androgen resistance: Receptor deficiency 5α-reductase deficiency

gestation, androgen causes only clitoral hypertrophy. With earlier exposure, there is some fusion of the labioscrotal folds, and the degree of fusion depends on the level, duration, and timing of androgen exposure. Even with complete virilization of the external genitalia, the uterus and oviducts are present because there is no source of müllerian-inhibiting factor (Fig. 11–6). The mother can also be a source of excess androgen if she has an androgen-secreting tumor or is taking certain synthetic steroids. In the past, synthetic progestational steroids were prescribed to help maintain problem pregnancies. However, since these steroids have intrinsic androgenic activity and occasionally virilized a female fetus, this practice has been discontinued.

Male pseudohermaphrodism is usually caused by hypoandrogenism *in utero* because of either low testicular androgen production or androgen insensitivity of target tissues (Table 11–2). Low androgen production can be due to an abnormal testicular responsiveness to LH and hCG or a defect in one of the enzymes needed for testosterone synthesis. In either case, the genitalia are female or ambiguous and the male reproductive tract is absent or poorly developed. The degree of masculinization, however, can vary depending on the severity of the deficiency. A similar range of symptoms is seen in androgen-insensitive individuals. In the most severe instance (complete androgen resistance or testicular feminization), androgen receptors are either absent or nonfunctional. These individuals have testes and elevated testosterone levels but are phenotypically female (female genitalia and secondary sexual characteristics). Male reproductive tracts fail to develop, but female tracts are also absent because müllerian-inhibiting factor production is normal. This condition is often first discovered because of amenorrhea at puberty. Partial androgen resistance can also occur with considerable variability in the degree of masculinization of both genitalia and reproductive tracts. A different type of partial androgen resistance is caused by 5α-reductase deficiency; in this case, only the external genitalia are affected (Figure 11–6). Finally, a few otherwise normal males have oviducts and a uterus, indicating a defect in either the production of or responsiveness to müllerian-inhibiting factor.

It is essential that pseudohermaphrodism (male or female) be diagnosed correctly as early as possible after birth. For some types of congenital adrenal hyperplasia, replacement therapy must be started immediately. However, even if the condition is not life-threatening, correct diagnosis allows for an appropriate assignment of sex for rearing so that gender identity crises at puberty can be avoided. Once a sex is assigned, it can be reinforced with surgical and hormonal treatment, if necessary, so that psychosexual development is relatively normal.

REFERENCES

Beard, R.W. and Nathanielsz, P.W.: Fetal Physiology and Medicine, 2nd ed. Marcel Dekker, Inc., New York, 1984.

Fisher, D.A.: Fetal Endocrinology: Endocrine Disease and Pregnancy. In Endocrinology, L.J. DeGroot, editor. Grune and Stratton, New York, p. 1649, 1979.

Fisher, D.A., Dussault, J.H., Sack, J., and Chopra, I.J.: Ontogenesis of hypothalamic-pituitary-thyroid function and metabolism in man, sheep, and rat. Rec. Prog. Horm. Res. 33:59, 1977.

Grumbach, M.M. and Conte, F.A.: Disorders of sexual differentiation. In Williams' Textbook of Endocrinology, 7th ed. J.D. Wilson and D.W. Foster, editors. W.B. Saunders Company, Philadelphia, p. 312, 1985.

Kaplan, S.L., Grumbach, M.M., and Aubert, M.L.: The ontogenesis of pituitary hormones and hypothalamic factors in the human fetus: Maturation of central nervous system regulation of anterior pituitary function. Rec. Prog. Horm. Res. 32:161, 1976.

Naftolin, F. and Butz, E.: Sexual dimorphism. Science 211:1263, 1981.

Seron-Ferre, M. and Jaffe, R.B.: The fetal adrenal gland. Ann. Rev. Physiol. 43:141, 1981.

PART IV

ENDOCRINE
REGULATION
OF
METABOLISM

12

PANCREATIC HORMONES

Coauthored with
Penelope A. Longhurst, Ph.D.

INTRODUCTION

The pancreas is an organ that has both endocrine and nonendocrine functions. The acinar or exocrine portion of the pancreas is concerned primarily with the regulation of gastrointestinal function. Scattered among the pancreatic acini are the endocrine units of the pancreas, the **islets of Langerhans** (Fig. 12–1). The islets are composed of four major types of cells, each having a different endocrine function. The most abundant cell type in the islets is the β cell, the site of **insulin** synthesis and secretion. **Glucagon** is produced by the α cells of the islets, and the D cells are the pancreatic site of **somatostatin** synthesis. A relatively minor cellular constituent of the islets, the F or PP cell, secretes **pancreatic polypeptide**. It is possible that some functional relationship exists between the various cells of the islets because, for example, it is

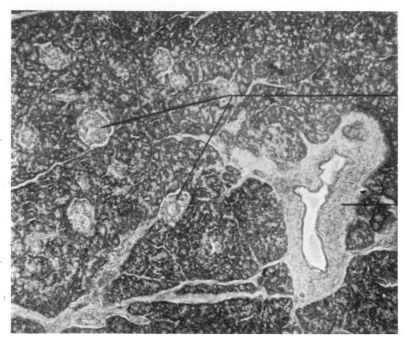

Pancreatic
acini

Islets of
Langer-
hans

Interlobu-
lar connec-
tive tissue
with duct

FIGURE 12–1. Photomicrograph of the human pancreas showing several islets. (From Bloom, W. and Fawcett, D.W.: A Textbook of Histology, 8th ed. W.B. Saunders Company, Philadelphia, p. 491, 1962.)

known that both glucagon and somatostatin affect insulin secretion by the β cell and that somatostatin also influences glucagon secretion by the α cell. However, the physiological significance of any direct interactions among the various types of cells of the islets of Langerhans has not yet been clearly defined.

Although the specific functions of each islet cell hormone are different, they are all involved in the regulation of fuel metabolism. The maintenance of glucose homeostasis is a particularly important function of the pancreas. Glucose is a major energy source for all cells and is supplied to tissues by the blood. Accordingly, normal blood glucose levels are essential for the maintenance of normal cellular function. Circulating glucose concentrations are determined by the balance existing among the following processes: glucose absorption from the intestinal tract, glucose utilization by cells, cellular (primarily hepatic) glucose production, and urinary excretion of glucose (Fig. 12–2). The relative constancy of blood glucose levels despite perturbations in any of these variables is the result of hormonal control of glucose production and utilization. Among the most important hormonal factors in the regulation of blood glucose concentrations are the pancreatic hormones, insulin and glucagon.

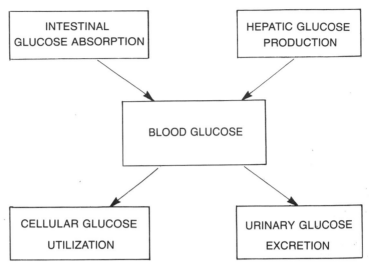

FIGURE 12–2. Factors affecting blood glucose levels.

INSULIN

In 1889 von Mering and Minkowski first demonstrated that pancreatecto-mized dogs showed many signs and symptoms characteristic of diabetes melli-tus. They suggested that diabetes was caused by the absence of some pancre-atic factor. Approximately 30 years later, Banting and Best devised methods for extraction of the active principle from the pancreas and then demonstrated that administration of the isolated factor reversed the symptoms of diabetes in dogs and in severely diabetic humans. Their pioneering work provided the basis for establishing a cause-and-effect relationship between insulin defi-ciency and diabetes. Several years later insulin was prepared in crystalline form by Abel, and its amino acid sequence was determined by Sanger in 1960. Insulin was first synthesized in the laboratory about 25 years ago. Insulin re-placement therapy has been used in the clinical management of diabetes for over 50 years and remains the most important approach for treating the dis-ease.

Insulin Biosynthesis

Chemistry of Insulin. The insulin molecule is a protein with a molecular weight of about 6000, consisting of 51 amino acids arranged as two polypep-tide chains, an A chain and a B chain (Fig. 12–3). The A chain contains 21 amino acids and the B chain 30 amino acids. Disulfide linkages connect the two chains of the molecule and are essential for the biological activity of the hormone.

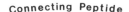

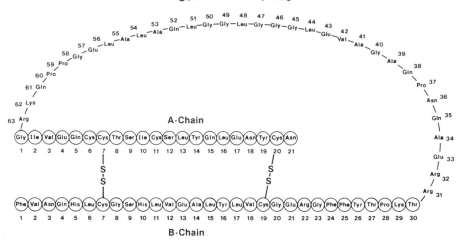

FIGURE 12–3. Primary structure of human proinsulin and variations in the amino acid sequence of insulin in several mammalian species. The amino acids of the insulin molecule are circled.

Insulin can exist as a monomer, dimer, or hexamer, the latter representing three dimers complexed with two molecules of zinc. The monomer is believed to be the active form of the hormone. There are species differences in the amino acid sequences of insulin (Fig. 12–3), but biological activities are not species-specific. Bovine, porcine, and ovine insulins differ only slightly from human insulin and have been used in the treatment of diabetes. Because of the structural similarities among these insulins, relatively few immunological problems are associated with the administration of animal insulins to humans. The porcine insulin is most similar to the human hormone and can be chemically modified to produce human insulin. In addition, human insulin produced by bacterial strains through the application of genetic engineering techniques is now available for therapeutic use.

Pathway of Insulin Biosynthesis. As already noted, insulin is synthesized by the β cells of the pancreatic islets of Langerhans. At one time it was generally believed that insulin was synthesized in the β cell by a process involving the fusion of separately formed A and B chains. However, it has now been clearly established that insulin is derived from larger polypeptide precursors. The immediate precursor to insulin is a single-chained polypeptide known as **proinsulin** (Fig. 12–3), which in turn is derived from an even larger molecule, **preproinsulin**. Preproinsulin, like other peptide hormone precursors, is synthesized in the rough endoplasmic reticulum and is converted to proinsulin at the same site (see Chapter 1). Proinsulin migrates to the Golgi apparatus where packaging of the peptide into developing storage granules occurs and conversion to insulin is initiated. With further development of the granules, the conversion of proinsulin to insulin by proteolytic enzymes is completed. The peptide fragment resulting from the cleavage of proinsulin is known as the **connecting or C-peptide** (Fig. 12–3). The C-peptide has no known function. The granules containing the insulin and C-peptide may be degraded by lysosomes, may be stored, or may be secreted by the process of exocytosis if an appropriate stimulus is provided.

Secretion and Distribution of Insulin

The control of insulin secretion by the β cell is complex, involving the coordinated actions of various nutrients, hormones, and neural input. Within the β cell, both cyclic AMP and Ca^{++} enhance the release of insulin (Fig. 12–4), probably by activating the microtubule-microfilament system involved in

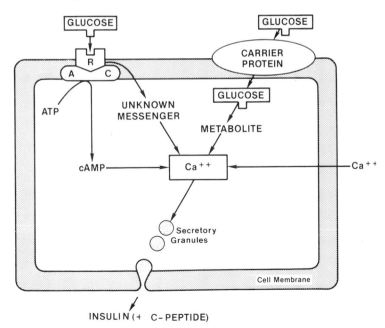

FIGURE 12–4. Proposed mechanisms of action of glucose on insulin secretion by the β cell.

moving secretory granules to the cell membrane and promoting exocytosis. Accordingly, many of the factors affecting insulin secretion act by altering intracellular cyclic AMP or Ca^{++} levels in the β cell, but other mechanisms may also be involved. Because secretion is by the process of exocytosis, insulin and C-peptide are released into the blood in equimolar quantities.

Insulin secretion by the β cell in response to appropriate stimuli appears to follow **biphasic kinetics** (Fig. 12–5). There is an initial burst of secretion that quickly reaches a maximum and begins to decline. A second secretory peak then slowly develops that persists for as long as the stimulus continues. This pattern of secretion has given rise to the theory of the existence of two different secretory pools of insulin, a rapidly releasable pool and a more slowly releasable pool. The second phase of secretion has been shown to require protein synthesis and therefore may involve new hormone production.

The peripheral plasma concentration of insulin during fasting is approximately 500 pg/ml. Although some insulin in plasma is associated with proteins, most circulates as free hormone.

Actions of Insulin

The overall effects of insulin are to lower blood levels of glucose, fatty acids, and amino acids and to promote their conversion to the storage form of each: glycogen, triglycerides, and protein, respectively. These effects are the results of insulin actions at multiple sites in the metabolic pathways for carbohydrate, lipid, and protein metabolism. Some of the major metabolic effects of insulin will be described and are summarized in Table 12–1 and in Figure 12–6.

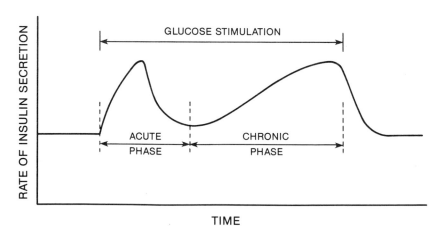

FIGURE 12–5. Kinetics of insulin secretion by the β cell in response to a continuous glucose stimulus.

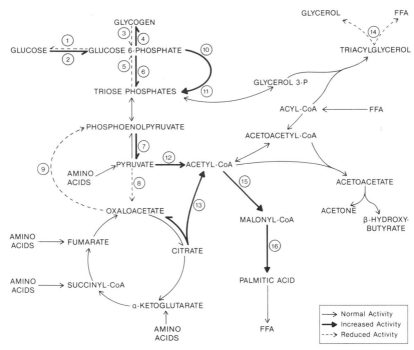

FIGURE 12–6. Metabolic pathways affected by insulin. The numbers correspond to each of the following enzymes: (1) glucose-6-phosphatase; (2) glucokinase; (3) phosphorylase; (4) glycogen synthase; (5) fructose–1,6-bisphosphate aldolase; (6) 6-phosphofructokinase; (7) pyruvate kinase; (8) pyruvate carboxylase; (9) phosphoenolpyruvate carboxykinase; (10) glucose-6-P-dehydrogenase; (11) 6-phosphogluconate dehydrogenase; (12) pyruvate dehydrogenase; (13) ATP-citrate lyase; (14) hormone-sensitive lipase; (15) acetyl-CoA carboxylase; (16) fatty acid synthase.

Carbohydrate Metabolism (Table 12–1 and Fig. 12–6)

GLUCOSE TRANSPORT. Glucose cannot readily penetrate most cell membranes in the absence of insulin. A few tissues are freely permeable to glucose. These include the brain, liver, renal medullae, red blood cells, and white blood cells, most of which require a constant supply of glucose for their minute-to-minute energy needs. However, most tissues are highly dependent upon insulin for the uptake of glucose from the blood and for its subsequent utilization. In these tissues it has been proposed that insulin increases the movement of a glucose transport protein from within the cell to the plasma membrane, but additional research is needed to substantiate this hypothesis. Inadequate amounts of insulin or interference with insulin action results in the metabolic disorder diabetes mellitus; this disease is characterized by abnormally high blood glucose concentrations and altered cellular metabolism, which are partially results of the inability of glucose to enter cells.

TABLE 12–1.   Sites of Action and Effects of Insulin on Carbohydrate, Lipid, and Protein Metabolism

Liver	Muscle	Adipose	Process Affected	Net Result
			Carbohydrate Metabolism	
	X	X	↑ glucose transport	
X	X	X	↑ glycogen synthesis	↓ blood glucose
X	X	X	↓ glycogenolysis	↑ glucose utilization
X			↓ gluconeogenesis	
			Lipid Metabolism	
X		X	↑ lipogenesis	↓ plasma free fatty acids
X		X	↓ lipolysis	↓ ketogenesis
			Protein Metabolism	
	X		↑ amino acid uptake	↓ plasma amino acids
	X		↑ protein synthesis	↓ urinary nitrogen
	X		↓ protein degradation	positive nitrogen balance
X			↓ gluconeogenesis	

GLYCOLYSIS. Several of the major enzymes involved in glycolysis (the oxidation of glucose to pyruvate and lactate) are induced by insulin. These enzymes include glucokinase, phosphofructokinase, and pyruvate kinase. The net effect of induction of these enzymes by insulin is to increase glucose metabolism.

GLYCOGEN SYNTHESIS AND DEGRADATION. In skeletal muscle, liver, and adipose tissue, insulin increases glycogen synthase activity, resulting in an accelerated rate of conversion of glucose to glycogen. In addition, glycogen phosphorylase activity declines, decreasing glycogenolysis. The net effect of both changes is to increase tissue glycogen content and decrease glucose production.

GLUCONEOGENESIS. The production of glucose from amino acids and other noncarbohydrate precursors by the liver is decreased by insulin. This effect is the result of two distinct actions of the hormone. Insulin, by promoting protein synthesis in peripheral tissues, decreases the amounts of amino acids available to the liver for gluconeogenesis. In addition, insulin decreases the activities of fructose-1,6-bisphosphate aldolase, pyruvate carboxylase, phosphoenolpyruvate carboxykinase, and glucose-6-phosphatase, which are hepatic enzymes required for the conversion of amino acids to glucose (Fig. 12–6). Therefore, inadequate amounts of insulin or interference with insulin action increases the net production of glucose from protein.

Lipid Metabolism (Table 12–1 and Fig. 12–6)

TRIGLYCERIDE SYNTHESIS. Insulin increases triglyceride synthesis in adipose tissue via several actions including the following: (1) increasing the transport of glucose into adipose tissue, which results in increased intracellular pyruvate for acetyl-coenzyme A (acetyl-Co-A) and fatty acid synthesis and increased glycerol-3-phosphate for esterification of fatty acids; (2) activating pyruvate dehydrogenase and acetyl-Co-A carboxylase, resulting in increased fatty acid synthesis from pyruvate and acetyl-Co-A; and (3) increasing the activity of lipoprotein lipase, an enzyme present in the capillary endothelia of extrahepatic tissues, which promotes the entry of free fatty acids into adipocytes.

LIPOLYSIS. Insulin decreases hormone-sensitive lipase activity in adipose tissue. This action is probably caused by a decrease in intracellular levels of cyclic AMP, resulting from inhibition of adenylate cyclase or stimulation of phosphodiesterase by insulin. Thus, insulin decreases the conversion of triglycerides to free fatty acids and glycerol. This antilipolytic effect requires less insulin than most of the other actions of the hormone. In the absence of adequate amounts of insulin, such as in diabetes mellitus, lipolysis increases and large amounts of free fatty acids are liberated into the blood. These fatty acids are extracted by the liver and oxidized to acetyl-Co-A. The acetyl-Co-A may in turn be converted to acetoacetate, β-hydroxybutyrate, and acetone, the **ketone bodies**. Thus, insulin, by decreasing the amounts of free fatty acids available to the liver as substrates for ketone body production, lowers plasma ketone levels.

Protein Metabolism (Table 12–1 and Fig. 12–6)

AMINO ACID UPTAKE. Insulin promotes the active transport of amino acids from blood into muscle and various other tissues. Thus, circulating amino acid levels decrease, and substrates for protein synthesis are provided to muscle. Insulin does not directly affect hepatic amino acid uptake, but indirectly it decreases hepatic uptake by lowering plasma amino acid levels.

PROTEIN SYNTHESIS AND DEGRADATION. Insulin increases the rate of amino acid incorporation into protein in various tissues, including muscle, and also inhibits protein degradation. The net result of these insulin actions is an anabolic effect or production of a positive nitrogen balance. As already noted, these anabolic actions of insulin also decrease gluconeogenesis by lowering the amount of circulating amino acids available to the liver as substrates. In diabetes mellitus, inadequate insulin action results in net protein degradation or a negative nitrogen balance. Circulating levels of amino acids are elevated in diabetes and serve as substrates for hepatic gluconeogenesis, contributing to the increase in blood glucose levels.

Mechanism(s) of Action of Insulin

Despite many years of intensive research, the mechanism of action of insulin has not yet been fully resolved. It is known that the actions of insulin are initiated by the interaction of the hormone with specific high-affinity receptors on the outer surface of cell membranes in target tissues. The **hormone-receptor** interaction is reversible, saturable, and apparently does not alter the insulin molecule. The insulin receptor has been purified and found to be composed of two polypeptide components, an α subunit with a molecular weight of about 135,000 and a β subunit having a molecular weight of about 90,000. It is the α subunit that appears to be most important in insulin binding. Recent studies indicate that insulin binding induces the phosphorylation of the β subunit of its own receptor, but any relationship between the phosphorylation and subsequent actions of insulin is unknown.

Once insulin binds to its receptor, the hormone-receptor complex is internalized by an endocytotic mechanism (Fig. 12–7). It is generally believed that the fate of the internalized insulin is degradation, probably by lysosomal enzymes. Thus, **internalization** of the hormone is probably not involved in the actions of insulin. In contrast to the fate of insulin, the internalized receptor appears to escape degradation and is recycled to the cell membrane for further use. The number of insulin receptors on the cell membrane is regulated, at least in part, by insulin itself through a process known as **down regulation**. Exposure of various types of cells to insulin results in a concentration- and

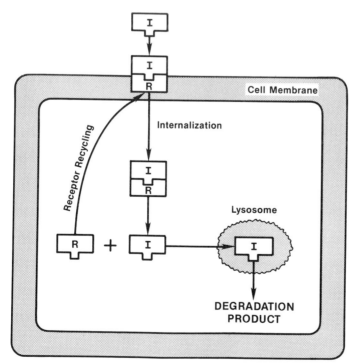

FIGURE 12–7. Fate of insulin and of the insulin receptor after binding occurs in target cell membranes.

time-dependent decrease in the number of functional membrane receptors. Thus, in conditions associated with high circulating insulin levels such as obesity, receptor binding activity in target tissues is reduced. Since there are normally more receptors ("spare receptors") present on target cell membranes than are needed for maximal effects of insulin, a decrease in the number of receptors would not necessarily decrease the maximal response to insulin. However, fewer receptors would tend to shift the insulin dose-response curve to the right, requiring more insulin to produce a given effect.

Since insulin apparently does not have to enter cells to exert its effects, considerable attention has been focused on possible **intracellular mediators** of insulin action. Any such mediator(s) would, of course, have to account for the wide variety of effects of insulin in different target tissues. Mediators apparently exist, because extracts of insulin-treated tissues contain substances that mimic some of the actions of insulin. The possible roles of cyclic nucleotides or ions or both have been investigated, but the results obtained have been inconclusive. Under certain circumstances, insulin lowers cyclic AMP and increases cyclic GMP levels in target cells. However, changes in cyclic nucleotide levels alone cannot adequately account for the various actions of insulin. Although the results of some studies suggest the existence of a peptide or phospholipid messenger for insulin, neither hypothesis has received widespread acceptance. Clearly, far more investigation is needed in this important area of research before the intracellular mechanism of action of insulin will be fully understood.

Metabolism of Insulin

Circulating insulin is rapidly degraded; its plasma half-life is less than 10 minutes in humans. Although insulin is degraded in all target tissues, the principal sites of metabolism are the liver and kidneys. Approximately 40 to 50 per cent of the insulin secreted by the pancreas is removed from the hepatic portal vein in a single pass through the liver; therefore, it never reaches the general circulation. Two major enzyme systems are involved in the hepatic metabolism of insulin. Glutathione-insulin transhydrogenase catalyzes the reduction of the disulfide bonds of insulin to yield separated A and B chains. There is also an insulin-specific protease that cleaves insulin to peptides and amino acids. Although both enzymes are widely distributed, the highest activities are found in the liver. Approximately 40 per cent of the insulin delivered to the kidneys by the blood is filtered through the glomeruli, but most is reabsorbed from the proximal tubule and degraded by tubular cells. Normally, little intact insulin is excreted in the urine.

Regulation of Insulin Secretion

Some of the substances known to influence insulin release by the pancreas are listed in Table 12-2. The most important physiological regulator of

TABLE 12–2.   Factors Affecting Insulin Secretion

Stimuli	Inhibitors
Glucose	Somatostatin
Amino acids	Epinephrine
Fatty acids	Norepinephrine
Gastrin	Alloxan
Pancreozymin-cholecystokinin	Streptozotocin
Secretin	
Gastric inhibitory polypeptide	
Glucagon	
Acetylcholine	

insulin secretion is the **glucose concentration** in the blood. Glucose stimulates insulin synthesis and release by the β cells, and thus blood insulin and glucose levels are usually directly related. Since insulin decreases blood glucose concentrations, a control system exists that maintains a relatively constant supply of glucose to tissues. The mechanism(s) through which glucose promotes insulin release has yet to be fully explained.

There are two prevalent hypotheses concerning the actions of glucose on the β cell (Fig. 12–4). One cites a direct interaction of the glucose molecule with receptors (glucoreceptors) on the β cell membrane, which in turn initiates a series of events culminating in insulin secretion. It is likely that cyclic AMP or Ca^{++} or both is involved as an intracellular mediator in that model. The second model hypothesizes the uptake and metabolism of glucose by the β cell, resulting in the generation of some intracellular signal for insulin release. A change in the $NADPH/NADP^+$ ratio resulting from glucose metabolism is one of the signals that has been proposed. It is, of course, possible that both the "glucoreceptor" and "glucose metabolism" hypotheses are valid and that multiple mechanisms may be involved in the regulation of insulin secretion by glucose.

It has been known for many years that the route of glucose administration influences the rate of insulin secretion, independent of blood glucose concentrations. Glucose given orally elicits a greater insulin secretory response than intravenous glucose, even though the latter may produce higher blood glucose levels. This suggests that the pancreas receives some signal from the gastrointestinal tract. Indeed, it is now well established that several **gastrointestinal hormones** including gastrin, pancreozymin-cholecystokinin, secretin, gastric inhibitory polypeptide (GIP), and "gut glucagon" stimulate insulin secretion. Thus, after glucose ingestion, gastrointestinal hormones probably act in concert with the glucose absorbed to enhance insulin secretion. **Amino acids** and **fatty acids,** although less potent stimuli than glucose, also promote insulin secretion; the effects of these nutrients on insulin release may also be mediated in part by gastrointestinal hormones.

A number of other hormones also affect insulin secretion by the β cells.

Glucagon, which is secreted by the α cells of the pancreas, acts directly on the β cell to stimulate insulin release. Glucagon is believed to interact with a membrane-bound receptor on the β cell, resulting in the activation of adenylate cyclase and an increase in intracellular cyclic AMP levels. **Somatostatin,** by contrast, acts on the β cell to block the release of insulin, probably by decreasing adenylate cyclase activity, thereby lowering cyclic AMP levels. The adrenal medullary hormone epinephrine also decreases insulin secretion. Although **catecholamines** may under some circumstances increase insulin release by selectively activating β-adrenergic receptors, the predominant interaction of epinephrine is with α-adrenergic receptors on the β cell, which inhibits insulin secretion. Several hormones including growth hormone, glucocorticoids, thyroid hormones, estrogens, and progesterone may also affect insulin secretion, but by indirect means rather than by direct effects on the β cell. It is believed that these hormones interfere with the peripheral actions of insulin. This requires that a greater amount of insulin be secreted to maintain normal blood glucose levels.

The islets of Langerhans are richly innervated by both adrenergic and cholinergic components of the **autonomic nervous system.** Activation of the sympathetic input to the pancreas or infusion of norepinephrine decreases insulin secretion, probably due to activation of α-adrenergic receptors on the β cell (Fig. 12–8). In contrast, an increase in vagal activity or acetylcholine infusion stimulates insulin release. Thus, the autonomic nervous system appears to participate in the regulation of insulin secretion.

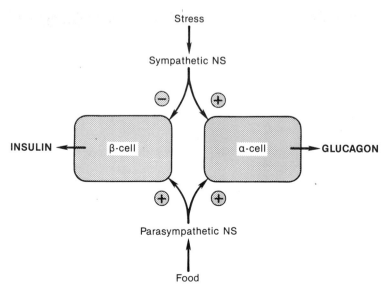

FIGURE 12–8. Regulation of insulin and glucagon secretion by the autonomic nervous system.

Alloxan and streptozotocin are compounds that selectively destroy the β cells of the pancreas and are used experimentally to produce severe forms of diabetes.

Diabetes Mellitus

Diabetes mellitus is by far the most common of all endocrine disorders. It has been estimated that approximately 5 per cent of the population of the United States may be affected by diabetes. Improved treatment of diabetes has substantially increased the life expectancy of diabetics. However, diabetes remains a significant health problem, representing one of the leading causes of death by disease and the second leading cause of blindness in the United States. Although considerable progress has been made in recent years toward understanding the etiology of diabetes, the fundamental mechanisms involved in the pathogenesis of the syndrome have not yet been determined.

Symptoms of Diabetes Mellitus. The acute symptoms of diabetes mellitus are all attributable to inadequate insulin action; the sequences of metabolic changes leading to their development are summarized in Table 12–3. As a result of insufficient insulin, glucose removal from plasma by muscle and adipose tissue decreases, glycogen synthesis decreases, and glycogenolysis and gluconeogenesis increase, all contributing to an increase in blood glucose levels (**hyperglycemia**). When the amount of blood glucose filtered by the kidneys exceeds the capacity of the tubular cells for reabsorption, glucose appears

TABLE 12–3. Acute Effects of Insulin Deficiency on Carbohydrate, Lipid, and Protein Metabolism

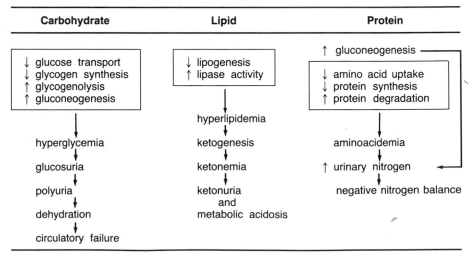

Carbohydrate	Lipid	Protein
↓ glucose transport ↓ glycogen synthesis ↑ glycogenolysis ↑ gluconeogenesis	↓ lipogenesis ↑ lipase activity	↑ gluconeogenesis ↓ amino acid uptake ↓ protein synthesis ↑ protein degradation
hyperglycemia	hyperlipidemia ketogenesis	aminoacidemia
glucosuria	ketonemia	↑ urinary nitrogen
polyuria	ketonuria and metabolic acidosis	negative nitrogen balance
dehydration		
circulatory failure		

in the urine (**glucosuria**). The osmotic effect of the glucose in the filtrate causes an osmotic diuresis (**polyuria**). In the absence of adequate fluid intake, water and accompanying electrolyte loss may result in dehydration and ultimately peripheral circulatory failure.

Insulin deficiency also decreases triglyceride synthesis and stimulates lipase activity in adipose tissue, resulting in an increase in the release of free fatty acids into the circulation. The fatty acids are taken up by the liver, converted to triglycerides, and released into the circulation, causing **hyperlipidemia**. With large amounts of circulating free fatty acids available to the liver as substrate, hepatic production and release of ketone bodies into the blood increases, causing **ketonemia**. Since the ketone levels exceed the capacity for renal reabsorption, ketone bodies appear in the urine (**ketonuria**).

The effects of insulin lack on protein metabolism result in a net shift toward catabolism; amino acid uptake and incorporation into protein by muscle decrease, and protein degradation increases. Thus, circulating levels of amino acids are increased (**aminoacidemia**), providing additional substrate for hepatic gluconeogenesis. The resulting increase in urinary nitrogen excretion causes a negative nitrogen balance. All of these acute metabolic changes in carbohydrate, lipid, and protein metabolism can be prevented or reversed by administration of adequate amounts of insulin.

There are also a number of **chronic complications** of diabetes that seem to account for the shorter life expectancy of diabetics. They include atherosclerotic changes involving the entire vascular system but especially the lower extremities, brain, kidneys, and heart. Cardiovascular lesions are the most common cause of premature death in diabetics. Microvascular lesions associated with thickening of capillary basement membranes are particularly prominent in the kidneys and retinas of diabetics. Renal disease is one of the most common findings in long-term diabetics, and diabetic retinopathy now represents one of the leading causes of blindness in the United States. Multiple neuropathies are also frequently found in diabetics, resulting in dysfunction of the peripheral nerves, spinal cord, and brain. Sensory impairment often results. Autonomic involvement may cause gastrointestinal or urinary bladder dysfunction, postural hypotension, impotence, and various other problems.

The mechanisms responsible for the development of the long-term complications of diabetes are still largely unknown. There is considerable disagreement about whether good management of the diabetic patient diminishes the incidence or frequency of the chronic abnormalities. Some investigators believe that the long-term complications of diabetes are caused by inadequate insulin and the resulting metabolic disturbances, but others believe that at least some of the lesions are genetic in origin and are associated with the genetic predisposition to diabetes. More research on the pathogenesis of the chronic complications of diabetes is needed before any definitive conclusions can be reached.

Types of Diabetes Mellitus. There are two major variants of diabetes mellitus, differing with respect to the capacity for pancreatic insulin production. **Type I, or insulin-dependent,** diabetes mellitus is characterized by inadequate secretion of insulin by the β cells of the pancreas and rapid onset of the disease. This type of diabetes was formerly known as juvenile-onset diabetes because of its prevalence in children. The disease may first be manifested at any age, making "type I" a more appropriate designation. Type I diabetics are prone to develop ketosis and require exogenous insulin for survival. The second major form of diabetes is now known as **type II, or noninsulin-dependent,** diabetes mellitus. This condition is associated with varying amounts of insulin production by the pancreas, with plasma insulin levels sometimes exceeding those in nondiabetics. The symptoms are usually slower in onset and less severe in type II than in type I diabetes. Type II diabetes was previously known as maturity-onset diabetes because it most commonly first appears in adults; however, this form of diabetes is also found in children. Patients with type II diabetes are not prone to develop ketosis and are often referred to as "ketosis-resistant." Type II diabetes is often associated with obesity. It may be treated by dietary control and oral hypoglycemic drugs or even dietary control alone. However, some type II diabetics may require insulin therapy to maintain normal blood glucose levels, although they may be asymptomatic without insulin.

Etiology of Diabetes Mellitus. Although both of the major types of diabetes appear to have **genetic** components to their etiologies, the genetic involvement seems to be greater in noninsulin-dependent diabetics. The genetic mechanisms are not understood but may be fully responsible for the development of type II diabetes. By contrast, studies with identical twins suggests that the etiology of insulin-dependent diabetes involves **environmental** as well as genetic factors. Although autoimmune and viral factors have been implicated in the pathogenesis of some types of diabetes, their overall significance is not clear. Conditions that antagonize the peripheral actions of insulin, such as obesity, pregnancy, and a number of endocrine disorders (Table 12–4), may precipitate diabetic symptoms, but mostly in individuals genetically

TABLE 12–4. Conditions or Drugs That Cause Insulin Resistance

Obesity	Acromegaly
Pregnancy	(growth hormone)
(estrogens)	Pheochromocytoma
Oral contraceptives	(epinephrine)
(estrogens)	Glucocorticoid therapy
Cushing's syndrome	Glucagon-secreting tumors
(glucocorticoids)	Insulin antibodies
Thyrotoxicosis	Starvation
(thyroid hormones)	Diabetes mellitus

predisposed to diabetes. Inappropriately high circulating levels of the hyperglycemic hormone, glucagon, have been implicated in some of the metabolic disturbances associated with diabetes, but abnormal glucagon secretion by the α cells of the pancreas may be secondary to insulin deficiency. Some investigators and clinicians think of diabetes not as a single disease but rather as a syndrome resulting from a number of different disease processes. If that point of view is correct, then multiple causes of diabetes would be expected.

It has been clearly established that pancreatic insulin production is grossly subnormal in type I diabetes and is associated with a decrease in the number of β cells. Accordingly, insulin secretion in response to glucose is also subnormal or even totally absent. However, basal insulin levels and insulin responses to glucose in type II diabetics are highly variable. In most cases, insulin secretion is delayed and reduced in magnitude. However, in many instances insulin levels may be normal or even higher than normal. Nonetheless, glucose metabolism is abnormal. These observations have led many investigators to conclude that **insulin resistance** is an important component of type II diabetes.

One of the problems of attempting to assess insulin resistance in type II diabetics is the prevalence of obesity. A large percentage of adult type II diabetics are overweight, and obesity in itself increases insulin resistance. Associated with obesity are hyperinsulinemia and a subnormal number of insulin receptors, the latter probably the result of down-regulation by insulin. The decrease in sensitivity to insulin with obesity can be overcome by secretion of greater amounts of insulin, and carbohydrate homeostasis is maintained in obese but otherwise normal individuals. However, it is believed that in individuals who are genetically predisposed to diabetes the sustained stress of obesity on the pancreas eventually exceeds the reserve secretory capacity of the β cell, and glucose intolerance results. It is important to appreciate that obesity-induced insulin resistance is reversible and that sensitivity increases with weight reduction. Accordingly, dietary control is extremely important in the treatment of type II diabetics and may, in some instances, be the only therapy required.

Stages and Diagnosis of Diabetes Mellitus. Diabetes is generally believed to progress through several stages of development before manifestation of the full-blown clinical syndrome (Table 12–5). Only those individuals with elevated fasting blood glucose levels and some or all of the symptoms of diabetes are classified as **diabetics**. The stage preceding diabetes is **impaired glucose tolerance**. This stage is symptom-free, and fasting blood glucose levels may be normal or mildly elevated. However, in response to a glucose load (glucose tolerance test), blood glucose will reach abnormally high levels and the return to normal will be delayed (beyond two to three hours). The **previous abnormality of glucose tolerance** stage precedes impaired glucose tolerance and is characterized by normal fasting blood glucose levels and a normal glucose tolerance test. Some defect may be demonstrable during this stage if

TABLE 12–5.   Stages of Development of Diabetes Mellitus

Stage	Fasting Blood Glucose	Glucose Tolerance Test	Cortisone-Glucose Tolerance Test
Potential abnormality of glucose tolerance	Normal	Normal	Normal
Previous abnormality of glucose tolerance	Normal	Normal	Abnormal
Impaired glucose tolerance	Normal or ↑	Abnormal	Abnormal*
Diabetes	↑	Abnormal*	Abnormal*

*Not necessary for diagnosis.

an additional stress is placed on the pancreas during the glucose tolerance test by simultaneously administering cortisone, a peripheral insulin antagonist. The earliest stage is known as **potential abnormality of glucose tolerance** and is representative of those individuals who are genetically predisposed to diabetes but who have no demonstrable abnormalities. This stage can be determined only retrospectively, that is, after progression to a more advanced stage of diabetes. The rate of progression from one stage to the next is highly variable; in fact, development of the disease may stop at any stage.

Treatment of Diabetes Mellitus

INSULIN. Insulin is the only treatment available for insulin-dependent (type I) diabetes mellitus and in many cases is the drug of choice for noninsulin-dependent (type II) diabetes mellitus. Most commercially available insulin is obtained by extraction of bovine or porcine pancreatic tissue. Human insulin can be produced by recombinant DNA techniques or by chemical modification of porcine insulin. Insulin is available in many different formulations, which differ with respect to onset of action, maximal activity, and duration of action. By conjugating insulin with zinc or with protamine, the normally rapid rate of absorption of insulin from injection sites is reduced, resulting in a longer duration of action. Insulin preparations are traditionally classified as fast, intermediate, and long-acting. The actions of fast-acting insulin preparations are evident from about 30 minutes after administration up to 24 hours, intermediate insulins from about 1 to 28 hours, and long-acting preparations from about 4 to over 36 hours. However, considerable variability may occur, depending on the site of injection, volume injected, physical activity of the patient, and many other factors.

FUTURE TRENDS IN INSULIN THERAPY. Several new developments in the treatment of insulin-dependent diabetes mellitus have the potential to improve therapy. Some data suggest that the incidence of vascular lesions and other chronic complications of diabetes is reduced if insulin (and glucose) levels are manipulated to mimic normal physiological concentrations as closely as possible. Therefore, it has become increasingly common for physicians to recommend the administration of **multiple doses** of insulin during the day. The simplest regimen is to administer a mixed dose of a regular insulin and an intermediate-acting insulin before breakfast. The regular insulin will be absorbed and peak with the increase in blood glucose following breakfast. The level of the intermediate-acting insulin will still be rising at lunchtime and will remain elevated for dinner. If necessary, a second much smaller dose of an intermediate-acting insulin may be given at bedtime to decrease fasting glucose levels. The regimens for multiple-dose therapies are becoming increasingly sophisticated and can mimic physiological control of blood glucose fairly well.

Constant plasma insulin levels can now be maintained throughout the day by the use of an electromechanical insulin delivery system. These **insulin pumps** are worn externally and deliver a constant infusion of insulin at a rate designed to match basal metabolic needs. The basal infusion can be supplemented by a bolus injection 15 to 30 minutes before each meal. At present, the rate of infusion must be manually adjusted by the physician or the patient. More sophisticated systems that automatically monitor blood glucose levels and adjust the rate of insulin infusion accordingly are under development.

Pancreatic transplantation represents still another potential approach to the treatment of diabetes. Transplantation of islets of Langerhans alone may be easier to accomplish than transplantation of the whole pancreas, since the transplanted islets seem to be less immunogenic than the whole pancreas.

ORAL HYPOGLYCEMIC AGENTS. Some of the less severe forms of noninsulin-dependent diabetes mellitus may be controlled by the use of oral hypoglycemic agents. Only the sulfonylureas are currently used in the United States. The use of the sulfonylureas is limited to those patients in whom the β cells of the pancreas are capable of secreting insulin. For this reason, oral hypoglycemics alone are of no use in insulin-dependent diabetes mellitus.

The mechanism of action of sulfonylureas was previously thought to involve only stimulation of insulin release from the β cells of the pancreas, since they are ineffective in pancreatectomized animals or insulin-dependent diabetics. Recently it has become obvious that the sulfonylureas also have extrapancreatic effects. An increase in the binding of insulin to peripheral receptors has been noted in diabetics following sulfonylurea treatment, which may account for the increase in glucose utilization and decrease in hepatic glucose production also observed.

GLUCAGON

Although glucagon was discovered within a few years of the discovery of insulin, research on pancreatic α cell function lagged considerably behind studies on the β cell. Only during the past couple of decades has the role of glucagon in the regulation of various metabolic processes become widely recognized and the mechanisms of action of the hormone determined. Many investigators now view the β and α cells as a coupled endocrine system whose combined secretory output (insulin plus glucagon) is a major factor in the regulation of intermediary metabolism.

Glucagon Biosynthesis

Chemistry of Glucagon. Glucagon is a single-chain polypeptide hormone consisting of 29 amino acids and having a molecular weight of approximately 3500 (Fig. 12–9). In contrast to other peptide hormones, very few species differences are seen in the structure of glucagon. Bovine, porcine, and human glucagons, for example, have the identical sequence of amino acid residues. Two glucagon-like substances produced in the gastrointestinal tract cross-react with antibodies to pancreatic glucagon. One of these compounds is produced by cells in the stomach that are quite similar to the pancreatic α cells. This peptide is structurally identical to pancreatic glucagon and is known as **gut glucagon.** The other gastrointestinal factor that is immunologically similar to glucagon is produced by cells in the small intestine and is known as **glicentin.** Glicentin is structurally similar to pancreatic glucagon, consisting of the 3500 molecular weight glucagon molecule with a C-terminal octapeptide extension having a molecular weight of about 1500. It has been found that glicentin circulates in plasma. However the regulation of glicentin secretion by the small intestine and of glucagon secretion by the pancreas are apparently independent of one another.

Pathway of Glucagon Synthesis. Glucagon, like most other peptide hormones, is synthesized as a larger precursor molecule, which is then converted to the active hormone. The glucagon precursor has a molecular weight of about 18,000 and is synthesized in the endoplasmic reticulum of the α cells in

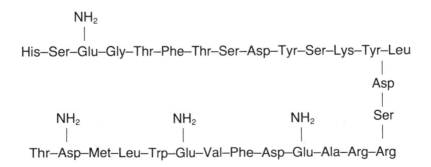

FIGURE 12–9. Amino acid sequence of human glucagon.

the islets of Langerhans. Several intermediates are generated in the course of glucagon synthesis, including a 9000 molecular weight species that has been found in human plasma. After the synthesis of glucagon precursors, further processing occurs within the endoplasmic reticulum and the Golgi apparatus of the cell. This processing ultimately results in the inclusion of glucagon within storage granules. The active form of the hormone is then ready to be secreted.

Secretion and Distribution of Glucagon

Less is known about the mechanism and kinetics of secretion of glucagon than of insulin. However, as for other peptide hormones, glucagon is secreted by the process of exocytosis (see Chapter 1). That is, the storage granules containing glucagon migrate toward the periphery of the α cell, fuse with the plasma membrane, and release their contents into the vasculature in response to appropriate stimuli. Increases in cyclic AMP levels within the α cell promote secretion of glucagon. In addition, calcium seems to be required for the normal release of glucagon. Thus, the mechanisms involved in the control of glucagon secretion may be quite similar to those described for insulin earlier in this chapter.

Glucagon circulates in the plasma primarily as the free 3500 molecular weight molecule. However, as already noted, a 9000 molecular weight species has also been identified in plasma and is believed to be a glucagon precursor. The physiological significance of the precursor is unknown. The measurement of plasma glucagon levels by radioimmunoassay has been complicated in the past by the cross-reactivity of structurally similar compounds with antibodies to glucagon. However, in recent years more specific antibodies have been developed, and basal plasma levels of glucagon are now believed to be approximately 50 pg/ml. Similar plasma levels have been obtained when measurements were done by bioassay rather than radioimmunoassay.

Actions and Mechanism of Action of Glucagon

Glucagon affects many of the same metabolic processes that are influenced by insulin. However, in most cases, the actions of glucagon are opposite to those of insulin (Table 12–6). The physiologically most important site of action of glucagon is the liver, where effects on carbohydrate, lipid, and protein metabolism are readily demonstrable. Effects of glucagon have also been demonstrated in adipose tissue, heart, pancreatic β cells, and skeletal muscle. However, the physiological significance of the latter effects is unclear because relatively high concentrations of glucagon are required to produce the extrahepatic effects. As for other hydrophilic hormones, glucagon cannot readily enter its target cells; therefore, it depends upon an intracellular mediator for its effects. That mediator is **cyclic AMP**. All of the actions of glucagon are the

TABLE 12–6.   Sites of Action and Effects of Glucagon

Site	Effect
Liver	↑ Glycogenolysis
	↑ Gluconeogenesis
	↑ Lipolysis
	↑ Ketogenesis
Adipose tissue	↑ Lipolysis
Heart	↑ Force of contraction
	↑ Cardiac output
Pancreatic β cells	↑ Insulin secretion

result of an increase in target cell cyclic AMP levels. Thus, as discussed in Chapter 1, glucagon interacts with membrane-bound receptors at its target cells, thereby activating the enzyme adenylate cyclase, which in turn catalyzes the conversion of ATP to cyclic AMP within the cell (Fig. 12–10). The cyclic AMP then activates a protein kinase. This brings about the phosphorylation of various enzymes, producing the metabolic effects of glucagon. Thus, glucagon is a classical example of a hormone whose effects are mediated via a second messenger—in this case, cyclic AMP.

Glucagon exerts a variety of effects on carbohydrate, lipid, and protein metabolism (Table 12–6). As noted, the major site of action of glucagon is the liver. The overall effects of glucagon on carbohydrate metabolism result in an

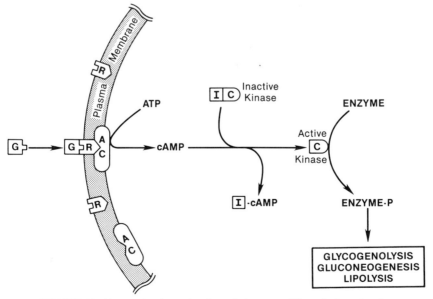

FIGURE 12–10. Mechanism of action of glucagon (G) on its target cells.

increase in hepatic glucose production and release, and thereby an increase in blood glucose levels. Thus, glucagon is a **hyperglycemic** hormone. The increase in hepatic glucose production is the result of the glucagon-stimulated increase in cyclic AMP levels within the hepatocyte. An increase in cyclic AMP decreases glycogen synthesis and promotes glycogenolysis. Cyclic AMP also stimulates hepatic gluconeogenesis, which further increases glucose production. The action of glucagon on each of these processes is opposite to that of insulin, and the resulting effect on blood glucose levels is also opposite to that produced by insulin. Thus, with respect to carbohydrate metabolism, the actions of glucagon oppose those of insulin.

The effects of glucagon on fat and protein metabolism also oppose those of insulin. Glucagon, acting via cyclic AMP, **promotes lipolysis** by stimulating lipase activity in the liver and in adipose tissue, resulting in the breakdown of triglycerides to free fatty acids. In addition, triglyceride synthesis is inhibited. Glucagon also enhances hepatic ketogenesis, promoting the conversion of free fatty acids to ketone bodies. Thus, under the influence of glucagon, plasma levels of free fatty acids and ketones increase (Table 12–6). The effects of glucagon on hepatic protein metabolism can be categorized as **catabolic**. Glucagon inhibits hepatic protein synthesis and promotes the degradation of protein. The stimulation of gluconeogenesis by glucagon further contributes to the catabolic effects of the hormone.

At high concentrations, glucagon increases the force of contraction of cardiac muscle, thereby increasing cardiac output. The effect of glucagon on the heart is also mediated by cyclic AMP, but it probably represents a pharmacological rather than physiological effect of the hormone. Glucagon has also been shown to increase insulin secretion by the pancreatic β cells. Although the physiological significance of this effect is unknown, it represents a direct action of glucagon on the β cell because the increase in insulin secretion precedes any change in blood glucose levels. The effect of glucagon on the β cell is apparently also mediated via cyclic AMP.

Metabolism of Glucagon

Circulating glucagon is rapidly metabolized and has a plasma half-life of only about five minutes. Although some degradation of the hormone may occur in the plasma, the principal sites of metabolism are the liver and kidney. It has been estimated that about 50 per cent of the circulating glucagon is removed in a single passage through the liver. The metabolic clearance rate in humans is approximately 10 ml/min × kg. Unaltered glucagon is not excreted by normal human subjects but may be found in the urine of patients with some types of kidney disease. Glucagon metabolism by liver and kidney involves proteolytic degradation of the hormone, but it is not clear whether a specific enzyme is involved in the metabolism. Metabolism of glucagon results in the formation of biologically inactive products.

Regulation of Glucagon Secretion

A number of factors have been shown to influence glucagon secretion by the α cells. However, the major physiological regulator of α cell function is **plasma glucose concentration**. An inverse relationship exists between plasma glucose levels and glucagon secretion. Thus, as plasma glucose levels fall, glucagon secretion increases in an attempt to restore blood glucose to normal levels. Conversely, an increase in plasma glucose concentrations such as occurs after a meal inhibits glucagon secretion, which tends to restore glucose levels to normal. Since glucose stimulates insulin secretion, opposite changes in circulating levels of glucagon and insulin result. Thus, although glucagon and insulin exert opposing effects on carbohydrate metabolism, they act in concert to preserve normoglycemia in the face of any perturbations that might tend to elevate or lower blood glucose concentrations (Fig. 12–11). The normal regulation of glucagon secretion by blood glucose levels requires the presence of insulin. As a result, in diabetics plasma glucagon concentrations may be inappropriately high for the prevailing blood glucose levels. It appears that glucose uptake by the α cell is an insulin-dependent process. Thus, insulin is required for the α cells to be able to monitor blood glucose levels and adjust glucagon secretion accordingly.

Many of the substances that influence insulin secretion also affect glucagon secretion but usually in the opposite direction (Table 12–7). The opposite effects on secretion are appropriate because in many instances the actions of insulin and glucagon on various metabolic processes also oppose one another. However, a **high protein meal** or amino acid infusion has similar effects on the secretion of glucagon and insulin, stimulating secretion of both hormones. Arginine is a particularly potent stimulus. The effects of protein ingestion on

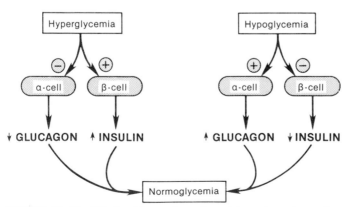

FIGURE 12–11. Effects of hyperglycemia and hypoglycemia on the secretion of insulin and glucagon by the pancreatic β cells and α cells, respectively.

TABLE 12–7.   Comparison of the Effects of Various Factors on Insulin and Glucagon Secretion by the Pancreas

Factor	Insulin Secretion	Glucagon Secretion
Nutrients		
Glucose	I	D
Amino acids	I	I
Fatty acids	I	D
Hormones		
Gastrin	I	I
Secretin	I	D
Pancreozymin-cholecystokinin	I	I
Gastric inhibitory polypeptide	I	I
Somatostatin	D	D
Transmitters		
Catecholamines	D	I
Acetylcholine	I	I
Stress	D	I

I = increases; D = decreases

both glucagon and insulin secretion seem reasonable if one considers the concomitant effects of the two hormones on blood glucose levels. If amino acids increased insulin secretion only, hypoglycemia might result. However, the simultaneous increase in glucagon secretion increases hepatic glucose production and helps to maintain normal blood glucose levels.

Fatty acids also affect glucagon secretion, but in an inverse relationship. Increases in plasma free fatty acid levels inhibit glucagon output by the pancreas, whereas decreases in circulating free fatty acids stimulate glucagon secretion. Since glucagon stimulates lipolysis, thereby increasing free fatty acid levels, the effects of free fatty acids on glucagon secretion form the basis of a negative feedback control system. Some of the **intestinal hormones** that increase insulin secretion have also been found to increase glucagon secretion. Thus, the intestinal hormones that are secreted in response to various ingested nutrients may interact with those nutrients in regulating glucagon secretion. The secretion of glucagon, like that of insulin, is inhibited by **somatostatin,** the hormone produced by the D cells of the pancreas. The effects of various chemical agents that influence pancreatic β cell function such as alloxan, streptozotocin, and the sulfonylurea drugs are apparently specific for the β cell, because glucagon secretion is unaffected by these compounds.

The **autonomic nervous system** seems to play a role in the regulation of glucagon as well as insulin secretion by the pancreas (see Fig. 12–8). The catecholamines, epinephrine and norepinephrine, and activation of the sympathetic nervous system increase glucagon secretion by the α cell. Stress, probably by acting through the sympathetic nervous system, also raises blood glucagon levels. Acetylcholine, or activation of the parasympathetic input to the pancreas, also increases glucagon secretion.

Overall Significance of Glucagon

For a number of years, the physiological importance of glucagon in the regulation of metabolism was questioned. However, today it is generally acknowledged that glucagon plays an important role in the regulation of carbohydrate, lipid, and protein metabolism. Since insulin and glucagon exert opposing effects on various metabolic processes, many investigators like to think of the **insulin-to-glucagon ratio** in the plasma as an important determinant of the overall metabolic status. Thus, when there is a high ratio of insulin to glucagon, the effects of insulin would dominate, producing a relatively anabolic state. That is, conversion of glucose, fatty acids, and amino acids to their storage forms (glycogen, triglycerides, and protein, respectively) is favored. When the ratio of insulin to glucagon is low, a catabolic state exists and the breakdown of glycogen to glucose, of triglycerides to free fatty acids, and of protein to amino acids is favored.

The effects of feeding and fasting on insulin and glucagon secretion may serve to illustrate the importance of the hormonal ratio in controlling overall metabolic status. After a meal, increasing blood glucose levels stimulate insulin secretion and inhibit glucagon secretion. The changes in the secretion of both hormones promote the incorporation of glucose into glycogen, of amino acids into protein, and of fatty acids into triglycerides, changes similar to those illustrated in Figure 12–6. Thus, the increase in the insulin-to-glucagon ratio produces an anabolic state that is appropriate when nutrients are in abundance. Between meals or during short periods of fasting, the opposite changes occur. That is, a small decrease in blood glucose inhibits insulin secretion and stimulates glucagon secretion. The decrease in the insulin-to-glucagon ratio under those circumstances produces a relatively catabolic state, promoting the breakdown of the storage forms of nutrients to generate glucose, free fatty acids, and amino acids, which is appropriate when these molecules are in short supply. Thus, the relative amounts of insulin and glucagon may be a more important determinant of overall metabolic status than the absolute amount of either hormone alone.

SOMATOSTATIN

Biosynthesis and Secretion of Somatostatin

Somatostatin was first isolated from the hypothalamus; its role in the regulation of neuroendocrine function is discussed in Chapter 5. After its identification in hypothalamic tissue, somatostatin was found in other cells of the brain, in various parts of the gastrointestinal tract, and in the D cells of the pancreas. Somatostatin is apparently synthesized at each of these as well as other sites in the body. Somatostatin is a cyclic peptide containing 14 amino acids including a 12-membered ring joined by disulfide bonds between two cysteine residues (see Fig. 5–3). In recent years, it has become apparent that somatostatin and structurally related peptides constitute a family of compounds that includes an amino terminal-extended form of somatostatin known as somatostatin-28, and several other larger molecules, some of which are precursors to somatostatin. Somatostatin-28 and some of the larger precursor molecules, as well as somatostatin, are secreted and have biological activity. The pathway of somatostatin biosynthesis in the D cell is similar to that for other peptide hormones. That is, larger precursor molecules are processed in the endoplasmic reticulum and Golgi apparatus of the cell, and the somatostatin, once formed, is sequestered in storage or secretory granules. Some prohormone as well as somatostatin-28 may also be found in the secretory granules. The forms of somatostatin that are found in the granules vary somewhat from cell type to cell type, and this may be of some physiological significance since the different molecules have somewhat different biological activities. Since secretion is believed to occur by exocytosis, the entire contents of the granule are released into the circulation and the different forms of somatostatin may be found in the blood. Little is known about the mechanisms involved in regulation of somatostatin release by the D cells, and the role of possible second messengers is yet to be determined.

Actions and Mechanism of Action of Somatostatin

Like other peptide hormones, somatostatin appears to exert its effects through interactions with membrane-bound receptors in target cells. As a result of the interaction of somatostatin with its receptor, intracellular levels of cyclic AMP are reduced. However, evidence indicates that the decrease in cyclic AMP content cannot fully account for the effects of somatostatin. It has been proposed that somatostatin effects on calcium permeability in target cells may be important in its mechanism of action. Additional investigations are needed to further clarify the mechanisms involved in the effects of somatostatin.

Somatostatin exerts a wide range of inhibitory effects in a number of different tissues (Table 12–8). Its effects on neuroendocrine function were discussed in Chapter 5. Since somatostatin can influence the function of cells adjacent to its site of production in both the pancreas and gastrointestinal tract, it may be serving a paracrine function in those tissues. In addition, since there is evidence to indicate that somatostatin can inhibit its own secretion by the D cells of the pancreas, it can also serve an autocrine function. Some of the cell-to-cell interactions proposed in the pancreatic islets are illustrated in Figure 12–12. The overall effects of somatostatin on gastrointestinal function are to **decrease nutrient absorption** as well as to **inhibit digestion** of nutrients.

TABLE 12–8.   Inhibitory Effects of Somatostatin in Various Target Organs

Organ	Process Inhibited
Stomach	Motility, acid secretion, pepsin secretion
Small intestine	Absorption, motility
Exocrine pancreas	Enzyme secretion, bicarbonate secretion
Gastrointestinal endocrine cells	Gastrin secretion, secretin secretion, GIP secretion, motilin secretion, VIP secretion, CCK secretion
Splanchnic vasculature	Blood flow
Endocrine pancreas	Insulin secretion, glucagon secretion, pancreatic polypeptide secretion, somatostatin secretion
Pituitary gland	Growth hormone secretion, TSH secretion
Gallbladder	Contraction

Motility of the stomach and small intestine is inhibited by somatostatin, and splanchnic blood flow is decreased. The secretion of a wide variety of hormonal substances required for normal gastrointestinal function is also inhibited by somatostatin (Table 12–8).

Both the exocrine and endocrine functions of the pancreas are inhibited by somatostatin. Within the islets of Langerhans, somatostatin inhibits the function of all of the major cell types. Thus, **secretion of insulin, glucagon, pancreatic polypeptide, and somatostatin itself is decreased by somatostatin.** Within the pancreatic islets, somatostatin may have an important role in the

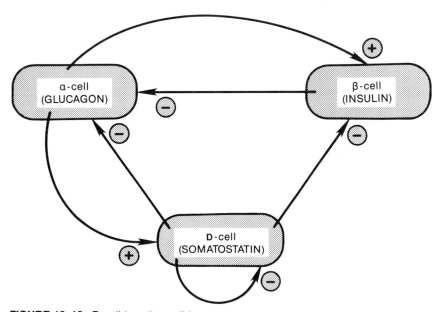

FIGURE 12–12. Possible cell-to-cell interactions in the pancreatic islets.

local regulation of hormone secretion, but its physiological significance has not yet been determined. Because the α cell is more sensitive than the β cell to the inhibitory effects of somatostatin, somatostatin may play a more important role in the regulation of glucagon secretion than of insulin secretion.

Distribution and Metabolism of Somatostatin

Blood levels of somatostatin in normal humans have been estimated at 40 to 100 pg/ml. In addition to somatostatin itself, somatostatin-28 and other larger forms apparently also circulate in the blood and may contribute to the observed biological effects. Circulating somatostatin is rapidly metabolized, having a plasma half-life of less than five minutes in normal persons. Some degradation occurs directly in plasma, but the liver and kidney are probably also important sites of metabolism. Since somatostatin is produced at a number of different sites within the body, the source of circulating somatostatin is not clear. Little is known about the specific enzymatic reactions involved in the metabolism of somatostatin and its related peptides.

Regulation of Somatostatin Secretion

Although the physiological control of somatostatin secretion is not fully understood, a number of factors are known to affect somatostatin production by the pancreas (Table 12–9). Nutrients such as glucose and amino acids stimulate somatostatin secretion, as do the neurotransmitters, acetylcholine, norepinephrine, and epinephrine. The hormones of the pancreatic islets also influence somatostatin secretion. Insulin has not been shown to have a direct effect on somatostatin production, but in some insulin-deficient states so-

TABLE 12–9. Factors Affecting Pancreatic Somatostatin Secretion

Substance	Effect on Secretion
Nutrients	
Glucose	I
Amino acids	I
Hormones	
Insulin	D
Glucagon	I
Somatostatin	D
Transmitters	
Epinephrine	I
Norepinephrine	I
Acetylcholine	I

I = Increases; D = Decreases

matostatin secretion increases, suggesting an inhibitory effect of insulin on somatostatin secretion. As already noted, somatostatin itself inhibits somatostatin production, and glucagon stimulates secretion of somatostatin. The relationship between glucagon and somatostatin secretion may represent a negative feedback loop. Increasing amounts of glucagon stimulate somatostatin output, which in turn inhibits glucagon production. The various effects of the pancreatic islet hormones on the secretion of one another suggest a local control system within the pancreas, but the nature of such a system has yet to be fully resolved.

Clinical Use of Somatostatin

There is no evidence to indicate that somatostatin is involved in the etiology of any human disease state. However, somatostatin may be of some therapeutic value for several disorders. Somatostatin may be useful in the treatment of some diabetics by inhibiting glucagon secretion, thereby providing better control of the blood glucose levels. In addition, somatostatin may be useful for several gastrointestinal disorders, including acute gastrointestinal hemorrhage and pancreatitis. The potential therapeutic value of somatostatin is now being studied in a variety of clinical trials, and definitive information should be available within a few years.

PANCREATIC POLYPEPTIDE

Very little is known about the function of the hormonal product of the F cells of the islets of Langerhans, pancreatic polypeptide. In mammals, the pancreas appears to be the only source of pancreatic polypeptide. The hormone is a linear peptide containing 36 amino acids with a molecular weight of about 4200. There are species differences in the amino acid sequences of the hormone.

The effects of pancreatic polypeptide seem to be concerned primarily with **gastrointestinal function**. The hormone inhibits pancreatic enzyme secretion and gallbladder contraction in humans but seems to have no direct effects on carbohydrate, lipid, or protein metabolism. It has been reported that pancreatic polypeptide increases gut motility and gastric emptying.

Basal levels of pancreatic polypeptide in plasma, as measured by radioimmunoassay, are about 80 pg/ml in humans. Ingestion of protein markedly increases plasma levels of the hormone, whereas carbohydrate or lipids have little effect. A number of gastrointestinal hormones including gastrin, secretin, and cholecystokinin also increase pancreatic polypeptide secretion. Plasma levels of pancreatic polypeptide increase with aging from the third to the seventh decade of life and are increased in a number of disease states. As mentioned previously, secretion of pancreatic polypeptide is inhibited by somatostatin. Stimulation of the vagus nerve rapidly increases secretion of pancreatic polypeptide; therefore, metabolic signals affecting the vagus also influence pancreatic polypeptide production.

REFERENCES

Ellenberg, M. and Rifkin, H.: Diabetes Mellitus. Theory and Practice, 3rd ed. Medical Examination Publishing Co., Inc., New York, 1983.

Fain, J.N.: Insulin secretion and action. Metabolism 33:672, 1984.

Flier, J.S.: Insulin receptors and insulin resistance. Ann. Rev. Med. 34:145, 1983.

Hansen, B., Lernmark, A., Neilsen, J.H., Owerbach, D., and Welinder, B.: New approaches to therapy and diagnosis of diabetes. Diabetologia 22:61, 1982.

Jacobs, S. and Cuatrecasas, P.: Insulin receptors. Ann. Rev. Pharmacol. Toxicol. 23:461, 1983.

Porte, D. and Halter, J.B.: The endocrine pancreas and diabetes mellitus. In Textbook of Endocrinology, R.J. Williams, editor, 6th ed. W.B. Saunders Company, Philadelphia, p. 716, 1981.

Sakamoto, N. and Alberti, K.G.M.M.: Current and Future Therapies with Insulin. Excerpta Medica, Princeton, 1982.

13

ADRENAL MEDULLA

INTRODUCTION

The adrenal medulla, the innermost portion of the adrenal gland, comprises approximately 10 to 20 per cent of the total adrenal mass. As early as 1895 it was recognized that extracts of the adrenal glands produced effects on the cardiovascular system, suggesting that the adrenals produced a secretory product. The active substance released from the adrenal medulla was named **epinephrine** shortly thereafter. Pure epinephrine (Fig. 13–1) was synthesized in 1901, the first hormone to be produced synthetically. A few years later it was suggested that epinephrine was also released from sympathetic nerve endings, because the cardiovascular responses to adrenal stimulation and to sympathetic nerve stimulation were similar. However, it was not until 1946 that **norepinephrine** (Fig. 13–1) was identified as the neurotransmitter of the sympathetic nervous system.

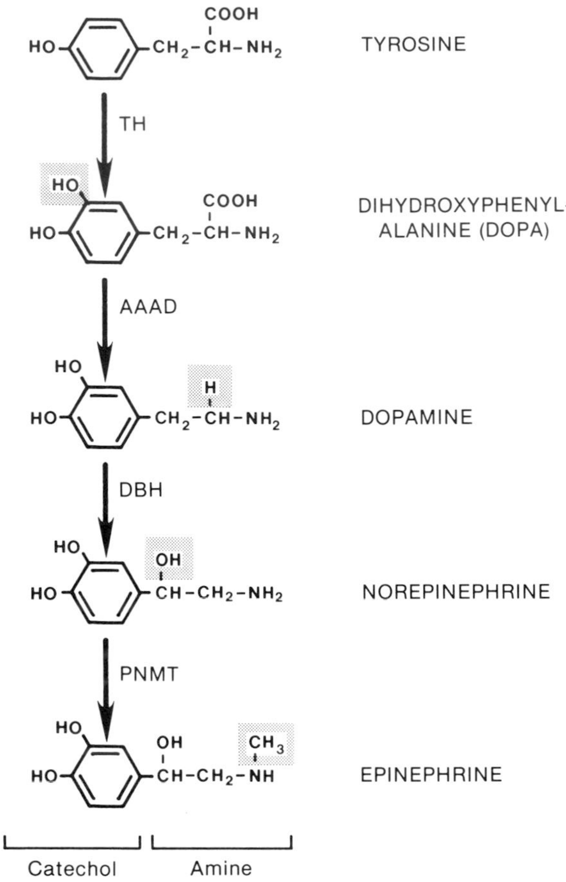

FIGURE 13–1. Pathway of catecholamine synthesis in the adrenal medulla. Shaded areas denote the structural changes occurring at each step. (TH, tyrosine hydroxylase; AAAD, aromatic-L-amino acid decarboxylase; DBH, dopamine-β-hydroxylase; PNMT, phenylethanolamine-*N*-methyltransferase.)

The adrenal medulla is structurally and functionally analogous to a postganglionic sympathetic neuron in several ways. Both are derived from neuroectoderm, are innervated by preganglionic sympathetic neurons, and synthesize and secrete catecholamines. Because the adrenal medulla stores large amounts of catecholamines, it is included among the **chromaffin** tissues. Individual adrenal medullary cells synthesize and store either epinephrine or norepinephrine. A prominent feature of all chromaffin cells is the abundance of granules called **chromaffin granules** in which the catecholamines are stored. The epinephrine- and norepinephrine-containing cells have different types of chromaffin granules, which are histologically distinct from one another.

When the preganglionic nerve fibers to the adrenal medulla are stimulated, epinephrine and norepinephrine are released into the circulation to exert their far-reaching effects. Both epinephrine and norepinephrine are secreted by the adrenal medulla; however, in the human, epinephrine comprises about 80 per cent of the total catecholamine secretion. Most of the circulating norepinephrine is derived from sympathetic nerves. Adrenal medullary hormones are not essential for life, but they play important roles in the regulation of intermediary metabolism and in the responses to stress (sometimes referred to as "fight or flight" responses). They influence a host of other processes as well. Virtually all organs in the body are affected by catecholamines.

BIOSYNTHESIS AND STORAGE OF CATECHOLAMINES

Pathway of Catecholamine Biosynthesis

The pathway for the biosynthesis of catecholamines is similar in all chromaffin cells and is illustrated in Figure 13–1. The initial substrate for the pathway may be either phenylalanine or tyrosine. Phenylalanine is converted to tyrosine by the enzyme phenylalanine hydroxylase. However, since tyrosine is a naturally occurring amino acid, its synthesis is not required for catecholamine production. In fact, most of the catecholamine synthesis in the adrenal medulla begins with tyrosine as substrate. The oxidation of tyrosine to dihydroxyphenylalanine (DOPA) is catalyzed by tyrosine hydroxylase and is the rate-limiting step in the synthesis of the catecholamines. The enzyme is located in the cytosol of the cell and is found only in those tissues that synthesize catecholamines. Tyrosine hydroxylase requires molecular oxygen, tetrahydropteridine, and NADPH for activity. Activity of the enzyme is inhibited by its end products (DOPA, dopamine, norepinephrine, and epinephrine), all of which compete for the pteridine co-factor binding site on the enzyme (Fig. 13–2). This negative feedback regulation of tyrosine hydroxylase activity maintains adrenal catecholamine levels within a relatively constant range despite short-term changes in secretion. Acute neural stimulation of catecholamine release causes a decrease in intracellular catecholamine concentrations, releasing tyrosine hydroxylase from end-product inhibition, which increases catecholamine synthesis. In contrast, prolonged activation of the sympathoadrenal system also stimulates the synthesis of tyrosine hydroxylase as a means of increasing catecholamine production.

Once DOPA is produced, it is converted to dopamine by the cytosolic enzyme, aromatic-L-amino acid decarboxylase (DOPA decarboxylase). This enzyme has a broad specificity toward all aromatic amino acids and requires pyridoxal phosphate as a co-factor. Dopamine-β-hydroxylase (DBH), which catalyzes the conversion of dopamine to norepinephrine, is the only enzyme involved in the synthesis of catecholamines that is not located in the cytosol of the chromaffin cell. DBH is located in the chromaffin granules; therefore,

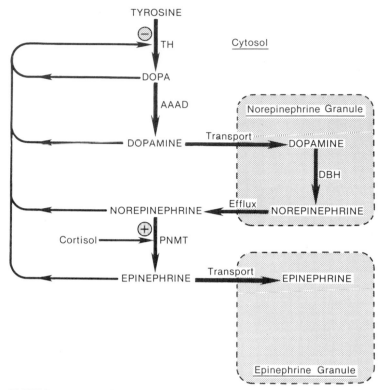

FIGURE 13–2. Regulation of catecholamine biosynthesis in the adrenal medulla. Abbreviations are the same as for Figure 13–1.

dopamine must be taken up into the granules before its conversion to norepinephrine. DBH is a mixed-function oxidase enzyme that requires molecular oxygen and a reducing agent, such as ascorbic acid, as co-factors. The enzyme is not specific for dopamine and will also oxidize other phenylethylamines to their β-hydroxylated derivatives.

The final enzyme in the pathway for catecholamine biosynthesis, phenylethanolamine-N-methyltransferase (PNMT), catalyzes the conversion of norepinephrine to epinephrine. The enzymatic reaction involves the transfer of a methyl group from S-adenosyl-methionine to the primary nitrogen group of norepinephrine or other phenylethanolamines (Fig. 13–1). PNMT is located in the cytosol of only the epinephrine-producing cells in the adrenal medulla and of a few epinephrine-containing neurons in the central nervous system. It is the selective localization of PNMT to these cells that restricts epinephrine production to the same sites. Since PNMT is a cytosolic enzyme, norepinephrine must leave the chromaffin granules and enter the cytosol for epinephrine production to take place.

The chromaffin cells of the adrenal medulla are located near the portal venous sinuses draining the adrenal cortex. As a result, the medullary cells are perfused with blood containing high concentrations of glucocorticoids. This anatomical relationship is of functional significance since glucocorticoids stimulate the synthesis of PNMT (Fig. 13–2). Hypophysectomy decreases the amount of PNMT present in the adrenal medulla, and enzyme activity can be restored by glucocorticoid administration. Thus, the relatively selective localization of epinephrine to the adrenal medulla may be the result of the juxtaposition of the cortex and medulla.

Catecholamine Storage

As noted earlier, norepinephrine and epinephrine, once produced in adrenal medullary cells, are stored in **chromaffin granules**, which are similar to the vesicles found in sympathetic nerve endings. Norepinephrine and epinephrine are stored in distinctly different types of granules. The ratio between these types of granules approximates the relative amounts of epinephrine and norepinephrine secreted by the gland.

The chromaffin granules have a very efficient catecholamine uptake system. As a result, the concentration of epinephrine in the chromaffin granules is at least 25,000 times greater than that in the cytosol. Uptake of dopamine into chromaffin granules for conversion to norepinephrine, and of norepinephrine and epinephrine into the granules for storage, is an active process requiring Mg^{++} and ATP. The Mg^{++}-dependent ATPase of the granule membrane breaks down ATP into ADP and inorganic phosphate at the same time that it drives protons from the cytosol of the chromaffin cell into the chromaffin granule. This transfer of charge across the granule membrane produces an electrical gradient that drives the uptake of catecholamines into the granule. Transport of catecholamines across the granule membrane probably involves a carrier protein; the identity of this protein has not been determined. Sequestration of catecholamines in the granules serves to protect them from oxidative degradation by cytosolic enzymes. In addition, as discussed later in this chapter, the granules participate directly in the secretion of epinephrine and norepinephrine by the process of exocytosis.

The chromaffin granules contain a variety of transmitter substances and proteins in addition to the catecholamines (Table 13–1). All of the substances in the chromaffin granules are released with the catecholamines upon stimulation of the adrenal medulla. The electrochemical gradient responsible for catecholamine uptake into the chromaffin granules also promotes ATP transport into the granules, producing a concentration of ATP in the granules that is approximately 30 times greater than that in the cytosol. It has been proposed that ATP interacts with the catecholamines in the granule to produce a storage complex, thereby preventing the osmotic rupture of the granule membrane that might occur if the high levels of catecholamines were free in solution.

Chromaffin granules also contain the analgesic neuropeptides, enkepha-

TABLE 13–1.   Functions of the Contents of Chromaffin Granules

Substance	Function
Epinephrine	Hormone
Norepinephrine	Hormone
ATP	Catecholamine storage complex
Enkephalins	Analgesic?
Acidic proteins	Unknown
Calcium	Exocytosis
DBH	Conversion of dopamine to norepinephrine
Ascorbic acid	Co-factor for DBH

lins, and larger molecules that appear to be enkephalin precursors. The function of these substances in the adrenal medulla is not known. However, they may provide some analgesic effects during stress, when they are released with the other contents of the granules. The functions of chromogranin A, the most abundant protein present in the chromaffin granules, and of the other related acidic proteins are not known.

High concentrations of calcium are found in the adrenal chromaffin granules, mostly bound to intracellular matrix proteins, ATP, and inner membrane surfaces. During prolonged stimulation of the chromaffin cell, the calcium concentration of the remaining granules increases. This suggests that the granules act as a sink for calcium entering the cell during depolarization. Calcium uptake into the granules is thought to take place via a Na^+/Ca^{++} exchange mechanism.

As noted earlier, the enzyme DBH is present in the chromaffin granules, where it catalyzes the conversion of dopamine to norepinephrine. Chromaffin granules contain high concentrations of ascorbic acid, which probably serves as a co-factor for DBH. It seems likely that ascorbic acid acts as an electron donor for DBH and in the process is converted to semidehydroascorbate. A cytochrome that is present in the granule membrane transfers electrons into the vesicles to regenerate ascorbate from the semidehydroascorbate, thereby ensuring a continuous supply of co-factor for DBH.

SECRETION AND DISTRIBUTION OF CATECHOLAMINES

Secretion of catecholamines by the chromaffin cell into the circulation takes place by **exocytosis**; therefore, it is analogous to peptide hormone secretion. Upon stimulation of the medulla, the chromaffin granules move toward the chromaffin cell membrane, the granule membrane and the cell membrane fuse, and the entire contents of the granule are released into the extracellular space. Thus, in addition to epinephrine and/or norepinephrine, ATP, DBH, enkephalins, proteins, and other substances located in the granule are simultaneously secreted. Following exocytosis, the granule membrane is recycled by **endocytosis**. The fused membrane is pinched off into a new vesicle and returns to the interior of the chromaffin cell where it can again function in the storage of catecholamines.

The process by which activation of the sympathetic input to the adrenal medulla leads to the release of catecholamines is called **stimulus-secretion coupling** (Fig. 13–3). Stimulation of the preganglionic nerve fibers innervating the adrenal medulla causes release of the transmitter acetylcholine, which binds to receptors on the chromaffin cell membrane. The mechanism(s) linking receptor binding to catecholamine secretion is not clear but seems to involve elevation of cytosolic calcium levels in the chromaffin cells. It has been proposed that calcium could enter the cells (1) through nonselective ionic acetylcholine channels in a manner analogous to that which occurs at the neuromuscular junction, or (2) through specific voltage-sensitive channels. Since cytosolic calcium is required for exocytosis, the influx of calcium may provide a crucial link between neural input and hormone release by the adrenal medulla. However, more recent evidence indicates that sodium entry into the chromaffin cell may also play a role in stimulus-secretion coupling.

Plasma concentrations of norepinephrine are normally far greater than those of epinephrine; under basal conditions, plasma levels of norepinephrine are approximately 100 to 350 pg/ml and epinephrine approximately 20 to 50 pg/ml. Virtually all of the circulating epinephrine is derived from the adrenal medulla. Under basal conditions, only a very small amount of the norepinephrine in blood is of adrenal origin; most of it is catecholamine that has been released by sympathetic nerve endings. However, when the adrenal medulla is stimulated, sufficient amounts of norepinephrine may be secreted to comprise a significant portion of the total plasma pool. Approximately 50 per cent of the epinephrine and norepinephrine in the plasma are loosely bound to albumin, and the other 50 per cent circulates as free hormone. Since catecholamines are quite water-soluble, the significance of the protein binding is unclear.

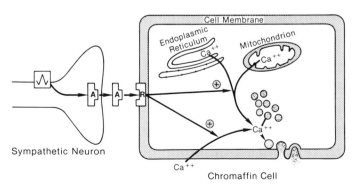

FIGURE 13–3. Stimulus-secretion coupling in the adrenal chromaffin cell. Note that cytosolic calcium may be derived from intracellular or extracellular sources. (A, acetylcholine; R, receptor.)

ACTIONS AND MECHANISMS OF ACTION OF CATECHOLAMINES

Catecholamines exert effects on most of the tissues of the body and influence a host of different processes. The diversity of catecholamine actions and sites of action makes it difficult to summarize their overall functional role. Cannon characterized adrenal medullary activation as producing a "fight or flight" response, meaning that the actions of catecholamines tend to mobilize the individual to meet an emergency. Although this description may be an oversimplification, the effects of catecholamines are generally appropriate for a "fight or flight" response.

Mechanisms of Action

Types of Receptors. Catecholamine actions are mediated through interactions with specific adrenergic receptors on target cell membranes. Binding of the catecholamines to these receptors initiates a chain of intracellular events that result in a target tissue response. There are two major types of adrenergic receptors, known as α- and β-**receptors**. The α- and β-receptor classification is further divided into at least two subtypes of each, α_1 and α_2, and β_1 and β_2. Each type of receptor has its own unique pattern of distribution throughout the body. The relative number of each receptor type in each target organ determines, in part, the nature of the response of the organ to the catecholamines. α_1-Receptors predominate at postsynaptic nerve endings, while α_2-receptors are presynaptic, where they control catecholamine release from sympathetic nerve endings. β_1-Receptors predominate in the heart, while β_2-receptors are involved in the control of smooth muscle contraction and intermediary metabolism.

Epinephrine and norepinephrine have different relative affinities for α- and β-receptors. However, neither hormone is totally specific for either receptor type, and each stimulates both α- and β-receptors to some extent. Whereas epinephrine has an affinity for α_1-receptors that is equal to or greater than that of norepinephrine, the opposite pertains for α_2-receptors. Although stimulation of α-receptors by the catecholamines produces a wide variety of effects (Table 13–2), in general, the responses are excitatory. At β_1-receptors epinephrine and norepinephrine are equipotent, but at β_2-receptors epinephrine is at least 10 times more potent than norepinephrine. Stimulation of β_1-receptors generally causes responses that are excitatory in nature, whereas the responses to stimulation of β_2-receptors tend to be inhibitory (Table 13–2). The specific mechanisms involved in the actions of catecholamines are dependent on the type of receptor mediating the action. Discussion of the mechanisms will begin with β-receptor activation because this process is more fully understood than either of the α-receptor–mediated mechanisms. The mechanisms are illustrated in Figure 13–4.

TABLE 13–2. Responses of Target Tissues to Catecholamines

Target Tissue	Receptor Type	Response
Liver	β_2	Glycogenolysis, lipolysis, gluconeogenesis
Adipose tissue	β_2	Lipolysis
Skeletal muscle	β_2	Glycogenolysis
Pancreas	α_2	Decreased insulin secretion
	β_2	Increased insulin secretion
Cardiovascular system	β_1	Increased heart rate, increased contractility, increased conduction velocity
	α	Vasoconstriction
	β_2	Vasodilation in skeletal muscle arterioles, coronary arteries, and all veins
Bronchial muscle	β_2	Relaxation
Gastrointestinal tract	β_2	Decreased contractility
	α	Sphincter contraction
Urinary bladder	α	Sphincter contraction
	β_2	Detrusor relaxation
Uterus	α	Contraction
	β_2	Relaxation
Male sex organs	α	Ejaculation, detumescence
	β_2	Erection?
Eye	α_1	Radial muscle contraction
	β_2	Ciliary muscle relaxation
CNS	α	Stimulation
Skin	α	Piloerection, sweat production
Renin secretion	β_1	Stimulation

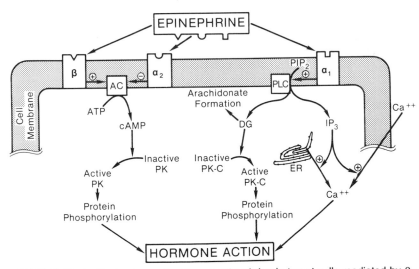

FIGURE 13–4. Mechanisms of action of epinephrine in target cells mediated by β-, α_2-, and α_1-adrenergic receptors. (PIP$_2$, phosphatidylinositol-4,5-biphosphate; PLC, phospholipase C; DG, diacylglycerol; IP$_3$, inositol-1,4,5-triphosphate; AC, adenylate cyclase; PK, protein kinase; PK-C, protein kinase C; ER, endoplasmic reticulum.)

β-Receptor–Mediated Actions. Activation of the β-receptor requires binding of a β-agonist to the three-component **adenylate cyclase** system. The catecholamine binds to the β-receptor on the outer surface of the target cell membrane, and guanosine triphosphate (GTP) interacts with the Mg-dependent coupling or guanine nucleotide regulatory protein on the inside of the membrane. These interactions result in the activation of the catalytic subunit of adenylate cyclase and the subsequent formation of the second messenger cyclic AMP from adenosine triphosphate (ATP). Increases in intracellular cyclic AMP activate protein kinases, resulting in protein phosphorylation. Phosphorylation either activates or inactivates the latter proteins, producing the characteristic responses associated with the target organs.

α$_2$-Receptor–Mediated Actions. The mechanisms responsible for producing the effects of catecholamines resulting from stimulation of α$_2$-receptors are poorly understood. However, some evidence suggests that activation of α$_2$-receptors **inhibits** the enzyme, **adenylate cyclase**, thereby decreasing intracellular cyclic AMP levels. The interaction of an α$_2$-agonist with adenylate cyclase is postulated to involve the inhibitory guanine nucleotide regulatory protein. Stimulation of this protein inhibits the activity of the catalytic subunit of adenylate cyclase and thus decreases cyclic AMP formation.

α$_1$-Receptor–Mediated Actions. The effects of catecholamines that are mediated by activation of α$_1$-receptors involve an intracellular cascade that is completely different from the one just described for β- and α$_2$-receptors. It is well established that stimulation of α$_1$-receptors has no effect on intracellular cyclic AMP levels and that calcium is required for an effect to be manifested. Activation of α$_1$-receptors in smooth muscle is associated with an **increase in intracellular calcium and a rapid breakdown of membrane polyphosphoinositides,** primarily phosphatidylinositol-4,5-bisphosphate (PIP$_2$), which is derived from phosphatidylinositol (PI). The hydrolysis of PIP$_2$ is associated with α$_1$-receptors but not α$_2$-receptors and appears to increase as the dose of the catecholamine increases. Inositol-1,4,5-triphosphate (IP$_3$), one of the hydrolysis products of PIP$_2$, is thought to cause intracellular calcium mobilization; therefore, IP$_3$ may act as a second messenger for compounds that stimulate PIP$_2$ hydrolysis. In addition, diacylglycerol, another hydrolysis product of polyphosphoinositides, activates calcium-dependent and phospholipid-dependent protein kinase C. The latter enzyme may then act in concert with intracellular calcium to effect the target organ response. Diacylglycerol may also be converted to arachidonic acid, which in turn may increase intracellular cyclic GMP levels by activating guanylate cyclase. However, the role of cyclic GMP in α$_1$-receptor–mediated processes has not been clearly established.

Effects of Catecholamines

Metabolic Effects. Catecholamines exert a number of effects on the processes involved in intermediary metabolism (Fig. 13–5). Most of these "meta-

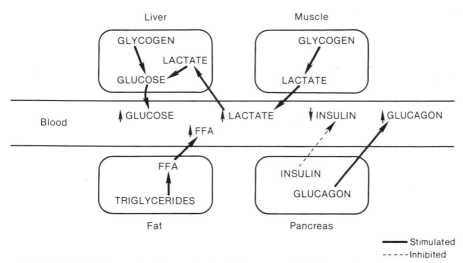

Liver   Muscle

GLYCOGEN   GLYCOGEN
        LACTATE
GLUCOSE   LACTATE

Blood   ↑GLUCOSE   ↑LACTATE   ↓INSULIN   ↑GLUCAGON
                  ↑FFA

        FFA   INSULIN

TRIGLYCERIDES   GLUCAGON

Fat   Pancreas

——— Stimulated
- - - - Inhibited

FIGURE 13–5. The major effects of epinephrine on carbohydrate and lipid metabolism.

bolic" effects are mediated by β_2-receptors; consequently, the effects of epinephrine on ′ intermediary metabolism are far greater than those of norepinephrine. The metabolic effects of epinephrine are quite similar to those of glucagon and in most instances opposite to those of insulin. Thus, catecholamines promote the breakdown of the storage forms of carbohydrate and lipid and tend to produce an overall catabolic effect (Fig. 13–5).

Epinephrine **increases blood glucose** levels primarily by increasing hepatic glucose production. Hepatic glycogenolysis increases in response to epinephrine as a result of its stimulatory effect on phosphorylase activity. In addition, hepatic gluconeogenesis is stimulated by epinephrine, further increasing glucose production.

In contrast to the actions of glucagon, epinephrine stimulates glycogenolysis in skeletal muscle as well as in liver. Since glucose-6-phosphatase is not present in skeletal muscle, glycogen cannot be converted directly to glucose. Instead, the glucose-6-phosphate produced by glycogenolysis is converted to lactate. Thus, epinephrine increases muscle lactate production and release into the blood. The lactate is then removed from the circulation by the liver and converted to glucose. In this way, the actions of epinephrine on skeletal muscle indirectly contribute to an increase in blood glucose levels. In addition, metabolism of lactate is probably responsible in large part for epinephrine's stimulation of oxygen consumption (i.e., its calorigenic effect).

The **inhibitory actions of catecholamines on pancreatic insulin secretion** are mediated by α-receptors and potentiate the hyperglycemic effects of epinephrine. Thus, epinephrine, in addition to stimulating hepatic production of glucose, inhibits secretion of the hormone primarily responsible for glucose removal from the blood. Epinephrine also stimulates the secretion of glucagon by the pancreatic α-cells, which further contributes to raising blood glucose levels. These effects of epinephrine on blood glucose levels are appropriate for "fight or flight" situations, since additional glucose would be made available to the brain as a source of energy.

Epinephrine is a potent **lipolytic** hormone, acting through β$_2$-receptors (and cyclic AMP) to increase hormone-sensitive lipase activity in adipose tissue. As a result, triglycerides are broken down, and free fatty acids are released into the blood. Since insulin is an antilipolytic hormone, inhibition of insulin secretion by epinephrine further enhances its lipolytic actions. As noted in Chapter 7, glucocorticoids potentiate the effects of epinephrine on lipolysis. Although not essential for epinephrine-induced lipolysis, glucocorticoids increase the magnitude of the effect of catecholamines.

Cardiovascular System. Epinephrine and norepinephrine are potent cardiac stimulants. Through their actions on β$_1$-receptors, both hormones increase the force of contraction of the heart (**positive inotropic effect**), and increase the rate of diastolic depolarization, resulting in an increase in heart rate (**positive chronotropic effect**). Epinephrine and norepinephrine exert approximately equipotent effects on cardiac function but differ in their effects on reflex vagal activity. Both epinephrine and norepinephrine promote **arteriolar constriction** through interactions with α-receptors. However, because of its high affinity for β$_2$-receptors, epinephrine also causes **dilation of skeletal muscle and coronary blood vessels**. As a result, epinephrine produces an overall decrease in total peripheral resistance, often resulting in a decline in diastolic blood pressure. Mean blood pressure rises only slightly if at all. The increase in heart rate caused by epinephrine, accompanied by a decrease in total peripheral resistance, results in an increase in cardiac output. In contrast, norepinephrine causes increases in systolic and diastolic blood pressure that are attributable to its effects on α-receptors but with little effect on β$_2$-receptors. The increase in blood pressure is accompanied by an increase in total peripheral resistance and a reflex decrease in heart rate. Because of the increase in total peripheral resistance, norepinephrine produces no change in cardiac output, or a decrease in it.

The cardiovascular actions of epinephrine just noted may be viewed as appropriate responses in "fight or flight" situations. Thus, at times of stress, epinephrine secretion by the adrenal medulla results in constriction of the arterioles of the skin and various other organs, while skeletal muscle and coronary blood vessels dilate, preparing the body for movement and action in response to the stress.

Smooth Muscle. Epinephrine, but not norepinephrine, has a potent **relaxant effect on bronchial smooth muscle** as a result of interactions with β$_2$-receptors, an effect that is most pronounced when the bronchial muscle is already contracted, as occurs in asthma. Both epinephrine and norepinephrine increase the rate and depth of respiration, probably as a result of effects on the central nervous system.

In general, **gastrointestinal smooth muscle is relaxed** by epinephrine through activation of β_2-receptors. As a result, the tone and frequency of peristaltic contractions are reduced. The sphincters of the gastrointestinal tract contain α-receptors that mediate contraction when tone is low.

The detrusor (body) of the urinary bladder contains predominantly β_2-receptors, which mediate relaxation, while the trigone (base) and neck contain predominantly α-receptors, which mediate contraction. Epinephrine, therefore, has the ability to **contract the bladder base and relax the bladder body**. These effects may contribute to urinary retention, which might be helpful in "fight or flight" situations. The effects of norepinephrine are primarily on the α-receptors of the trigone.

The response of the **uterus** to epinephrine is species-dependent and varies with the stage of the ovarian cycle or pregnancy. In general, α-receptors mediate contraction and β_2-receptors mediate relaxation. Norepinephrine has been found to cause contraction of the uterus in pregnant women, while epinephrine can produce either relaxation or contraction.

The sympathetic nervous system is probably involved in both the **erectile and ejaculatory responses** in the male. Although the parasympathetic nervous system is principally responsible for erectile function, low doses of epinephrine may stimulate β_2-receptors to cause vasodilation and erection. Larger amounts of epinephrine or norepinephrine cause ejaculation or detumescence or both, as a result of α-receptor stimulation and corporal vasoconstriction.

Stimulation of the β_2-receptors in the ciliary muscles of the eye by epinephrine causes relaxation and a decrease in the curvature of the lens (mydriasis). In addition, epinephrine, by activating α-receptors, causes contraction of the radial (dilator) muscle of the iris to produce **dilation of the pupil** and mydriasis. Epinephrine also affects the intraocular pressure of the eye by decreasing the rate of aqueous humor production, probably through actions mediated by β_2-receptors. In addition, epinephrine increases the efflux of aqueous humor from the eye through the trabecular mesh; this effect is probably mediated by α-receptors.

Central Nervous System. The effects of catecholamines on the central nervous system can be generally classified as excitatory and are associated with states of **arousal**, alertness, and mood elevation. Such effects are appropriate for fight or flight situations. Depletion of brain catecholamines, on the other hand, tends to cause sedation and depression. Many drugs that are used as stimulants or sedatives probably act by altering catecholamine levels in the central nervous system. It is the actions of locally produced catecholamines rather than adrenomedullary secretions that are normally important in the regulation of the central nervous system.

Other Effects. Epinephrine and norepinephrine cause **sweating and piloerection** as a result of interactions with α-receptors in the skin.

As discussed in Chapter 7, infusion of catecholamines or stimulation of the renal nerves **increases renin secretion** by the juxtaglomerular cells of the kidney. This effect appears to be mediated by β_1-receptors. The physiological significance of catecholamines in the regulation of the renin-angiotensin system has not yet been resolved.

REGULATION OF CATECHOLAMINE SECRETION BY THE ADRENAL MEDULLA

Catecholamine secretion by the adrenal medulla is controlled entirely by the sympathetic nervous input to the gland. All of the conditions known to stimulate adrenomedullary secretion do so by **increasing sympathetic impulses to the medulla.** Since each preganglionic neuron innervates many chromaffin cells in the medulla, activation of the sympathetic input can produce massive increases in hormone secretion. Although control of adrenomedullary secretion seems relatively simple, the complexity of the sympathetic nervous system has made it difficult to define many of the neural afferent pathways affecting catecholamine secretion. In addition, the various components of the sympathetic nervous system may be independently affected by various physiological stimuli. Thus, the overall activity of the sympathetic nervous system is not always an accurate index of adrenomedullary secretion.

Some of the major factors influencing adrenal catecholamine secretion are listed in Table 13–3. One of the most potent stimuli to adrenomedullary secretion is **hypoglycemia.** A decrease in blood glucose levels may increase adrenal secretion 10- to 50-fold. The magnitude of the increase in catecholamine secretion is in proportion to the severity and duration of the hypoglycemia. Changes in epinephrine secretion occur in response to decreases in blood glucose within the physiological range of blood glucose levels. In contrast to the activation of the adrenal medulla, overall sympathetic nervous system activity is depressed when blood glucose levels are below normal.

The effects of hypoglycemia on adrenal catecholamine secretion are apparently mediated by glucose-sensitive neurons in the central nervous system. Epinephrine secretion is certainly an appropriate response to hypoglycemia, since the effects of the hormone would help to restore blood glucose levels to normal. Fasting also increases adrenal catecholamine secretion, probably as a result of the small decrease in blood glucose that occurs. Epinephrine secretion may contribute to the metabolic adaptations required during fasting, such

TABLE 13–3. Conditions Stimulating Adrenomedullary Secretion

Hypoglycemia	Exercise
Physical or psychological trauma	Illness
Circulatory failure (hemorrhage)	Hypoxia
Stress	Cold exposure

as an increase in lipolysis. Increases in epinephrine secretion may also occur between meals when blood glucose levels decline slightly.

It has long been recognized that adrenomedullary secretion is stimulated by intense or prolonged **exercise**. An increase in catecholamines during exercise might serve to maintain blood pressure and cerebral blood flow by causing constriction of the splanchnic and renal vasculature, offsetting the vasodilation in skeletal muscle and skin. These cardiovascular effects of catecholamines probably increase exercise tolerance (i.e., the capacity for prolonged exercise). The actions of epinephrine also assist with the increased fuel needs during exercise by increasing glycogenolysis and lipolysis, thereby generating glucose and free fatty acids, respectively.

Trauma (whether physical or psychological), **illness, hypoxia, circulatory failure**, and most other types of **stress** elicit increases in catecholamine secretion by the adrenal medulla. Adrenal secretion tends to be greatest in response to acute stresses and decreases somewhat with more chronic stimulation. As noted earlier, virtually all of the actions of catecholamines are helpful in "fight-or-flight" situations, and should, therefore, be appropriate during periods of extreme stress. The cardiovascular effects may be particularly important at times of severe blood loss (e.g., hemorrhage) to help maintain adequate blood pressure. Prolonged **exposure to cold** also stimulates the adrenal medulla; the resulting secretion of epinephrine may serve to increase formation of the metabolic fuels needed for heat production.

METABOLISM OF CATECHOLAMINES

Circulating catecholamines turn over quite rapidly. Norepinephrine has a plasma half-life of 2.0 to 2.5 minutes and a metabolic clearance rate of approximately 40 ml/min $\times$ kg of body weight. Plasma epinephrine is cleared even more rapidly than norepinephrine; its metabolic clearance rate is approximately 90 ml/min $\times$ kg. Following release from the adrenal medulla or from sympathetic nerve endings, catecholamines are removed from the active pool by three methods: (1) enzymatic conversion to inactive products, (2) neuronal and extraneuronal uptake, and (3) excretion. Circulating catecholamines are metabolized primarily by enzymatic modification in the liver and kidneys, whereas re-uptake processes are more important in the local disposition of catecholamines at sites of release.

Enzymatic Modification

Two major enzymatic reactions are important in the degradation of catecholamines. They are **deamination** by the enzyme monoamine oxidase (MAO), and **3-O-methylation** by the enzyme catechol-O-methyltransferase (COMT). The principal pathways involved in catecholamine metabolism are illustrated in Figure 13–6.

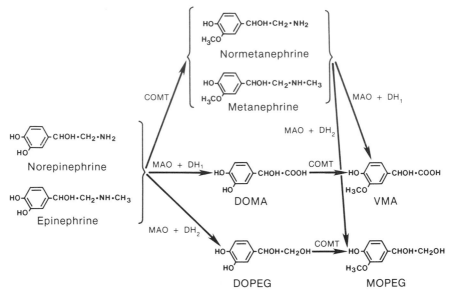

FIGURE 13–6. Pathways of epinephrine and norepinephrine metabolism. (COMT, catechol-O-methyltransferase; MAO, monoamine oxidase; DH$_1$, aldehyde dehydrogenase; DH$_2$, alcohol dehydrogenase; DOMA, 3,4-dihydroxymandelic acid; VMA, 3-methoxy-4-hydroxymandelic acid; DOPEG, 3,4-dihydroxyphenylglycol; MOPEG, 3-methoxy-4-hydroxyphenylglycol.)

Deamination. Monoamine oxidase catalyzes the oxidative deamination of primary, secondary, and tertiary amines that contain an unsubstituted methylene group. Deamination of the amine produces the corresponding aldehyde (Fig. 13–6), which is then metabolized to the corresponding carboxylic acid by aldehyde dehydrogenase (DH$_1$) or to the corresponding alcohol by alcohol dehydrogenase (DH$_2$). MAO is found in the outer mitochondrial membrane of most tissues; high concentrations are found both intraneuronally and extraneuronally in liver, kidney, stomach, and intestine. Recent studies indicate that more than one form of MAO exists.

MAO acts in combination with two dehydrogenases to catalyze the deamination of epinephrine and norepinephrine to 3,4-dihydroxymandelic acid (DOMA) and 3,4-dihydroxyphenylglycol (DOPEG) (Fig. 13–6). MAO also catalyzes deamination of the O-methylated metabolites (metanephrines) of epinephrine and norepinephrine to 3-methoxy-4-hydroxymandelic acid (vanillylmandelic acid, VMA), the major urinary metabolite, and to 3-methoxy-4-hydroxyphenylglycol (MOPEG) (Fig. 13–6).

O-Methylation. Catechol-O-methyltransferase catalyzes the 3-O-methylation of epinephrine and norepinephrine to metanephrine and normetanephrine, respectively, and of DOMA and DOPEG to VMA and MOPEG, respectively (Fig. 13–6). The presence of a catechol group is required for O-methylation to take place, but the enzyme is not stereoselective. Enzyme activity requires the methyl donor, S-adenosyl-methionine, and a divalent cation as co-factors. Although COMT is widely distributed in all mammalian tissues, activity is almost exclusively extraneuronal, and the highest activities are found in liver and kidney.

Tissue Uptake

The most important process in the termination of the local actions of catecholamines is uptake into sympathetic nerve endings (neuronal uptake) and into target tissues (extraneuronal uptake). The uptake process is physiologically important because catecholamines are removed from the target cells, thus terminating their actions. In addition, following neuronal uptake the catecholamines are recycled. This contributes to the maintenance of fairly constant catecholamine stores despite variation in neural activity.

Neuronal Uptake. The neuronal uptake of catecholamines occurs in two distinct stages. The catecholamines are first taken up into the nerve ending from the synapse and are then transported into the chromaffin granule, as described earlier in this chapter. Neuronal uptake is a sodium-dependent, energy-requiring process that is stereoselective and has specific structural requirements for substrate uptake. The process is saturable and has a very high affinity for epinephrine and norepinephrine. Following neuronal uptake, catecholamines may be deaminated by MAO or taken up into chromaffin granules for storage and subsequent release.

Extraneuronal Uptake. Extraneuronal uptake of catecholamines occurs in many tissues and results in the formation of various metabolites. The metabolites are produced by reactions involving MAO or COMT or both. Extraneuronal uptake has a much lower affinity for epinephrine and norepinephrine than neuronal uptake, but the capacity (V_{max}) is much greater. Extraneuronal uptake is neither stereoselective nor substrate specific and will transport those catecholamines that are not taken up by the more specific neuronal transport system.

Excretion

Epinephrine, norepinephrine, and various metabolites are excreted in urine. Epinephrine and norepinephrine are excreted principally as the deaminated metabolites **VMA** and **MOPEG**. Small amounts of unchanged epinephrine and norepinephrine and of the O-methylated metabolites metanephrine and normetanephrine, respectively, are also excreted. Some glucuronide or sulfate conjugates are also found in the urine.

DISEASES OF THE ADRENAL MEDULLA

Adrenomedullary dysfunction is extremely rare. The most common disorder of the gland is a functional catecholamine-secreting tumor, known as a

pheochromocytoma. The incidence of pheochromocytoma is about 1 to 4 per 100,000 persons, and these tumors, although usually not malignant, are invariably fatal if left untreated. The deaths are attributable to the large amounts of catecholamine (mostly epinephrine) that may be secreted by these tumors. There appears to be a genetic component associated with the development of pheochromocytoma.

The normal human adrenal medulla contains 0.9 to 1.5 mg of catecholamines per gm of tissue, but pheochromocytomas may contain up to 20 mg/gm of tissue. In addition, not all of the catecholamines that are produced are stored in the chromaffin granules; some continuously leak out of the pheochromocytoma cells. Release is not under neuronal control and may be influenced by mechanical events, such as squeezing the tumor when bending. The relative amounts of epinephrine and norepinephrine in pheochromocytoma cells are highly variable. They may depend on the amounts of PNMT present.

The clinical symptoms associated with pheochromocytomas are directly attributable to the actions of the large amounts of catecholamines released by the tumor (Table 13–4). The most common signs and symptoms are hypertension, headache, excessive sweating, palpitations, gastrointestinal disturbances, and hyperglycemia. The hypertension, which is frequently paroxysmal, may cause a lethal hypertensive crisis. It should be noted that less than 1 per cent of patients with essential hypertension have pheochromocytoma.

The diagnosis of pheochromocytoma is usually made by measuring plasma or urinary levels of free catecholamines, metanephrines, or VMA, or all of these. In general, the urinary excretion of catecholamines in patients with pheochromocytoma is greater than twice the upper limit of normal values. Such measurements will identify 90 per cent of patients with pheochromocytoma. Increases in epinephrine levels would tend to localize the lesion to the adrenal medulla and exclude tumors in other chromaffin tissues. There are also a number of pharmacological tests available for the diagnosis of pheochro-

TABLE 13–4. Symptoms of Pheochromocytoma

Symptom	Frequency of Occurrence (%)
Hypertension (paroxysmal or intermittent)	90
Severe headache	80
Excessive perspiration	70
Palpitations with or without tachycardia	65
Nausea	40
Tremor	30
Weakness, exhaustion, fatigue	30
Anxiety, nervousness	25
Abdominal pain	20
Blurred vision	10

mocytoma. However, because these tests may be potentially dangerous to the patient, in general they are not recommended.

Treatment of pheochromocytoma is by surgical removal of the tumor. Use of adrenergic antagonists preoperatively is recommended for these patients to prevent crises caused by catecholamine release during surgical manipulation. Short-term treatment of severe hypertensive episodes is also accomplished by administration of α-adrenergic antagonists.

REFERENCES

Birnbaumer, L., et al.: Regulation of hormone receptors and adenylyl cyclases by guanine nucleotide binding N proteins. Rec. Prog. Horm. Res. 41:41, 1985.

Carmichael, S.W. and Winkler, H.: The adrenal chromaffin cell. Sci. Am. 253:40, 1985.

Cryer, P.E.: Diseases of the adrenal medulla and sympathetic nervous system. *In* Endocrinology and Metabolism, P. Felig, et al., editors. McGraw-Hill Book Company, New York, p. 511, 1981.

Hokin, L.E.: Receptors and phosphoinositide-generated second messengers. Ann. Rev. Biochem. 54:205, 1985.

Landsberg, L. and Young, J.B.: Catecholamines and the adrenal medulla. *In* Williams' Textbook of Endocrinology, 7th ed. J.D. Wilson and D.W. Foster, editors. W.B. Saunders Company, Philadelphia, p. 891, 1985.

Nishizuka, Y., et al.: Phospholipid turnover in hormone action. Rec. Prog. Horm. Res. 40:301, 1984.

Stiles, G.L., Caron, M.G., and Lefkowitz, R.J.: β-adrenergic receptors: Biochemical mechanisms of physiological regulation. Physiol. Rev. 64:661, 1984.

Ungar, A. and Phillips, J.H.: Regulation of the adrenal medulla. Physiol. Rev. 63:787, 1983.

NORMAL GROWTH
  Fetal Growth
  Postnatal Growth

GROWTH HORMONE
  Biosynthesis and Chemistry
  Secretion and Distribution
  Actions
  Mechanism of Action
  Metabolism
  Regulation of Secretion
  Clinical Application

OTHER HORMONES AFFECTING GROWTH
  Insulin
  Thyroid Hormones
  Androgens
  Estrogens
  Glucocorticoids

PEPTIDE GROWTH FACTORS
  Insulin-like Growth Factors
    (Somatomedins)
  Platelet-Derived Growth Factor
  Fibroblast Growth Factors
  Epidermal Growth Factor
  Erythropoietin
  Nerve Growth Factor
  Thymic Peptides
  Interleukins

14

HORMONAL CONTROL OF GROWTH

NORMAL GROWTH

Growth is an extremely complex process influenced by genetics, nutritional status, endocrine function, and various other factors. The height of an individual is determined by skeletal growth, but the overall process of growth also includes increases in the sizes and numbers of cells in a variety of tissues throughout the body. The final size achieved depends upon both the rate and duration of growth, factors that are controlled in part by various hormones. Among the hormones that influence growth are growth hormone, thyroid hormones, androgens, estrogens, insulin, and glucocorticoids. This chapter will first describe the normal patterns of fetal and postnatal growth in humans and then concentrate on the actions of those endocrine factors participating in the regulation of normal growth. In addition, the actions of several peptide growth factors, which may also be involved in the overall control of growth or the growth of specific cells, are discussed.

Fetal Growth

Organ development in the fetus is nearly completed by about the 10th week of gestation, but the fetus weighs only approximately 3 gm and the crown-to-rump length is only approximately 3 cm. A period of rapid growth begins at about this time (Fig. 14–1), which reaches its maximal rate near the 20th week of development. Increases in fetal weight lag somewhat behind the increases in linear growth. The rate of growth decreases dramatically toward the end of gestation (Fig. 14–1).

Fetal growth seems to be largely independent of hormonal control, although as discussed later in this chapter, a role for insulin has been proposed. Size at birth is determined principally by genetic and environmental factors, neither of which is well understood. Infant size at birth tends to be proportional to maternal size, but when the first pregnancy is at a relatively advanced maternal age, infants tend to be smaller than average. First-born infants generally tend to be smaller than others, and on the average males are larger than females at birth. Altitude is one of the environmental factors that seems to affect fetal growth; infants born at high elevations tend to be smaller than those born at lower altitudes. Many other factors also seem to influence fetal growth, but the mechanisms responsible are generally not well understood.

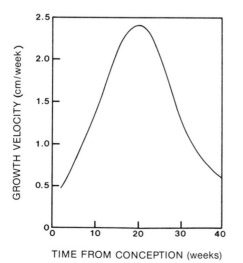

FIGURE 14–1. Rate of linear growth of the human fetus throughout gestation.

Postnatal Growth

Prepubertal Growth. After birth, hormonal factors begin to play an important role in the regulation of growth. The function of individual hormones is discussed later in this chapter. Genetic and nutritional factors also have significant impact on growth during this period. The first year of life is characterized by a quite rapid growth rate, with occurrence of approximately a 50 per cent increase in body length. During the next one or two years of life there is a relatively sharp decline in the rate of linear growth, and the rate then continues to slowly decline until puberty. There is little sexual difference in height or weight before puberty (Fig. 14–2).

Pubertal and Postpubertal Growth. One of the principal characteristics of puberty is acceleration of linear growth. Puberty occurs approximately two years earlier in girls than in boys, beginning at about the ages of 11 and 13, respectively. As a result of this difference, boys have, on the average, two more years of prepubertal growth than girls. Thus, at the start of their respective pubertal growth spurts, boys are usually several inches taller than girls (Fig. 14–2). This difference, plus a greater pubertal growth spurt in boys than in girls, is responsible for the average height differences between men and women. The pubertal growth spurt lasts for an average of two years and peaks at about age 12 in girls and 14 in boys (Fig. 14–2).

The mechanisms responsible for the pubertal growth spurt are not well understood. Apparently, both hormonal and genetic factors are involved.

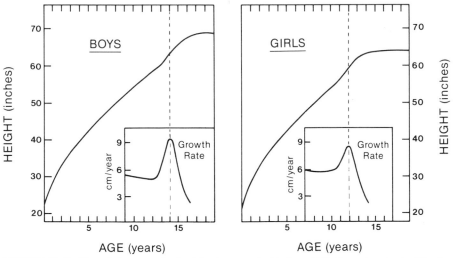

FIGURE 14–2. Cumulative growth chart for boys and girls from birth through puberty. The inserts indicate the relative growth velocities during periods that include the pubertal growth spurts. The dashed lines indicate the ages at which the maximal growth velocities occur. (Modified from Rosenfield, R.L.: Endocrinology, Volume 3, L. deGroot editor. Grune and Stratton, New York, p. 1811, 1979.)

Some evidence indicates that growth hormone secretion increases at the time of puberty and thus may contribute to the pubertal growth spurt. The anabolic effects of androgens, whose secretion increases dramatically at this time, also contribute to the pubertal growth spurt. It is testicular testosterone that is of greatest importance in boys and adrenal androgens that are most likely significant in girls. Although estrogens may also contribute to the pubertal growth spurt in girls, their precise role has not yet been defined. However, it must be borne in mind that both androgens and estrogens also promote bone maturation, bringing about the closure of the epiphyses and the cessation of long bone growth after puberty.

GROWTH HORMONE

A number of different hormones are known to affect human growth. The principal actions of the classical hormones on growth are summarized in Table 14–1. The actions of some of these hormones have been described in other chapters and will be described only briefly in this chapter. The present section will focus on **growth hormone**, the hormone that is probably most important in the control of postnatal growth.

Biosynthesis and Chemistry

As described in Chapter 4, growth hormone is produced by the somatotropic cells of the anterior pituitary gland. These growth hormone–producing cells comprise more than one third of the total gland, and growth hormone accounts for approximately 25 to 30 per cent of the total protein in these cells. Thus, the anterior pituitary in humans normally contains substantial amounts (about 5 to 10 mg) of growth hormone.

Like other protein hormones, growth hormone is synthesized by the

TABLE 14–1. Hormones Influencing Normal Growth and Their Principal Actions

Hormone	Action(s)
Growth hormone	Major stimulus of postnatal somatic growth
Thyroid hormones	Promote CNS development; are permissive for growth hormone actions; enhance growth hormone secretion
Androgens	Accelerate linear growth (pubertal spurt); increase muscle mass (anabolic); promote epiphyseal closure
Estrogens	Decrease somatic growth; promote epiphyseal closure; increase plasma growth hormone levels but decrease somatomedin levels
Insulin	Stimulates fetal somatic growth; enhances postnatal somatic growth; increases somatomedin production
Glucocorticoids	Inhibit somatic growth

post-translational modification of a larger precursor molecule. The human growth hormone is a single-chain protein containing 191 amino acids with two intramolecular disulfide bonds and a molecular weight of about 22,000. Because of species differences in the amino acid sequences of growth hormones, only certain primate growth hormones are biologically active in humans. Consequently, until recently, the only growth hormone available for treatment of growth hormone–deficient individuals was that obtained from human pituitaries at autopsy. However, the development of recombinant DNA technology has resulted in the large-scale bacterial synthesis of human growth hormone. Thus, large amounts of human growth hormone are now available for clinical use.

In addition to the 22,000 molecular weight growth hormone, several structural variants are found in the pituitary gland. A few smaller molecules, which are apparently derived from the 22,000 molecular weight growth hormone, have considerable biological activity. Because they have not been identified in plasma, their physiological significance is not known. A 45,000 molecular weight compound is also found in the pituitary and apparently represents an aggregated form of human growth hormone. Several large molecules are also found in plasma, including those known as "big" human growth hormone (40,000 to 70,000 molecular weight), "big-big" human growth hormone (molecular weight greater than 100,000), and an 80,000 molecular weight compound that has some biological activity. The physiological significance of these compounds is unknown.

There is one structural variant of growth hormone having a molecular weight of 20,000 that may be of physiological importance. This compound comprises approximately 5 to 10 per cent of the total growth hormone content of the pituitary as well as of plasma. It has biological activity equal to that of the 22,000 molecular weight growth hormone except that it does not exert the early insulin-like effects of growth hormone. The molecule differs structurally from the 22,000 molecular weight human growth hormone in that it lacks the 32 through 46 amino acid residues.

Secretion and Distribution

Like most of the peptide hormones, growth hormone is stored in vesicles and secreted by the process of **exocytosis** in response to appropriate stimuli. In normal adults, approximately 1 to 2 mg of growth hormone are secreted daily by the pituitary gland. The average plasma concentration of growth hormone in adults is approximately 2 to 4 ng/ml. As discussed later in this chapter, values are somewhat higher during puberty than at other times postnatally. Growth hormone is believed to circulate only as the free hormone in plasma. As already described, several structural variants of growth hormone have also been identified in plasma, but their physiological functions, if any, have not yet been determined.

Actions

Growth hormone exerts a variety of effects, some of which are summarized in Table 14–2. The effects most commonly associated with growth hormone are **stimulation of skeletal and soft tissue growth**. Growth hormone promotes long bone growth by stimulating the proliferation of epiphyseal cartilage, thereby widening the epiphyses and providing more matrix for bone formation. The increase in the width of the epiphyses has in fact been used as a bioassay for growth hormone. Once long bones have matured and the epiphyses have been sealed after puberty, growth hormone can no longer stimulate linear growth. In addition to affecting bone, growth hormone promotes the proliferation of connective tissues throughout the body. Similarly, the growth of many organs is enhanced as a result of the overall anabolic effects of growth hormone.

A number of specific metabolic effects are clearly attributable to growth hormone (Table 14–2). Growth hormone **stimulates lipolysis** in adipose tissue resulting in an elevation of plasma free fatty acid levels. As a result, there is an increase in fatty acid oxidation by the liver, leading to increased formation of ketone bodies. Thus, growth hormone promotes ketogenesis. The effect of growth hormone on fat metabolism is seen clinically as a loss of subcutaneous fat when growth hormone–deficient individuals are treated with growth hormone.

The effects of growth hormone on protein metabolism can be generally categorized as **anabolic**. In muscle as well as in other tissues, growth hormone stimulates protein synthesis, in part by promoting amino acid uptake into muscle (Table 14–2). Growth hormone also influences carbohydrate metabolism. There are some transitory insulin-like effects of growth hormone, but these effects are believed to be pharmacological in nature and of little physiological or clinical significance. The more important effect of growth hormone is to **antagonize the peripheral actions of insulin**. Growth hormone interferes with the actions of insulin on carbohydrate metabolism in muscle and in liver,

TABLE 14–2.   Effects of Growth Hormone on Various Target Tissues

Target Tissue(s)	Action(s)
Bone	Proliferation of epiphyseal cartilage
Connective tissue	Stimulates proliferation
Viscera	Stimulation of growth
Adipose tissue	↑ Lipolysis
Muscle	↑ Amino acid transport
	↑ Protein synthesis
	Antagonizes insulin effects on glucose metabolism
Liver	↑ Glucose output
	↑ Fatty acid oxidation
	↑ Ketogenesis

which increases hepatic glucose output and decreases glucose uptake by muscle. Such effects tend to raise blood glucose levels. In normal individuals, such antagonism can be overcome by an increase in insulin secretion by the β cells of the pancreas so that normal blood glucose levels are maintained. However, in individuals with limited pancreatic reserve, prolonged hypersecretion of growth hormone may result in the development of diabetes mellitus.

Mechanism of Action

Growth hormone, like other protein hormones, initiates its effects by interacting with specific receptors on target cell membranes. However, very little is known about the postreceptor mechanism(s) of action of growth hormone. Most of the available evidence suggests that at least the growth-promoting effects of growth hormone are mediated by secondary peptides whose synthesis is induced by growth hormone. These peptide mediators are known as **somatomedins, or insulin-like growth factors**. The somatomedin hypothesis of growth hormone action is based in part upon the observation that direct addition of growth hormone to cartilage *in vitro* does not promote proliferation, whereas serum obtained from growth hormone–treated animals does. It is now generally believed that growth hormone stimulates the production of somatomedins, which in turn exert direct effects on bone to promote growth (Fig. 14–3). As discussed later, the somatomedins may also be involved in the feedback regulation of growth hormone secretion by the anterior pituitary gland.

Although the principal site of production of the somatomedins appears to

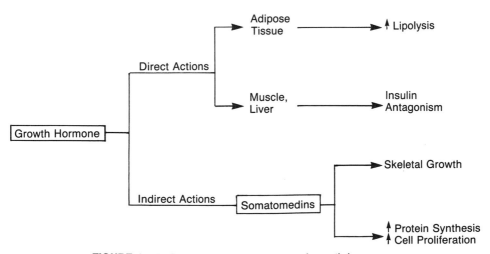

FIGURE 14–3. Direct and indirect actions of growth hormone.

be the liver, production in a variety of other tissues has also been demonstrated. Two different somatomedin peptides known as insulin-like growth factors I and II have been isolated and purified. The characteristics of these somatomedins are described more fully in the section of this chapter dealing with peptide growth factors. In contrast to the indirect effects of growth hormone on cellular proliferation and growth, its effects on carbohydrate and lipid metabolism appear to result from direct actions in target tissues (adipose tissue, muscle, liver) (Fig. 14–3). The mechanism of action of growth hormone in these tissues is not understood.

Metabolism

Circulating growth hormone is metabolized quite rapidly in humans. Its plasma half-life is about 20 to 25 minutes and its clearance rate has been estimated to be 100 to 150 ml/min $\times$ m^2 body surface. Metabolism occurs by proteolytic digestion of the hormone, and the major site of metabolism appears to be the liver. The clearance rate of growth hormone is similar in males and females and does not appear to be affected by age. Certain disease states such as diabetes mellitus and hypothyroidism have been found to decrease the rate of metabolism of growth hormone.

Regulation of Secretion

The overall regulation of growth hormone secretion is summarized in Figure 14–4. As discussed in Chapters 4 and 5, two hypophysiotropic hormones,

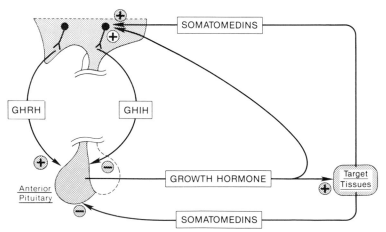

FIGURE 14–4. Regulation of growth hormone secretion by the anterior pituitary gland. (GHIH, growth hormone inhibiting hormone; GHRH, growth hormone releasing hormone.)

growth hormone–releasing hormone (GHRH, somatocrinin) and **growth hormone–inhibiting hormone** (GHIH, somatostatin), are involved in the control of growth hormone secretion by the anterior pituitary gland. Both peptides interact with membrane receptors on the somatotropic cells of the anterior pituitary gland to effect changes in growth hormone release. The effects of GHRH to stimulate growth hormone secretion are calcium-dependent and may involve activation of both adenylate cyclase and the phosphatidylinositol system. In addition to stimulating growth hormone secretion, GHRH promotes the synthesis of new growth hormone within the somatotropes. The effect of somatostatin to inhibit growth hormone secretion may also involve more than one action of the hormone on the somatotropes. Although somatostatin has been shown to decrease the concentrations of cyclic AMP within somatotropic cells, this effect cannot fully account for the actions of somatostatin. Apparently, somatostatin also decreases somatotrope membrane permeability to calcium, which seems to be more important for its inhibition of growth hormone release. (Some of the other effects of somatostatin related to gastrointestinal and pancreatic function are discussed in Chapter 12.)

In addition to the hypothalamic input to the somatotropes, **feedback effects of growth hormone and of somatomedins** participate in the regulation of growth hormone secretion (Fig. 14–4). Recent evidence suggests that both growth hormone and the somatomedins, which are produced in response to growth hormone, inhibit pituitary secretion of growth hormone by stimulating somatostatin release from the hypothalamus. The somatomedins may also exert direct effects on the anterior pituitary to inhibit the effects of GHRH on growth hormone release.

Interacting with or overriding the basic control system just described are a number of factors that influence growth hormone secretion (Table 14–3). There is, for example, a well-characterized **diurnal rhythm** in growth hormone secretion (Fig. 14–5). Throughout most of the day plasma growth hormone levels tend to be fairly constant, although some increases after meals

TABLE 14–3. Factors Affecting Growth Hormone Secretion

Stimuli	Inhibitors
Somatocrinin	Somatostatin
Sleep (stages III and IV)	Corticosteroids (high doses)
Stress	Somatomedins
Hypoglycemia	Hyperglycemia
Amino acids	High free fatty acid levels
Low free fatty acid levels	Obesity
α-Adrenergic agonists	α-Adrenergic antagonists
β-Adrenergic antagonists	β-Adrenergic agonists
Estrogens	

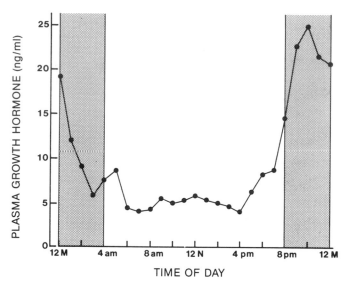

FIGURE 14–5. Diurnal rhythm in plasma growth hormone concentrations in humans. Shaded areas represent approximate sleep time in these subjects.

may occur. However, approximately one hour after the onset of deep sleep, growth hormone secretion markedly increases (Fig. 14–5). This surge in growth hormone secretion is highly correlated with the onset of stage III or IV sleep. The mechanisms responsible for this pattern of growth hormone secretion and its physiological significance are not understood.

Exercise and various types of nonspecific **stress** stimulate growth hormone secretion (Table 14–3). The release of growth hormone under such circumstances may serve to provide free fatty acids and glucose as energy sources. **Metabolic and nutritional factors** also directly influence growth hormone release (Table 14–3). For example, hypoglycemia stimulates growth hormone secretion, a response that seems appropriate because growth hormone tends to raise blood glucose levels. Hyperglycemia, on the other hand, decreases growth hormone secretion. A number of amino acids, particularly arginine and leucine, also enhance growth hormone secretion. Thus, at times of amino acid abundance such as after a high protein meal, the anabolic actions of growth hormone promote the utilization of those amino acids for protein synthesis. High levels of plasma free fatty acids inhibit growth hormone secretion, whereas a decline in free fatty acid levels stimulates the release of growth hormone. Because of the lipolytic actions of growth hormone, such regulation contributes to maintaining fairly constant plasma levels of free fatty acids. The secretion of growth hormone in response to various stimuli tends to be diminished in obese individuals; the mechanism responsible for this inhibition and its physiological significance have not been determined.

Plasma growth hormone levels vary as a function of **age**. Growth hormone levels are very high in the fetus, although growth hormone is not required for fetal growth. During early childhood, a period of quite rapid linear growth, plasma growth hormone levels are similar to those found in normal adults. Growth hormone secretion increases at about the time of puberty, which contributes to the pubertal growth spurt. Plasma growth hormone levels decline after puberty to basal levels of about 3 to 5 ng/ml and remain in that range until old age, when a gradual decrease in concentration occurs.

Several pharmacological agents affect pituitary growth hormone secretion (Table 14–3). Norepinephrine and other α-adrenergic agonists such as clonidine stimulate growth hormone secretion. Conversely, α-adrenergic antagonists decrease pituitary release of growth hormone. In contrast, β-adrenergic agonists inhibit growth hormone secretion, whereas β-adrenergic blockers such as propranolol enhance growth hormone release. Pharmacological amounts of estrogens also stimulate growth hormone secretion. However, the significance of estrogens in the physiological regulation of growth hormone secretion is not clear.

Clinical Application

Diagnostic Procedures. As with all endocrine systems, disease states associated with growth hormone are the result of hypersecretion, hyposecretion, or failure of tissues to respond to the hormone. Diagnostic procedures include, of course, measurement of plasma growth hormone levels. However, because of the diurnal variation in growth hormone secretion as well as the pulsatile nature of growth hormone release (see Chapter 4), it is difficult to reliably assess basal serum growth hormone concentrations. Measurement of serum insulin-like growth factor I (IGF I) levels is often used as a screening method because it is a relatively reliable index of overall growth hormone secretion. Thus, IGF I concentrations are elevated under conditions of growth hormone hypersecretion and depressed by growth hormone hyposecretion. In addition, since IGF I concentrations tend to be relatively constant throughout the day, multiple blood samples are not usually necessary. However, since abnormal plasma levels of IGF I may have causes other than abnormal growth hormone secretion, it is necessary to confirm any suspected defect in growth hormone secretion with other tests. Those most commonly used are provocative tests of growth hormone secretion. The provocative agents most often employed in the clinical evaluation of growth hormone secretion are listed in Table 14–4. In normal individuals, each of these agents would be expected to increase growth hormone levels in plasma. The effects of sleep on growth hormone secretion are not routinely evaluated because the procedure involves taking blood samples from an indwelling venous catheter at approximately 30 minute intervals, without disturbing the individual's normal sleep.

Growth Hormone Deficiency. Growth hormone deficiency may occur as

TABLE 14–4. Provocative Stimuli Used in the Clinical Evaluation of Growth Hormone Secretion

Insulin	Arginine
Exercise	Sleep
Propranolol (β-adrenergic antagonist)	Clonidine (α-adrenergic agonist)
Glucagon	L-Dopa

an isolated entity or may be associated with deficiencies in other hormones. In this section, only the characteristics of growth hormone deficiency alone will be considered. Inadequate growth hormone secretion may be caused by hypothalamic dysfunction or by a primary pituitary lesion. In addition, abnormal growth may result from the failure of tissues to respond normally to growth hormone. The latter is well illustrated by the syndrome known as **Laron dwarfism**. In this condition, plasma growth hormone levels are high, but tissues do not respond normally to growth hormone because of either receptor or postreceptor defects. Serum levels of IGF I are below normal in these dwarfs, and the symptoms resemble those of severe growth hormone deficiency. African pygmies are similarly resistant to the growth-promoting effects of growth hormone.

Although growth hormone deficiency has relatively little effect on growth during fetal life, growth velocity declines soon after birth and continues at about half the normal rate through childhood. Because all bone growth may not be equally affected, some craniofacial deformities may occur. Bone maturation is usually retarded. Growth hormone–deficient children usually have excessive subcutaneous fat and underdeveloped musculature (Table 14–5). Pubertal development is usually delayed, and the normal maturational changes in body proportions are retarded. Relatively few symptoms result from the development of growth hormone deficiency in adults (Table 14–5). A decrease

TABLE 14–5. Major Disorders of Growth Hormone Secretion and the Symptoms of Each

Disorder	Symptoms
Growth Hormone Deficiency	
Children (Dwarfism)	Decreased growth velocity; retarded skeletal development; poorly developed musculature; excess subcutaneous fat; delayed pubertal development
Adults	Increased insulin sensitivity; decreased muscle strength; decreased bone density
Growth Hormone Excess	
Children (Gigantism)	Increased growth velocity
Adults (Acromegaly)	Connective tissue proliferation; dermal overgrowth; enlargement of the extremities; skull deformities; peripheral neuropathy; insulin resistance

in growth hormone in adults tends to increase tissue sensitivity to insulin, which may at times result in hypoglycemia. In addition, there may be decreases in muscle strength and tone as well as a decrease in the density of bone.

The diagnosis of growth hormone deficiency can usually be established by showing an inadequate growth hormone response to any of the provocative stimuli listed in Table 14–4. In addition, plasma IGF I levels are lower than normal in patients with inadequate growth hormone production. The availability of growth hormone–releasing hormone (GHRH) for clinical testing should allow for the differential diagnosis of hypothalamic versus primary pituitary disorders. Patients with hypothalamic disease should respond to GHRH with an increase in growth hormone secretion whereas those with primary pituitary disorders should not.

Children with growth hormone deficiency must be treated with human growth hormone. Availability of human growth hormone for such treatment is now less of a problem than in the past because bacterial production through the use of recombinant DNA technology has been achieved. Some clinicians recommend the combined treatment of growth hormone and low doses of androgens, which seems to produce a greater growth response than use of growth hormone alone. However, the effects of androgens on bone maturation and ultimately the cessation of growth must also be considered. The response of growth hormone–deficient children to growth hormone is frequently greatest during the first year of treatment and then gradually decreases with time.

Growth Hormone Excess. Hypersecretion of growth hormone is most often caused by a functional tumor of the pituitary gland but some ectopic tumors may also produce growth hormone. If growth hormone hypersecretion begins in childhood, before the sealing of the epiphyseal plates in bones, the principal manifestation of the disorder is a marked increase in growth velocity. This disease is known as **pituitary gigantism** (Table 14–5).

The hypersecretion of growth hormone after bone maturation, known as **acromegaly**, is characterized by connective tissue proliferation. This produces coarsening of the facial features and a number of other skeletal and connective tissue deformities. Peripheral neuropathy is a common symptom; it results from the entrapment of nerves by bone or connective tissue overgrowth or both. The neuropathy may also cause muscle weakness, and increases in the sizes of the liver and kidneys may result from excessive stimulation by growth hormone. The increase in insulin resistance caused by the elevated growth hormone levels may lead to impaired glucose tolerance. In those individuals with limited pancreatic reserve this may result in development of overt diabetes mellitus. The diagnosis of growth hormone hypersecretion can be made by measurement of plasma growth hormone or IGF I levels; both are markedly elevated in patients with acromegaly. In addition, the diurnal rhythm in growth hormone secretion is absent in such patients, and growth hormone levels are not suppressed by glucose loading. Growth hormone hypersecretion is treated by neurosurgery to remove the functional pituitary tumor, by radiation therapy, or by treatment with drugs such as bromocriptine that inhibit growth hormone secretion.

OTHER HORMONES AFFECTING GROWTH

Insulin

Some investigators believe that insulin, in addition to serving as the primary regulator of glucose metabolism, may also be an important growth-promoting factor. There is some evidence to suggest that insulin may be particularly important in the regulation of fetal growth. Fetuses exposed to large amounts of insulin, such as those with diabetic mothers, tend to be quite large, whereas those with insulin resistance or with insulin deficiency fail to grow normally. It has been proposed that insulin might stimulate fetal growth by increasing somatomedin production.

After birth, there is also a correlation between insulin levels and growth. In a variety of abnormal conditions, hyperinsulinism is associated with excessive growth, and growth failure often accompanies insulin deficiency. These growth-promoting effects of insulin may be the result of its structural similarity to IGF I and of interactions with the somatomedin (IGF I) receptor, which is quite similar to the insulin receptor.

Thyroid Hormones

Thyroid hormones are apparently not important for normal fetal growth because thyroid hormone–deficient infants are of approximately normal size at birth. However, the absence of adequate amounts of thyroid hormones during the fetal period retards development of bone and the central nervous system. Brain development is especially dependent upon thyroid hormones during the last part of gestation and the first several months after birth. If thyroid hormone levels are inadequate during this period, severe irreversible mental retardation occurs. Thus, early diagnosis and immediate replacement with thyroid hormones are essential. It is possible that the actions of thyroid hormones on the central nervous system may be mediated by nerve growth factor (NGF). The effects of NGF are discussed later in this chapter.

The thyroid hormones are required for normal growth in children. Growth is severely retarded in children suffering from hypothyroidism. It is generally believed that thyroid hormones play a permissive role in promoting skeletal growth. That is, the actions of growth hormone are fully manifested only in the presence of adequate amounts of thyroid hormones. The mechanism responsible for this interaction is not known. The influence of thyroid hormones on growth may also result from effects on pituitary secretion of growth hormone. In hypothyroid patients, growth hormone secretion in response to various stimuli is subnormal and normal responses are restored by treatment with thyroid hormones. Thus, thyroid hormones may promote growth both by stimulating growth hormone secretion and by enhancing the actions of growth hormone.

Androgens

Androgens are potent anabolic steroids that probably play an important role in the pubertal growth spurt. When given to children, androgens stimulate linear growth, promote weight gain, and increase muscle mass. The anabolic effects of androgens are dependent upon the presence of growth hormone. In the absence of growth hormone, androgens have virtually no effect on somatic growth. However, in the presence of growth hormone, androgens synergistically enhance linear growth. There is some evidence to suggest that androgens may also enhance growth by stimulating pituitary growth hormone secretion.

Although androgens stimulate growth, they also promote bone maturation, resulting in the sealing of the epiphyseal plates. Thus, the actions of androgens ultimately terminate the potential for further linear growth. Consequently, when androgens are used as a means of stimulating growth in children, the balance between the anabolic effects and the effects on bone maturation must be carefully considered. For a number of years, chemists have been attempting to develop synthetic androgens that are growth-promoting but that have little or no effect on bone maturation and little virilizing activity. Such agents would of course be useful for stimulating growth in growth-retarded children.

Estrogens

Estrogens, like androgens, stimulate the closure of the epiphyses of long bones and therefore ultimately terminate linear growth. However, the effects of estrogens on growth prior to bone maturation are not well understood. Pharmacological amounts of estrogens increase plasma growth hormone concentrations but decrease somatic growth. The inhibition of growth by estrogens may be the result of effects on somatomedin production. Estrogen administration decreases the amount of somatomedin produced in response to growth hormone. Because of the growth-inhibiting effects of large doses of estrogens, such treatment has been used to diminish the growth rates of exceptionally tall girls.

The results of several studies suggest that the nature of the effects of estrogens on growth may be dose-dependent. Although large doses of estrogens inhibit growth, several investigators have found that small amounts of estrogens may actually stimulate growth. The mechanism responsible for the growth-promoting effects of low doses of estrogens is unknown. It is also unclear what role estrogens may play in the pubertal growth spurt in girls.

Glucocorticoids

Glucocorticoids are potent catabolic agents (as discussed in Chapter 7); as a result, they exert inhibitory effects on growth. Inhibition of growth is commonly seen in children suffering from hypercortisolism. In addition to the inhibitory effects of glucocorticoids on linear growth, glucocorticoids also inhibit DNA synthesis in a number of tissues, including muscle, liver, and kidney. The growth-inhibiting effects of glucocorticoids appear to result principally from direct actions in target tissues because only extremely large amounts of glucocorticoids inhibit growth hormone secretion or influence plasma somatomedin concentrations. The mechanisms responsible for the actions of glucocorticoids on growth are not fully understood.

PEPTIDE GROWTH FACTORS

In recent years a number of peptide factors that stimulate cell proliferation have been isolated and identified. Many laboratories are now actively investigating the mechanisms of action and physiological functions of these compounds. At least some of these factors appear to be regulated by hormones and thus may serve as mediators of hormonal effects on growth. Because of the potential importance of these peptide growth factors in the overall regulation of growth, the characteristics of several of these factors are described in this section. Some of the actions of these peptides are summarized in Table 14–6.

Insulin-like Growth Factors (Somatomedins)

Chemistry, Biosynthesis, and Distribution. As discussed earlier in this chapter, the somatomedins or insulin-like growth factors (IGF) are believed to mediate the growth-promoting effects of growth hormone. Two somatomedins have been identified, IGF I and IGF II. IGF I is also known as somatomedin C. Both peptides have molecular weights of about 7500 and are structurally related to proinsulin. The names IGF I and IGF II are derived from some of the insulin-like actions of these compounds, which are described later in this section. IGF I appears to be far more growth hormone–dependent than IGF II.

Unlike most peptide hormones, the somatomedins circulate in plasma associated with a large carrier protein, which has a molecular weight of about 150,000. The carrier protein, like the somatomedins, appears to be growth hormone–dependent. Because of their protein binding, the somatomedins are

TABLE 14–6. Growth Factors and Their Principal Actions

Growth Factor	Target	Effect(s)
Somatomedins	Adipose tissue	Stimulate glucose uptake and inhibit lipolysis
	Bone	Epiphyseal cartilage proliferation
	Muscle	Myoblast proliferation and differentiation
		Stimulate glucose and amino acid uptake
	Connective tissue	Proliferation
Platelet-derived growth factor	Fibroblasts	Competence factor
	Smooth muscle cells	Competence factor
Fibroblast growth factors	Endodermal and mesodermal cells	Competence factor
Epidermal growth factor	Ectodermal (and mesodermal) cells	Epithelial cell proliferation
Erythropoietin	Bone marrow	Stimulates erythropoiesis
Nerve growth factor	Sympathetic ganglia	Stimulates ganglionic growth in embryo
Thymic hormones	Lymphocytes	Lymphocyte proliferation and maturation
Interleukins	Lymphocytes	Lymphocyte proliferation and maturation

metabolized more slowly and consequently have a longer plasma half-life than do most peptide hormones. Both somatomedins can be measured with specific radioimmunoassays, but the assay for IGF II is not routinely available for clinical use. In normal adults, plasma levels of IGF I and IGF II average about 200 and 650 ng/ml, respectively.

The liver appears to be the major site of synthesis and release of the somatomedins. However, production by many other tissues has also been demonstrated. After growth hormone administration, somatomedin levels increase far more rapidly in some tissues than in plasma. It has been proposed that somatomedins that are locally produced in target tissues and that act via autocrine or paracrine mechanisms may be responsible for at least some of the growth hormone–induced effects.

Actions. The biological effects of somatomedins appear to be mediated by two different membrane-bound receptors in target tissues. The type I receptor has a higher affinity for IGF I than IGF II and binds insulin weakly. The type II receptor preferentially binds IGF II and does not bind insulin. However, it has been demonstrated that insulin will increase the binding of IGF II to cells containing type II receptors, probably by increasing the number of receptors.

The physiologically important activities of the somatomedins have to do with their mitogenic and growth-promoting effects. The somatomedins stimulate cellular differentiation or proliferation or both in a variety of tissues, including connective tissues. Somatomedins mediate the actions of growth hormone on linear growth by stimulating the proliferation of epiphyseal cartilage in long bones. In muscle, the somatomedins stimulate the differentiation of myoblasts into myotubules and, in addition, promote myoblast proliferation. It is generally believed that the full effects of the somatomedins on DNA synthesis in various tissues depend upon interactions with other growth factors and that the somatomedins alone are only weakly mitogenic. It has been demonstrated that administration of IGF I or IGF II to animals *in vivo* will stimulate growth. As discussed in the previous section of this chapter, the actions of somatomedins may also include a role in the feedback regulation of growth hormone secretion by the anterior pituitary gland.

The insulin-like effects of somatomedins are manifested principally in adipose tissue and muscle. In adipose tissue, the somatomedins stimulate glucose uptake and inhibit lipolysis. In muscle, both glucose and amino acid transport are stimulated by the somatomedins. The insulin-like effects of IGF II are somewhat more potent than those of IGF I, but both peptides are far less potent than insulin. It is generally believed that these insulin-like actions of the somatomedins are mediated by insulin receptors in muscle and adipose tissue. Although these effects are demonstrable in isolated tissue preparations *in vitro*, most investigators do not believe that the somatomedins play a significant role in regulation of carbohydrate or lipid metabolism *in vivo*.

Regulation. A number of factors influence plasma somatomedin levels in humans, including **age** (Fig. 14–6). Plasma somatomedin levels are relatively low at birth and remain low through the first several years of life despite the fact that growth is quite rapid during this period. It has been suggested that tissues may be more responsive to somatomedins at this time or alternately that local production of somatomedins in target tissues may be more important than delivery by the blood during this period. Plasma IGF I levels increase gradually from birth until puberty, and at puberty in both boys and girls a dramatic increase in IGF I levels occurs to approximately twice normal adult levels. Growth hormone may contribute to the pubertal rise in plasma IGF I levels since growth hormone secretion also appears to increase during puberty. It is not clear whether androgens or estrogens contribute to the pubertal increase in IGF I levels. This rise in somatomedin production at about the time of puberty may, of course, be an important factor in the pubertal growth spurt.

After puberty there is a decline in plasma somatomedin levels to normal adult values. IGF I concentrations in the plasma of normal adults are relatively constant throughout the day, showing no evidence of diurnal rhythm. A progressive decrease in plasma somatomedin levels tends to occur with aging. In elderly individuals, plasma IGF I levels are only about half those found in young adults. Sex also seems to influence circulating concentrations of IGF I. Plasma levels of IGF I appear to be somewhat higher in females than in males at all ages. Relatively little is known about the effects of age on

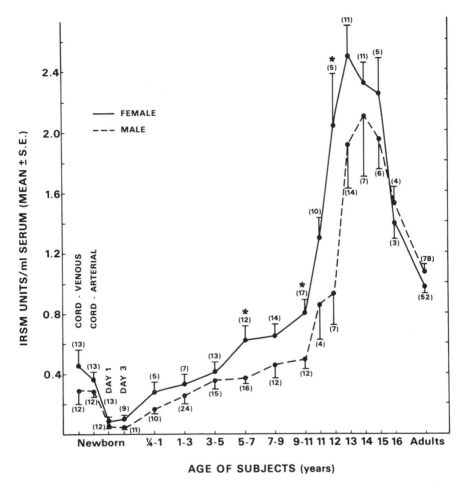

FIGURE 14-6. Effects of age on serum levels of immunoreactive somatomedin (IRSM) in males and females. (From Bala, R.M., Lopatka, J., Leung, A., McCoy, E. and McArthur, R.G., J. Clin. Endocrinol. Metab. 52:508, 1981.)

plasma IGF II concentrations. However, in contrast to IGF I levels, there does not appear to be an increase during puberty.

Hormonal and nutritional factors exert various effects on plasma somatomedin levels. IGF I levels are elevated in acromegaly and lower than normal in patients with growth hormone deficiency. Plasma IGF II levels, in contrast, are not affected by acromegaly and decrease only slightly as a result of growth hormone deficiency. Because of the close relationship between growth hormone secretion and plasma IGF I levels, the latter is commonly used as a screening procedure for diseases of growth hormone secretion. Plasma IGF I levels are elevated during pregnancy. However, as noted earlier, they are decreased by the administration of pharmacological amounts of estrogens. The increase during pregnancy is probably promoted by placental lactogen. In patients with hypothyroidism, plasma IGF I levels are markedly depressed, and they increase in response to thyroid hormone treatment.

Protein malnutrition in children causes a decrease in plasma IGF I levels. Fasting also decreases IGF I levels even though it increases growth hormone secretion. A number of diseases, including hepatic and renal failure, are also associated with a decline in serum IGF I concentrations. The mechanisms responsible for the decreases in plasma somatomedin levels in certain illnesses are not as yet understood.

Platelet-Derived Growth Factor

It has been recognized for a number of years that platelets produce growth factors that play a role in wound healing by promoting mitosis. One of those factors, the platelet-derived growth factor (PDGF), has been purified and found to be a peptide having two chains and a molecular weight between 28,000 and 35,000. This peptide promotes the growth of fibroblasts and smooth muscle cells.

PDGF is one of the growth factors that promotes cellular growth by acting as a "competence factor," that is, by initiating cellular processes essential for mitosis to occur. This process of initiation is manifested by PDGF-stimulation of membrane protein phosphorylation in target cells and by stimulation of protein synthesis. Once cells become competent, they are able to undergo mitosis in response to appropriate stimuli. Cytosol from PDGF stimulated cells is able to transfer this state of competence to cells that have not been exposed to PDGF.

It has been proposed that PDGF may be involved in the development of atherosclerosis. Damage to the walls of blood vessels caused by the formation of atherosclerotic plaques might attract platelets, and the subsequent release of PDGF might initiate proliferation of arterial smooth muscle cells, which could result in further narrowing of the arterial lumen. Consequently, investigators are now trying to find ways to inhibit the production or release of PDGF; they are also attempting to determine if such an approach would diminish the vascular damage resulting from atherosclerosis.

Fibroblast Growth Factors

Fibroblast growth factors (FGF), substances that have been isolated from pituitary glands and from brains, promote the proliferation of many different endodermal and mesodermal cells. FGF is a peptide having a molecular weight of approximately 13,000. Like PDGF, it seems to stimulate cell proliferation by acting as a competence factor. Little is known about the physiological significance of FGF or of the factors that influence its production.

Epidermal Growth Factor

Epidermal growth factor (EGF), which is produced in a variety of tissues, is a 53 amino acid peptide containing three disulfide bonds. It is derived from a larger precursor consisting of two molecules of EGF and two molecules of a binding subunit. The binding subunit also serves to cleave the larger precursor molecule, producing the active peptide. The structure of human EGF is quite similar to that of urogastrone, the peptide that has been isolated from the urine of pregnant women and that inhibits gastric secretion.

Although the effects of EGF are exerted primarily on ectodermal cells, some mesodermal cells are also affected. EGF stimulates epithelial cell proliferation. Since it has been identified in amniotic fluid, some investigators have proposed that EGF might be an important fetal growth factor having a role in epithelial proliferation and differentiation. EGF has been identified in human breast milk, and receptors for EGF are found in human placental membranes. The mitogenic effects of EGF are greatest in the presence of other growth factors such as somatomedins.

EGF initiates its effects by interactions with membrane receptors in target tissues. The EGF receptor is a tyrosine-specific kinase that upon activation phosphorylates its own tyrosine residues. The receptors for various other peptide growth factors have similar characteristics. After binding, the hormone-receptor complex is internalized by the process of pinocytosis. It is not yet known whether internalization plays any role in the actions of EGF, but at least some of the hormone-receptor complex is destroyed by lysosomal enzymes.

Little is known about the factors affecting EGF production in humans. Some animal studies indicate that androgens and thyroid hormones stimulate EGF production. Recent observations indicate that some tumors produce EGF-like factors that may be of significance in the tissue growth abnormalities associated with cancer.

Erythropoietin

Erythropoietin is a sialoprotein involved in the **regulation of erythropoiesis.** The compound has a molecular weight of approximately 39,000 and is produced primarily by the kidneys. Erythropoietin stimulates the proliferation of primitive hematopoietic stem cells as well as of proerythrocytes, resulting in the formation of mature cells able to produce hemoglobin.

The major factor in the regulation of erythropoietin production is tissue oxygenation. Hypoxia stimulates erythropoietin formation by the kidney. Production is also increased by some hormones, including androgens and growth hormone. As a result, androgens are useful in the treatment of patients suffering from aplastic anemia, a disease in which the bone marrow does not produce adequate numbers of erythrocytes.

Nerve Growth Factor

Nerve growth factor (NGF), a protein having a molecular weight of about 130,000, is made up of dimers, each of which consists of three subunits. The β subunit, a 118 amino acid peptide, is the biologically active component. The γ subunit is believed to have a role in cleaving the active β subunit from the larger precursor molecule. The function of the third component, the α subunit, is unknown.

It is generally believed that the actions of NGF are of greatest importance during fetal life, during which time the growth of ganglia is stimulated. It has also been proposed that NGF functions postnatally in maintaining the sympathetic nervous system. Since mitogenic effects have not been demonstrated, NGF is generally considered to be a differentiating factor rather than a mitogenic agent.

A number of tissues have been found to produce NGF. Although little is known about the regulation of NGF production in humans, in animal studies it has been found that NGF production is stimulated by androgens. In addition, thyroid hormones increase NGF concentrations in brain. This has led to the hypothesis that the effects of thyroid hormones on brain development may be mediated by NGF.

Thymic Peptides

Peptides known as thymosins and thymopoietins have been isolated from the thymus gland and have been shown to promote the growth and maturation of lymphoid cells. Thymopoietin is a single-chain peptide containing 49 amino acids; it stimulates the differentiation of prothymocytes into mature T cells. Thymosin, a smaller peptide containing 28 amino acids, stimulates lymphocyte proliferation. Although the physiological significance of these peptides has not yet been established, both may be of use in the treatment of certain types of immune disorders.

Interleukins

The interleukins are peptides that are produced by lymphocytes and that are involved in the proliferation and maturation of lymphocytes. Three different interleukins, known as interleukins I, II, and III, have been identified. Interleukin I is produced by monocyte macrophages and is also known as lymphocyte-activating factor. A single-chain peptide, it has been found to exert several effects, including stimulation of thymocyte mitosis and of the growth of activated T cells, and induction of T cell reactivity and of lymphocyte rejection capabilities. The production of interleukin I is stimulated by endotoxin or by exposure of macrophages to antigen.

Interleukin II is produced by lymphoid and spleen cells, and its formation is stimulated by interleukin I. Interleukin II has a molecular weight of about 15,000; interleukin III is a glycosylated peptide having a molecular weight of about 28,000. The actions of interleukins II and III are similar; both compounds stimulate the growth and differentiation of lymphocytes. Even though little is known about the physiological significance or regulation of the interleukins, these peptides are of potential clinical value in the treatment of diseases involving the lymphoid system.

REFERENCES

Antoniades, H.N. and Owen, A.J.: Growth factors and regulation of cell growth. Ann. Rev. Med. 33:445, 1982.

Cooke, P.S. and Nicoll, C.S.: Hormonal control of fetal growth. The Physiologist 26:317, 1983.

Daughaday, W.H.: The anterior pituitary. In Williams' Textbook of Endocrinology, 7th ed. J.D. Wilson and D.W. Foster, editors. W.B. Saunders Company, Philadelphia, p. 568, 1985.

Isaksson, O.G.P., Eden, S., and Jansson, J.: Mode of action of pituitary growth hormone on target cells. Ann. Rev. Physiol. 47:483, 1985.

Raisz, L.G. and Kream, B.E.: Hormonal control of skeletal growth. Ann. Rev. Physiol. 43:225, 1981.

Rosenfeld, R.L.: Somatic growth and maturation. In Endocrinology, Vol. 3, DeGroot, L.J., et al., editors. Grune & Stratton, New York, p. 1805, 1979.

Underwood, L.E. and Van Wyk, J.J.: Normal and aberrant growth. In Williams' Textbook of Endocrinology, 7th ed. J.D. Wilson and D.W. Foster, editors. W.B. Saunders Company, Philadelphia, p. 155, 1985.

15

OVERVIEW OF FUEL METABOLISM

INTRODUCTION

Humans, like all living organisms, require energy to survive. Even at rest, the normal adult uses approximately 1800 Calories/day. This basal energy consumption is used for essential muscular activity (e.g., respiratory and cardiac muscle), for maintenance of cell structure and the intracellular environment (e.g., protein synthesis and ion transport), and for maintenance of extracellular homeostasis (e.g., synthesis and secretion of hormones). The amount of energy used by any individual in excess of the basal rate depends on the amount of physical activity; the total energy requirements of an adult average 2500 Calories/day, but can vary from 2000 to 5000 Calories/day.

To meet these energy needs, the body must take in the equivalent amount of energy in the form of organic molecules that can be metabolized. The major dietary source of energy for humans is **carbohydrate** (Table 15–1),

TABLE 15–1. Dietary Sources of Energy

Source	Energy Content (Cal/gm)	Dietary Intake (gm/day)	Average Total Energy Intake (Cal/day)
Carbohydrate	4.1	300–400	1400
Fat	9.3	60–100	750
Protein	4.4	70–90	350

which can come in the form of simple sugars (e.g., glucose) or more commonly as disaccharides (sucrose, lactose) or polysaccharides (starch). **Fat**, most of which consists of triglycerides, is the second major energy source; it is the most efficient source of energy, providing twice as many calories/gram as carbohydrate (Table 15–1). Although **protein** represents a relatively small percentage of the total dietary energy intake, it provides the amino acids that are essential components of enzymes and structural proteins.

At a superficial level, fuel metabolism appears relatively simple: the amount of energy in the diet must be sufficient to meet the energy needs of the body. This simple relationship, however, is complicated by two important considerations. First, dietary fuel intake is intermittent, not continuous. Consequently, the excess energy absorbed during a meal must be stored for use during periods when dietary sources are not available. There are three major forms of energy storage in the body (Table 15–2). Carbohydrates are stored as **glycogen** in liver and muscle. Glycogen, however, is a relatively small energy reservoir; the amount of energy stored as glycogen is not sufficient to meet a single day's needs. The major site of energy storage is adipose tissue, where there is sufficient **triglyceride** to provide energy for several weeks. Consequently, during any prolonged period of fasting, the free fatty acids released from adipose tissue serve as the primary source of energy for most tissues. There is also a significant amount of energy stored as **protein**, primarily in muscle (Table 15–2). Protein, however, is a relatively expensive source of energy because it serves other essential functions.

The second factor complicating fuel metabolism is that several tissues, most notably the **brain**, are normally dependent on **glucose** as a source of

TABLE 15–2. Major Sites and Forms of Energy Storage

Storage Form	Site of Storage	Amount Stored (gm)	Energy Content (Calories)
Glycogen	Liver	75	300
	Muscle	300	1200
Fat (triglyceride)	Adipose	15,000	140,000
	Muscle	300	2,800
Protein	Muscle	10,000	41,000

energy. Consequently, it is essential that blood glucose concentrations be maintained above a critical level. Hepatic glycogen is an important reservoir of glucose that can be used to maintain normoglycemia during a short fast. However, hepatic glycogen is depleted relatively quickly so that another source of glucose must be found. Protein can be readily converted to glucose via gluconeogenesis, whereas fat cannot. Once glycogen stores are depleted, catabolism of protein and conversion of amino acids to glucose becomes the primary means for meeting the energy requirements of glucose-dependent tissues.

As already noted, the disposition of organic molecules depends on the metabolic conditions. During a meal, ingested fuels are channeled into storage as glycogen, triglyceride, and protein. Between meals these energy stores are called upon to provide energy and to maintain plasma glucose concentrations. The flow along these metabolic pathways is influenced by a variety of hormones, including insulin, glucagon, epinephrine, cortisol, thyroid hormones, and growth hormone. The specific effects of each of these hormones on fuel metabolism have been considered in detail in previous chapters. This chapter will describe how these hormones interact in the overall control of fuel metabolism. First, some of the major actions of these hormones on fuel metabolism and their physiological significance will be reviewed. The interaction of these hormones will then be illustrated by describing the responses to different metabolic states.

HORMONAL REGULATION OF FUEL METABOLISM

Under most circumstances, **insulin** is the dominant hormonal regulator of fuel metabolism. Insulin can be thought of as an anabolic hormone; it lowers circulating concentrations of glucose, free fatty acids, and amino acids and promotes their storage as glycogen, triglyceride, and protein, respectively. Some of the major actions of insulin include stimulation of glucose uptake and conversion to glycogen in liver and muscle, inhibition of lipolysis in liver and adipose tissue, and stimulation of protein synthesis in muscle (Table 15–3). Although insulin promotes energy storage, all of its actions are readily reversible so that a fall in insulin concentrations will cause energy mobilization. In fact, changes in insulin secretion are important to fuel metabolism both during a meal (when plasma insulin levels are elevated) and between meals (when plasma insulin is low). The importance of insulin to normal fuel metabolism is perhaps best illustrated by the dramatic metabolic changes that occur in untreated diabetics (Chapter 12), changes that cannot be compensated for by any of the other hormones affecting fuel metabolism.

Glucagon is probably the second most important hormone, after insulin, in the normal control of fuel metabolism. The primary action of glucagon is to protect against hypoglycemia by stimulating liver glycogenolysis and glucone-

TABLE 15–3. Major Direct Metabolic Actions of Hormones

	Insulin	Glucagon	Epinephrine	Growth Hormone
Glycogenolysis	D	I	I	N
Gluconeogenesis	D	I	I	N
Blood glucose	D	I	I	N
Lipolysis	D	I	I	I
Blood FFA	D	I	I	I
Protein catabolism	D	N	N	D
Blood amino acids	D	N	N	D

D = Decreases; I = Increases; N = Not usually affected.
For simplicity only the catabolic actions are indicated. In most cases the hormones exert the opposite effect on anabolic reactions (e.g., insulin increases protein synthesis). Cortisol and thyroid hormones were not included because most of their actions on fuel metabolism are permissive.

ogenesis (Table 15–3). Glucagon also stimulates lipolysis in the liver but has no physiologically important effects on muscle or adipose tissue. Although the effects of glucagon are opposite to those of insulin, secretion of these two hormones is usually inversely related. Consequently, insulin and glucagon normally act in concert to maintain glucose homeostasis.

Epinephrine, like glucagon, stimulates hepatic glycogenolysis and gluconeogenesis. However, its more potent actions are on muscle and adipose tissue, in which it stimulates glycogenolysis and lipolysis, respectively (Table 15–3). The stimulation of lipolysis produces an increase in circulating free fatty acids, while glycogen breakdown in muscle leads to the release of lactate. The latter serves as a precursor for hepatic gluconeogenesis. Epinephrine plays only a minor role, at most, in the regulation of fuel metabolism under resting conditions but is important for the metabolic responses to stress and exercise.

Although **growth hormone** influences certain aspects of fuel metabolism, it is normally of little importance to the overall regulation of these processes. Growth hormone has protein anabolic effects in muscle but has catabolic effects on carbohydrate and fat metabolism. An increase in growth hormone can thus elevate plasma glucose and free fatty acid levels under some circumstances. However, circulating concentrations of these substances are not normally correlated with changes in growth hormone secretion.

The major metabolic effect of **cortisol**, and other glucocorticoids, is stimulation of hepatic gluconeogenesis. Cortisol also promotes protein catabolism in muscle, thus increasing the supply of gluconeogenic precursors. Most of the other actions of cortisol on fuel metabolism are permissive in that they allow other hormones to exert their full effects (e.g., epinephrine-induced lipolysis is enhanced by cortisol), but do not exert independent actions. Because of these permissive effects, adequate cortisol levels are a prerequisite for normal fuel metabolism; however, changes in cortisol secretion do not contribute significantly to the metabolic responses to feeding or fasting.

The actions of **thyroid hormones** are similar to those of cortisol in that they are permissive for normal metabolic responses. Thyroid hormones are generally catabolic; they tend to stimulate glycogenolysis, lipolysis, and protein catabolism. However, because their actions are quite slow in onset, changes in thyroid hormones are usually not important for fuel homeostasis.

It is interesting to note that, with the exception of the anabolic effects of growth hormone on protein metabolism, all of the actions of glucagon, epinephrine, cortisol, growth hormone, and thyroid hormones are opposite to those of insulin. Because of this insulin antagonism, these five hormones are often referred to as "counterregulatory hormones," with insulin being the "regulatory" hormone. However, as already noted for glucagon, the secretion of most of these hormones is also normally "counter," or inversely related, to insulin release. The net result is that these hormones usually act in concert with insulin to maintain normal fuel homeostasis.

METABOLIC RESPONSE TO STARVATION

The metabolic state that perhaps best illustrates the interplay of hormonal and nonhormonal factors in the regulation of metabolism is starvation. The metabolic changes that occur in starvation permit survival for months in the absence of any caloric intake. Some of those changes are mediated by hormones, most notably **insulin**, but other factors are also important. The metabolic adaptations that occur in starvation serve to meet the energy needs of normally glucose-dependent tissues such as the brain and at the same time minimize protein degradation.

Although starvation is not a major problem in the United States or in other western societies, in some parts of the world it is a very serious medical problem. In addition, starvation often accompanies certain debilitating diseases and, as a result of excessive protein wasting, may contribute to the cause of death. In this section, the changes in metabolism that occur in starvation will be described temporally beginning immediately after food intake and continuing through prolonged starvation. The role of various hormones in mediating these changes will also be discussed.

Metabolism in the Fed State

Immediately after a meal, absorption of the various nutrients results in high blood levels of glucose, fatty acids, and amino acids. The high circulating glucose concentration stimulates insulin secretion and decreases the secretion of glucagon (Fig. 15–1). Such a hormonal milieu, and in particular the high insulin levels, promotes the conversion of nutrients to their storage forms. Thus, glycogen synthesis is enhanced and glycogenolysis inhibited, resulting in an increase in **glycogen deposition** in the liver (Fig. 15–1). Similarly, in adi-

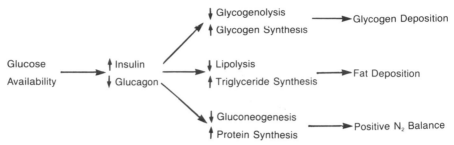

FIGURE 15–1. Metabolic and hormonal events during the fed state.

pose tissue there is relatively little lipolytic activity and a stimulation of triglyceride synthesis, resulting in **fat deposition**. Protein synthesis is also enhanced, as a result of a decrease in gluconeogenesis and an increase in amino acid uptake by muscle, creating a **positive nitrogen balance** (Fig. 15–1). Thus, at times of nutrient availability, metabolic fuels are stored for subsequent use when needed.

Metabolism in the Postabsorptive State

During the postabsorptive period (6 to 12 hours after food intake), a number of hormonal and metabolic changes occur; these represent the transition from the fed to the fasted state. The postprandial decline in blood glucose levels causes a decrease in insulin secretion and serves as a stimulus for glucagon secretion (Fig. 15–2). This change in hormonal environment has a variety of metabolic consequences that can generally be classified as catabolic (Fig. 15–3). **Glycogenolysis is enhanced** to meet the glucose needs of the brain and **glycogen synthesis decreases,** ultimately leading to depletion of hepatic glycogen. **Gluconeogenesis also increases,** with alanine being the principal amino acid substrate used by the liver for glucose production. During the postabsorptive period, the liver accounts for virtually all of the body's glucose production. Approximately 75 per cent is derived from glycogenolysis and 25 per cent from gluconeogenesis. The glucose produced is used principally by the brain.

The hormonal changes that occur during this period also have profound effects on fat and protein metabolism. **Triglyceride synthesis decreases and lipolysis is stimulated**, resulting in the increased release of free fatty acids. The free fatty acids are used to meet the energy needs of most tissues including muscle and heart, thus sparing glucose for those tissues that require it. With an increase in circulating levels of free fatty acids, production of ketone bodies by the liver also increases. The **increase in ketogenesis** is the result of both the increased availability of free fatty acids as substrates and the hormonal environment, which stimulates ketogenic pathways. The hormonal milieu also contributes to the **breakdown of protein**, as a result of the increase in gluconeogenic activity and a decrease in amino acid uptake by muscle.

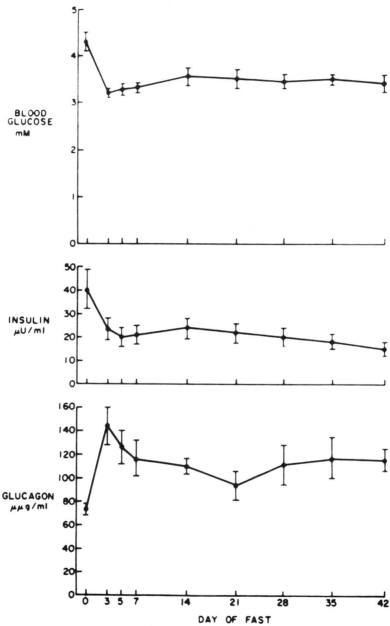

FIGURE 15–2. Blood glucose, serum insulin, and plasma glucagon levels during prolonged starvation. (From Marliss et al., J. Clin. Invest. 49: 2256, 1970.)

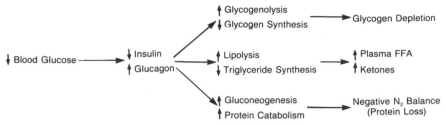

FIGURE 15–3. Metabolic and hormonal changes in response to short-term starvation.

Thus, relative to the fed state, a negative nitrogen balance exists during the postabsorptive period.

Short-Term Starvation

The metabolic changes that occur during periods of relatively short-term starvation (three to seven days) are a continuation and acceleration of the processes that began during the postabsorptive period (Fig. 15–3). The continuing decline in blood glucose levels further decreases insulin release and stimulates glucagon secretion by the pancreas. These hormonal changes in turn further **stimulate gluconeogenesis, lipolysis, and ketogenesis** (Fig. 15–3). With the depletion of hepatic glycogen stores, gluconeogenesis must provide for the glucose needs of the brain. Indeed, during this period, gluconeogenesis is two to three times greater than during the postabsorptive period and is responsible for virtually all of the glucose released by the liver. The decline in circulating insulin levels decreases glucose uptake by muscle, sparing the available glucose for the brain. The increase in gluconeogenesis during this period is associated with an **increase in protein degradation** and amino acid release by muscle. Many of the amino acids derived from protein catabolism are converted to alanine within muscle, so that there is a particularly large efflux of alanine from muscle. A corresponding increase occurs in the rate of hepatic uptake of alanine to serve as a gluconeogenic substrate. Thus, a substantial negative nitrogen balance exists, with most of the nitrogen being excreted in the urine as urea.

The other major metabolic change that occurs during short-term starvation is an **acceleration of ketogenesis**, resulting from increased circulating levels of free fatty acids and an increase in the oxidation of free fatty acids by the liver. As a result, plasma levels of ketones increase. Thus, overall metabolism during this period is characterized by high rates of protein catabolism, gluconeogenesis, and ketogenesis to meet the body's energy needs. However, because of the importance of the various functions of protein, it is a quite expensive source of carbohydrate. In fact, death resulting from starvation is not usually caused by hypoglycemia but rather by protein wasting. Thus, prolonged survival requires that gluconeogenesis be kept to a minimum while the energy needs of the brain are not compromised. As will be seen, the metabolic changes that occur during long-term starvation satisfy both require-ments.

Long-Term Starvation

The metabolic changes that occur during long-term starvation account for the ability to survive prolonged periods without any caloric intake. One major change is a **decrease in protein catabolism**. After approximately the first week of starvation, alanine release by muscle and circulating alanine levels decline (Fig. 15–4). As a consequence of the decreased availability of this gluconeo-genic substrate, hepatic glucose production decreases from about 200 gm/day during the postabsorptive period to approximately 50 gm/day during pro-longed starvation. Moreover, approximately 75 per cent of hepatic glucose production during this period is derived from non–amino acid sources (lactate, pyruvate, and glycerol). At the same time, gluconeogenesis in the kidneys be-comes an important source of carbohydrate, contributing about 40 gm/day. Most of the glucose produced by the kidneys is derived from amino acids, with the excess nitrogen being secreted as ammonia rather than urea. As a consequence of these changes, nitrogen loss progressively decreases during prolonged starvation.

It is important to note that the total hepatic and renal glucose production in prolonged starvation is substantially less than that in the postabsorptive pe-riod. Thus, if glucose consumption by the brain were unaltered, the decline in glucose production would ultimately lead to hypoglycemia and its severe consequences. However, in fact, blood glucose levels reach their minimum within about three days of starvation and subsequently remain relatively con-stant (Fig. 15–2), but, at the same time, brain function is not compromised. This apparent inconsistency is explained by the **use of ketones by the brain** as a major energy source during prolonged starvation, and a corresponding

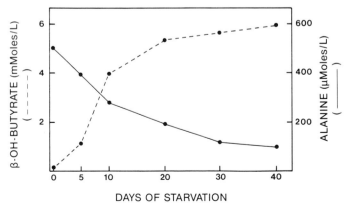

FIGURE 15–4. Plasma levels of alanine and β-OH-butyrate during starvation.

decrease in its use of glucose. Thus, glucose consumption is approximately equal to glucose production, maintaining blood glucose levels and still satisfying the energy needs of the brain.

Both of the major metabolic adaptations to prolonged starvation are attributable to high circulating ketone levels at that time (Fig. 15–5). Blood ketone levels continue to rise for several weeks during starvation (Fig. 15–4), although ketogenesis reaches its maximum within about one week. This apparent discrepancy is attributable to a progressive decline in ketone utilization by muscle with increasing duration of starvation, as well as an increase in the reabsorption of ketones by the kidney, decreasing ketone losses in the urine. The consequent increase in circulating ketone bodies does not produce ketoacidosis, because the ammonia production resulting from renal gluconeogenesis causes a compensatory increase in hydrogen ion excretion. One important consequence of the elevation of plasma ketone bodies is an increased utilization of ketones by the brain. The brain is capable of oxidizing ketones quite early in starvation, but only when blood levels become sufficiently high do ketones serve as a major energy source. The high blood levels of ketones also appear to be responsible for the decrease in gluconeogenesis that occurs in prolonged starvation. Ketones directly inhibit proteolysis in muscle and decrease alanine release by muscle, which decreases the amount of substrate available for gluconeogenesis. Thus, ketones both decrease hepatic glucose production and serve as an alternative energy source for the brain. As a result of these ketone-induced changes, the two major requirements for survival during prolonged starvation are met—namely, maintenance of blood glucose levels and conservation of protein.

Role of Hormones in the Metabolic Adaptation to Starvation

Insulin and Glucagon. The two hormones of greatest importance in the adaptation to starvation are insulin and glucagon. The roles of these hormones have been noted during the discussion of the metabolic changes that occur in starvation. Briefly, insulin secretion declines early in starvation and remains low throughout starvation (see Fig. 15–2). This initiates many of the metabolic responses that are characteristic of starvation, including **glycogenolysis, gluconeogenesis, proteolysis, and ketogenesis.** The increase in glucagon secretion early in starvation seems to be important for the maintenance of glycogenoly-

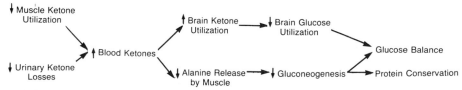

FIGURE 15–5. Metabolic adaptation to long-term starvation.

sis as well as for the stimulation of gluconeogenesis. Since plasma glucagon returns to control levels by about the third day of starvation (Fig. 15–2), it is unlikely that this hormone plays a significant role in the metabolic adaptation to more long-term starvation.

Growth Hormone. Growth hormone does not appear to be essential for either the increase in lipolysis occurring during starvation or for the protein conservation characteristic of late starvation. Although growth hormone levels are elevated in early starvation, they return to control values within about a week, whereas lipolysis continues to be increased. In addition, growth hormone deficiency does not diminish the lipolytic response to starvation. However, in growth hormone–deficient individuals, the fall in blood glucose levels in response to starvation is greater than in normal individuals. Thus, growth hormone appears to contribute to the **maintenance of blood glucose** concentrations during starvation.

Catecholamines. Catecholamines appear to be relatively unimportant in the metabolic adaptation to starvation. Plasma norepinephrine levels are elevated early in starvation, but plasma epinephrine concentrations do not change. As noted in Chapter 13, the effects of norepinephrine on metabolic processes are far less potent than those of epinephrine. Furthermore, β-adrenergic blocking agents have little effect on the increases in glycogenolysis and lipolysis that occur in response to starvation.

Glucocorticoids. Glucocorticoids do not appear to be important for the changes in protein metabolism that occur during starvation. Protein wasting is not accelerated in patients with Cushing's syndrome. Neither the increase in gluconeogenesis seen early in starvation nor the conservation of protein occurring in late starvation is correlated with changes in plasma cortisol levels. However, cortisol, like growth hormone, appears to contribute to the **maintenance of adequate blood glucose** levels during the course of starvation.

Thyroid Hormones. Starvation causes a dramatic decrease in plasma levels of free triiodothyronine (T_3) and a corresponding increase in reverse T_3 concentrations. These changes are caused by a **shift in the pattern of peripheral thyroxine (T_4) metabolism** in starvation, such that less of the T_4 is converted to the highly potent hormone T_3 and more to the inactive compound reverse T_3. Thus, this change in metabolism is probably responsible for the decrease in the basal metabolic rate that usually occurs with prolonged fasting.

METABOLIC RESPONSES TO STRESS AND EXERCISE

The endocrine and metabolic responses to stress and to exercise are similar. Although there are some significant differences, the responses to both stress and exercise involve activation of the sympathetic nervous system, alterations in insulin, epinephrine, and glucagon secretion, and increases in free fatty acid and glucose production.

Response to Stress

As noted in Chapter 13, the overall metabolic response to stress is appropriate for the "fight-or-flight" syndrome. Namely, there is an increase in circulating glucose and free fatty acids to provide additional energy for brain and muscle, respectively. The hyperglycemia and hyperlipidemia caused by stress represent the end result of a sequence of neuroendocrine events illustrated in Figure 15–6. Initially, exposure to a stressful situation **stimulates ACTH** secretion from the anterior pituitary and **activates the sympathetic nervous system**. The increase in circulating ACTH **stimulates cortisol** release from the adrenal cortex while the increase in sympathetic tone has three important actions: it **stimulates glucagon** and **inhibits insulin** secretion from the pancreas, and it produces a massive **outpouring of epinephrine** from the adrenal medulla.

These hormonal changes then act in concert to stimulate glucose production by the liver and free fatty acid release from adipose tissue. The decrease in insulin and increases in glucagon and epinephrine all promote hepatic glycogenolysis, and the changes in these hormones and cortisol favor hepatic gluconeogenesis (see Table 15–3). Consequently, glucose production by the liver increases and hyperglycemia results. At the same time, the fall in insulin and increase in epinephrine stimulate lipolysis in adipose tissue, increasing plasma free fatty acid concentrations. The increase in cortisol output also contributes to free fatty acid release by enhancing the lipolytic actions of epinephrine.

These hormonal changes have several other actions that potentiate their primary metabolic effects. Epinephrine stimulates glucagon and inhibits insulin secretion so that the initial changes in these two hormones induced by sympathetic nerves are maintained. In the absence of epinephrine secretion by the adrenal medulla, the hyperglycemia caused by stress would stimulate insulin and suppress glucagon release and the elevation in plasma glucose would not be sustained. Epinephrine also stimulates blood flow to muscle and brain, in which energy needs are greatest during stress. Finally, the hypoinsulinemia decreases glucose uptake by muscle, so that free fatty acids become the primary energy source for muscle, and glucose is spared for the brain.

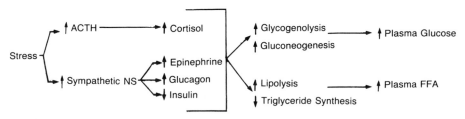

FIGURE 15–6. Metabolic response to stress.

Response to Exercise

The metabolic response to exercise depends upon the severity and duration of exercise. During mild exercise and the early stages of heavy exercise, local changes within muscle are dominant. The primary energy source used is muscle glycogen, possibly supplemented by muscle triglyceride. There is also an increase in blood flow to the exercising muscle, thus increasing the delivery of glucose and free fatty acids for oxidation.

During heavy exercise, blood glucose and free fatty acids replace local energy stores as the primary energy sources for muscle contraction. Heavy exercise activates the **sympathetic nervous system**, thus increasing **epinephrine** and **glucagon** secretion and inhibiting **insulin** release. The changes in these three hormones stimulate hepatic glucose production and mobilize free fatty acids from adipose tissue, as occurs in response to stress (Fig. 15–6). In this case, however, the increased production of these substances is balanced by increased utilization in muscle, so that marked changes in plasma glucose and free fatty acid levels do not occur.

CONCLUSION

This chapter has focused on the role of hormones in the regulation of fuel metabolism, but it is important to realize that other factors also contribute to the overall control of metabolism. For example, the rate of food intake, which is generally not under hormonal control, can obviously have a major impact on the body's energy stores. In fact, the most common clinical conditions resulting from abnormalities in fuel metabolism, malnutrition and obesity, are not usually the result of endocrine abnormalities.

The examples given to illustrate the interplay of various hormones in the regulation of metabolism are representative of the endocrine responses to a wide variety of different metabolic states. In general, an alteration in insulin secretion is the major determinant of the metabolic adaptation to any particular situation. In addition, secretion of one or more counterregulatory hormones (e.g., glucagon or epinephrine) usually changes in a direction opposite to that of insulin. Consequently, insulin and the counterregulatory hormones act in concert to achieve the appropriate metabolic response to the initial perturbation.

REFERENCES

Cahill, G.F.: Starvation in man. N. Engl. J. Med. 282:668, 1970.
Felig, P.: Starvation. In Endocrinology, Vol. 3, L.J. DeGroot, et al., editors. Grune and Stratton, New York, p. 1927, 1979.
Kinney, J.M. and Felig, P.: The metabolic response to injury and infection. In Endocrinology, Vol. 3, L.J. DeGroot, et al., editors. Grune and Stratton, New York, p. 1963, 1979.
Wahren, J.: Metabolic adaptation to physical exercise in man. In Endocrinology, Vol. 3, L.J. DeGroot, et al., editors. Grune and Stratton, New York, p. 1911, 1979.

16

CONTROL OF CALCIUM AND PHOSPHATE METABOLISM

INTRODUCTION

Calcium and phosphate metabolism encompasses the movement of these two ions into and out of the body, and among different compartments within the body, as well as the mechanisms regulating these movements. Of these two ions, calcium is much more tightly regulated than phosphate, and control of calcium metabolism will be the primary focus of this chapter. Calcium metabolism is regulated by three hormonal agents: **parathyroid hormone (PTH), calcitonin (CT)** and **vitamin D**. These agents participate in two types of control systems, each system regulating a different aspect of calcium metabolism. One system is responsible for **calcium homeostasis**, the minute-to-minute regulation of plasma calcium. Because this system is extremely sensitive, plasma calcium is one of the most tightly controlled variables in the body; plasma concentrations vary less than 5 per cent in normal adults. The other system is responsible for **calcium balance**. This system ensures that over the long term (i.e., weeks to months) calcium intake is equivalent to calcium excretion.

The tight regulation of plasma calcium is indicative of the physiological importance of this ion. Intracellular calcium concentrations control a variety of cellular processes including muscle contraction, stimulus-secretion coupling in nerves, exocytosis of hormones, and the activity of numerous enzymes. Plasma calcium is critical for such functions as the coagulation of blood, the maintenance of tight junctions between cells, and the stability of cell membranes. The latter action is particularly important for excitable tissue. Hypocalcemia causes spontaneous action potentials in muscles and nerves, which can lead to tetany in respiratory and other skeletal muscles and can result in death by asphyxiation. Finally, the calcium in bone and teeth is essential for the structural and functional integrity of these tissues.

Phosphates, which are regulated by the same endocrine systems that control calcium metabolism, are also critical for a number of physiological functions. Inorganic phosphate contributes to the structural integrity of bone and teeth and functions as a hydrogen ion buffer in plasma. Phosphate that is conjugated to organic molecules, however, is probably more important than inorganic phosphate. Organic phosphate is an essential component of a large number of biologically important molecules including nucleic acids (RNA and DNA), adenosine triphosphate (ATP), cyclic AMP, and membrane phospholipids. Because circulating inorganic phosphates serve primarily as substrates for the synthesis of organic phosphate, plasma phosphate concentrations need not be as finely regulated as plasma calcium levels.

OVERVIEW OF CALCIUM METABOLISM

Calcium Compartments in the Body

The body contains approximately one kilogram of calcium distributed among three major compartments: bone, intracellular fluid, and extracellular fluid. Approximately 99 per cent of this calcium is in **bone**, primarily in the form of **hydroxyapatite**, a complex crystal containing calcium, phosphate, and water. Hydroxyapatite comprises about 75 per cent of mature compact bone and is responsible for the compressional strength of bone. A small amount (less than 0.5 per cent) of the calcium in bone exists as amorphous crystals or is in solution. This small calcium pool is in dynamic equilibrium with calcium in the extracellular fluid and is important for the maintenance of plasma calcium concentrations.

The second largest pool of calcium in the body is **intracellular** calcium. There are about 10 gm of calcium in this pool, most of which is either bound to proteins or sequestered in the mitochondria and endoplasmic reticulum.

Under basal conditions, cytosolic calcium concentrations are quite low, ranging from 10^{-8} to 10^{-7} moles/liter. These low calcium levels are maintained by energy-dependent membrane pumps that actively transport calcium out of the cytosol into the extracellular fluid, mitochondria, and endoplasmic reticulum. In many cells, cytosolic calcium concentrations increase dramatically when the cell is stimulated, and the rise in calcium triggers a functional response characteristic of the particular cell (e.g., muscle contraction or hormone secretion).

Plasma calcium concentrations average 2.5 mmoles/liter in the normal adult. Approximately half of this calcium is either bound to plasma proteins or complexed with phosphate (Table 16–1). As with hormones, only the free calcium is biologically active and subject to regulation. Most of the protein-bound calcium is noncovalently attached to albumin; therefore, if serum albumin concentrations increase or decrease, total plasma calcium will change accordingly. However, under these conditions, hormonal regulation ensures that the biologically active free calcium is not affected. Because the free calcium in plasma can pass readily into the interstitial fluid, interstitial fluid and free plasma calcium are considered a single pool, usually referred to as **extracellular fluid (ECF)** calcium. Although this pool contains only about 1 gm of calcium, it plays a crucial role in calcium metabolism. Calcium in the ECF is in equilibrium with calcium in the other compartments, and it is the ECF calcium concentrations that are under tight hormonal control.

Calcium Exchanges

Regulation of calcium metabolism is achieved by controlling the movement of calcium between the ECF and three other compartments: the gastrointestinal tract, the kidneys, and bone. Calcium exchange also occurs between the intracellular compartment and the ECF, but this exchange is not under hormonal control and does not contribute to the maintenance of ECF calcium concentrations.

Intestinal Absorption of Calcium. Dietary intake of calcium varies widely among individuals but averages approximately 1 gm/day in normal adults. Approximately 0.4 gm of this calcium is absorbed, primarily in the ileum and jejunum (Fig. 16–1). However, 0.2 gm/day of calcium is also secreted into the intestine with the digestive enzymes. Consequently, the daily net absorption

TABLE 16–1.   States of Calcium in Plasma

Form	Concentration	Percentage of Total
Free ionized	1.1 mM	44
Protein-bound	1.2 mM	48
Complexed to anions	0.2 mM	8

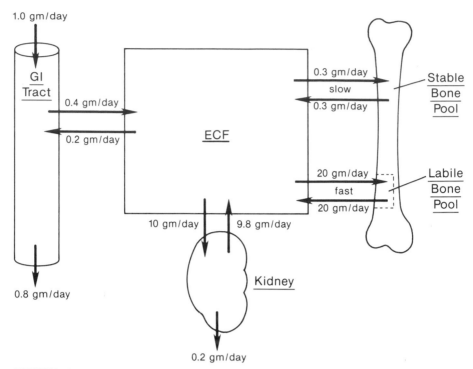

FIGURE 16–1. Average daily movements of calcium between extracellular fluid (ECF) and the gastrointestinal (GI) tract, kidney, and bone.

of calcium is 0.2 gm, with the rest of the calcium ingested (0.8 gm) being excreted in the feces.

Calcium absorption occurs via two mechanisms: passive diffusion and active transport. **Passive diffusion** is not saturable and occurs only at high intestinal calcium concentrations so that quantitatively it is less important than the active transport mechanism. **Active transport** of calcium occurs in two steps. Calcium first diffuses down its concentration gradient from the intestinal lumen into the intestinal cell, a process that is mediated by carrier proteins in the mucosal cell membrane. Calcium is then actively transported from the cell into the ECF by calcium pumps located on the serosal surface of this cell. This active transport system is saturable so that the intestinal absorption of calcium is self-limiting; if high levels of calcium are ingested, the transport system can handle only a small portion of the calcium and consequently the percentage of ingested calcium that is absorbed decreases. The rate of active transport also varies with dietary calcium, increasing with low calcium intake and decreasing with high dietary calcium. As described later, these changes in calcium absorption are mediated by vitamin D.

In contrast to calcium absorption, secretion of calcium into the gastrointestinal tract does not vary with calcium intake. Changes in secretion are thus not important in the regulation of calcium metabolism. However, under hypocalcemic conditions, calcium secretion into the gastrointestinal tract continues unabated. This can become an important route by which calcium is lost from the body.

Renal Excretion of Calcium. Approximately 10 gm of calcium per day are filtered by the renal tubules; 9.8 gm/day are reabsorbed, and 0.2 gm/day are excreted in the urine (Fig. 16–1). Note that the rate of calcium excretion in the urine equals the net rate of calcium absorption into the ECF. This state of calcium balance is generally found in normal adults but not in growing children, in whom calcium intake exceeds calcium excretion.

Between 50 and 60 per cent of the filtered calcium is reabsorbed in the **proximal tubule**. Reabsorption in the proximal tubule is not saturable and is not under hormonal control. Approximately 10 per cent of the filtered calcium is reabsorbed in the ascending loop of Henle and the remainder in the distal tubule. Calcium reabsorption in the **distal tubule** is an active process that becomes saturated when plasma calcium concentrations are greater than normal. The saturability of calcium reabsorption serves a homeostatic function; in hypercalcemia, urinary calcium excretion will automatically increase as the reabsorptive mechanisms in the distal tubule become saturated. Reabsorption in the distal tubule is also under hormonal control so that the rate of reabsorption increases in hypocalcemic conditions and decreases during hypercalcemia.

Calcium Exchange Between Bone and ECF. Two quantitatively distinct exchanges of calcium occur between bone and ECF. A **slow exchange**, 0.3 gm/day, occurs between ECF and most of the calcium in bone, whereas a **fast exchange** of 20 gm/day occurs between a small pool of bone calcium (about 4 gm) and ECF (Fig. 16–1). The latter pool is called **labile** bone calcium, whereas the rest of the calcium in bone comprises the **stable** pool.

The slow exchange represents a process known as **bone remodeling**, which occurs continuously in the adult. Bone remodeling allows mature bone to adapt to changes in the stress exerted on it and to repair fractures. The first step in this process is resorption of existing bone by **osteoclasts**. Osteoclasts release acids that dissolve hydroxyapatite crystals and enzymes that break down the organic matrix of bone. These cells usually operate in concert to create a tunnel several millimeters long and up to 1 mm in diameter. Bone is then deposited in this tunnel by **osteoblasts**. Osteoblasts lay down collagen, the organic matrix of bone, in concentric cylinders on the inner surface of the tunnel. Hydroxyapatite crystals then slowly mineralize these layers. As a consequence of this method of formation, most bone in the body is composed of parallel columns, referred to as **osteons** (or haversian systems). At the center of each osteon is a canal containing the blood vessels and nerves innervating that region of the bone (Fig. 16–2).

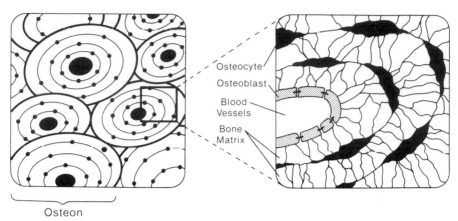

Osteon

FIGURE 16–2. Structure of the osteon, the functional unit of bone, shown in cross section at two magnifications.

To understand the fast exchange of calcium between bone and ECF, a more detailed description of the osteon is required. Once formation of an osteon is complete, the osteoblasts remain on the innermost surface of the tunnel, forming a cell layer between the bone matrix and blood vessels in the inner canal (Fig. 16–2). The other important cells in the osteon are the **osteocytes**, which are osteoblasts that were trapped within the bone matrix as it mineralized. The osteocytes and osteoblasts are connected by an extensive network of small canals that allows substances to be exchanged between osteocytes and the circulation. These small canals also contain cytoplasmic extensions of osteocytes and osteoblasts that are connected to each other by tight junctions. This cell network thus establishes a continuous membrane that separates the bone minerals from ECF. Movement of calcium across this "bone membrane" accounts for the fast exchange between bone and ECF. Although the mechanism of this calcium movement is not fully understood, it does not involve the breakdown or formation of bone. Instead, a small pool of calcium at the inner surface of the bone membrane is available for transport into the ECF. Because of the large surface area of osteocytes and osteoblasts, small movements of calcium across individual cells are amplified into large calcium fluxes between bone and ECF.

Both the fast and slow exchange of calcium between the bone and ECF are under hormonal control. Under normal conditions, the fast calcium exchange is much more important for the maintenance of plasma calcium concentrations than the slow exchange. Under conditions of chronic hypo- or hypercalcemia, however, hormonally induced alterations in the slow exchange can contribute to the processes that compensate for the calcium abnormality.

PARATHYROID HORMONE

Parathyroid hormone (PTH), one of the principal regulators of calcium and phosphate metabolism, is produced by the **parathyroid glands**. There are usually four parathyroid glands in humans, one located on the back surface of each of the upper and lower poles of the thyroid. Two major cell types, chief cells and oxyphil cells, are found in the parathyroid glands. **Chief cells** contain an extensive endoplasmic reticulum, a prominent Golgi apparatus, and numerous secretory vesicles. Chief cells are the primary source of PTH, while oxyphil cells are thought to be a degenerative form of chief cells that secrete little hormone.

Biosynthesis and Secretion of Parathyroid Hormone

PTH is a protein hormone containing 84 amino acids, with only the first 34 of these required for biological activity. Species variability exists in the structure of PTH, but most of the differences are not in the biologically active portion of the molecule. Consequently, there is little species specificity in the biological activity of PTH. However, because of the structural differences, antibodies against PTH are usually formed if PTH from one species is injected into another.

PTH is synthesized in the rough endoplasmic reticulum of chief cells as a preprohormone, containing 115 amino acids. The first 25 amino acids are rapidly cleaved at the site of synthesis to yield proPTH, which is then transported to the Golgi apparatus. In the Golgi, the 6 amino acid "pro" fragment is removed and PTH is packaged into secretory vesicles. Because this conversion is quite efficient, secretory vesicles contain PTH but very little of the pro fragment or proPTH. Once packaged in vesicles, PTH can be either secreted or degraded, and these two processes are inversely regulated. Specifically, stimuli for PTH secretion decrease the rate of intracellular degradation while inhibitors of secretion increase degradation.

Like other protein hormones, PTH is secreted by **exocytosis** as described in Chapter 1. In the parathyroid glands, changes in **cyclic AMP** levels appear to be particularly important in controlling exocytosis. In addition to PTH, secretory granules contain a protein called **parathyroid secretory protein**. This protein is released with PTH, but its biological significance is unknown.

Actions of Parathyroid Hormone

The overall effect of PTH is to increase plasma (ECF) calcium concentration. It does this directly by increasing calcium efflux from bone and calcium reabsorption by kidney and indirectly by enhancing calcium absorption in the gastrointestinal tract. PTH also acts to lower plasma phosphate concentration.

All of the effects of PTH appear to be mediated by the classic second messenger, cyclic AMP.

Actions of PTH on Bone. PTH has two major effects on bone. The earliest effect is a stimulation of **calcium efflux** from bone into the ECF. This calcium comes from the small, labile calcium pool, moves across the osteocytic-osteoblastic bone membrane, and is not accompanied by phosphate. A later effect of PTH is to trigger bone **resorption** by stimulating the activity of osteoclasts and inhibiting osteoblastic activity. This effect requires synthesis of new enzymes, involves resorption of stable bone, and increases both calcium and phosphate release into the ECF. There is still considerable controversy about which of these effects is more important for the maintenance of plasma calcium concentrations. Most investigators, however, believe that movement of calcium across the bone membrane plays the primary role in calcium homeostasis, since changes in bone resorption occur too slowly to contribute to the minute-to-minute regulation of plasma calcium. In addition, prolonged treatment with PTH actually increases osteoblastic activity and bone formation; however, the physiological significance of this effect is unclear.

Actions of PTH on Kidney. PTH stimulates **calcium reabsorption** by the kidney, thereby increasing plasma calcium and decreasing urinary calcium levels. This effect of PTH occurs rapidly and is due to increased calcium transport in the distal tubule. PTH increases urinary **phosphate excretion** by decreasing phosphate reabsorption, primarily in the proximal tubule. As a result, PTH causes a fall in plasma phosphate levels at the same time it increases calcium concentrations. The third important action of PTH on the kidney involves the activation of vitamin D and will be considered later. In addition to these major actions, PTH has a number of other effects on renal function, including decreasing bicarbonate and water reabsorption. The significance of these effects remains obscure.

Actions of PTH on the Gastrointestinal Tract. Although PTH has no direct effects on calcium movement in the intestine, increases in PTH secretion indirectly increase calcium absorption approximately 24 hours later. This increase in calcium absorption is mediated by PTH-induced vitamin D activation, which is described later in this chapter.

Metabolism of Parathyroid Hormone

PTH is rapidly metabolized primarily in the liver and kidneys and has a half-life of 5 to 10 minutes. The first steps in its metabolism appear to be cleavage at two sites between amino acid residues 34 and 38. The N-terminal (biologically active) fragment is then rapidly degraded to inactive forms, but the C-terminal fragments are metabolized more slowly. Consequently, significant amounts of the latter are found in the peripheral circulation. These C-terminal fragments have no biological activity and hence are not physiologically important. They are, however, detected by many radioimmunoassays for

"PTH," so that the "PTH levels" measured with such assays are not necessarily indicative of biologically active PTH.

Control of Parathyroid Hormone Secretion

The primary regulator of PTH secretion is the free ionized **calcium** concentration in plasma. Increases in plasma calcium decrease PTH release; decreases in plasma calcium increase PTH secretion. Since the actions of PTH increase plasma calcium levels, this relationship forms part of a classical **negative feedback loop** (Fig. 16–3). The mechanism by which calcium inhibits PTH secretion is not completely understood, but most evidence indicates that it acts by lowering cyclic AMP concentrations within chief cells. Since cyclic AMP stimulates PTH release, a fall in intracellular cyclic AMP will inhibit secretion of this hormone. The parathyroids are exquisitely sensitive to small changes in plasma calcium. It is this sensitivity that is primarily responsible for the tight regulation of plasma calcium concentrations.

Although calcium is the principal regulator of PTH secretion, other factors can also influence PTH release. Magnesium, in high concentrations, inhibits PTH secretion, although it is a far less potent inhibitor than calcium. Epinephrine stimulates PTH secretion by activating β-adrenergic receptors. This action accounts for the hypercalcemia associated with pheochromocytoma, but its physiological importance remains to be established. Finally, there is a circadian rhythm in PTH secretion, with PTH concentrations highest in the early morning hours. This increase in PTH secretion is sleep-related and appears to occur independently of plasma calcium concentrations.

CALCITONIN

The major actions of calcitonin (CT) on mineral metabolism are to lower plasma calcium and phosphate concentrations. This hormone was discovered in the early 1960s, some 40 years after the importance of PTH and vitamin D in calcium and phosphate metabolism had been established. CT is produced by the **parafollicular** cells or **C cells**, within the **thyroid** gland. These cells are

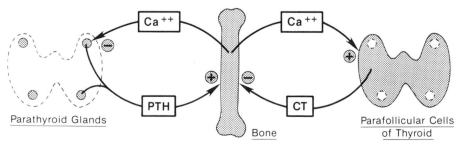

FIGURE 16–3. Negative feedback loops controlling PTH and CT secretion.

histologically and functionally distinct from the follicular cells that secrete thyroid hormones, and they are found scattered among the follicles.

Biosynthesis and Secretion of Calcitonin

Calcitonin is a 32 amino acid polypeptide with a proline-amide at the C-terminus and a ring structure at the N-terminus formed by a disulfide bridge between the first and seventh amino acids. There is considerable variability in the amino acid sequences of CT among species (up to 19 amino acids can differ) but all CTs have the 7 amino acid ring at one end and the proline-amide at the other. All 32 amino acids are required for significant biological activity, and there are considerable differences in the biological potencies of CTs from different species.

CT is synthesized as a preprohormone in the rough endoplasmic reticulum of the parafollicular cells, and the 25 amino acid "pre" segment is rapidly removed. CT is located in the middle of proCT so that two additional enzymatic cleavages are required to produce the final secretory product. This processing occurs in the Golgi apparatus but is not always complete at the time of packaging. Some proCT is found in the secretory vesicles.

Secretion of CT occurs by **exocytosis**, which results in the release of the entire contents of the secretory vesicles into the circulation. At a biochemical level, this process appears to be controlled by **intracellular calcium and by cyclic AMP**, both of which stimulate exocytosis. Since secretory vesicles contain CT and proCT, it is not surprising that both are found in plasma. In addition, some CT circulates as a dimer, which is apparently formed from the native hormone during its storage within the parafollicular cells. The larger circulating forms of CT are not physiologically important because they are biologically inactive. They are sometimes detected by radioimmunoassays for CT, and thus they may produce an overestimation of plasma CT concentrations.

Actions of Calcitonin

The hypocalcemic and hypophosphatemic effects of CT are due entirely to actions of this hormone on bone. Under some circumstances, CT can increase urinary excretion of calcium and phosphate, but these actions require pharmacological doses of CT. As described later, CT does have significant effects on gastrointestinal function, but these effects are not related to calcium or phosphate metabolism. All of the effects of CT appear to be mediated by cyclic AMP.

Actions of Calcitonin on Bone. Like PTH, CT has two effects on bone, but in this case, both effects decrease plasma calcium levels. Acutely, CT **decreases calcium efflux** across the osteoblast-osteocyte bone membrane. Chronically, CT **decreases bone resorption** by inhibiting the activity of osteoclasts. The suppression of bone resorption results in decreased release of calcium, phosphate, and hydroxyproline (one of the major constituents of the organic matrix of bone).

Although the mechanism by which CT lowers plasma phosphate concentration is not as well understood as its actions on calcium, it also appears to involve bone. The CT-induced decrease in bone resorption may account for part of this hypophosphatemic effect, but CT also increases the movement of phosphate from ECF into bone. The mechanism responsible for this increase in phosphate influx has not yet been determined.

Actions of Calcitonin on the Gastrointestinal Tract. CT inhibits a number of processes associated with digestion. The most prominent of these is gastric acid secretion. CT decreases the release of gastric acid directly, and it also does so indirectly by inhibiting gastrin secretion. Since gastrin stimulates CT secretion from the thyroids, a negative feedback loop may exist between the gastric mucosa and the parafollicular cells. CT has also been shown to decrease bile flow and the secretion of a number of pancreatic enzymes. The physiological significance of CT in the control of gastrointestinal function remains unclear.

Metabolism of Calcitonin

The removal of CT from the plasma appears to involve two exponential processes, one occurring with a half-life of about three minutes and the other with a half-life of 40 to 60 minutes. The kidneys are the primary site of metabolism, but significant metabolism also occurs in the liver. Although bone, thyroid, and plasma also degrade CT, they are of lesser importance than kidney and liver. The enzymes responsible for the metabolism of CT have not been identified.

Control of Calcitonin Secretion

The primary regulator of CT release is the free plasma calcium concentration. In contrast to its effects on PTH release, **calcium stimulates** CT secretion. Since CT decreases plasma calcium levels, this system forms a **negative feedback loop** analogous to that controlling PTH secretion (Fig. 16–3). These two negative feedback loops, however, operate in different ranges of plasma calcium concentrations. As illustrated in Figure 16–4, if calcium concentrations are below normal, CT release is totally inhibited while PTH secretion continues to respond to changes in calcium. Consequently, the PTH-calcium negative feedback loop is dominant during hypocalcemia. The opposite is true during hypercalcemia; PTH secretion stops while CT release continues. Thus, the CT-calcium negative feedback loop is more important during hypercalcemia.

Release of CT is also stimulated by a number of gastrointestinal hormones, including gastrin, cholecystokinin, secretin, and glucagon. Of these hormones, **gastrin** is the most potent and, as already discussed, may form part of a negative feedback loop with CT. There is also evidence that calcium ingestion stimulates gastrin release. The stimulation of CT by gastrin could thus

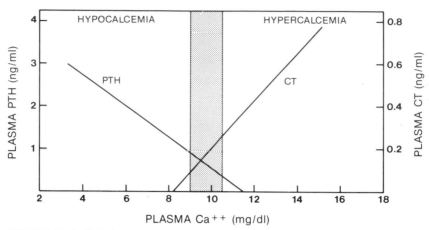

FIGURE 16–4. Relationship between serum concentrations of PTH, CT, and serum calcium levels. The shaded area depicts the normal range of serum calcium concentrations.

help protect against any possible hypercalcemia resulting from absorption of calcium after a meal.

VITAMIN D

Vitamin D, or **cholecalciferol**, is a steroid-like compound that is essential for calcium absorption in the gastrointestinal tract. Actually, vitamin D should be considered a hormone because it is usually synthesized by a tissue in the body and released into the blood. However, it was first discovered and isolated from a dietary source and is therefore traditionally considered a vitamin. Since vitamin D is a lipophilic substance it shares many characteristics with the steroid hormones, including its circulating forms and its mechanism of action.

Synthesis and Activation of Vitamin D

The immediate precursor to vitamin D is **7-dehydrocholesterol** (cholesterol with an additional double bond in the B-ring), which is synthesized from acetate and stored in the skin. Exposure of skin to ultraviolet light causes cleavage of the bond between the carbons at the C-9 and C-10 positions, giving rise to vitamin D (Fig. 16–5). For most individuals living in temperate or equatorial regions, the skin is an adequate source of vitamin D since over 75 per cent of the circulating vitamin D is probably derived from this source. However, if environmental conditions (e.g., winter months in higher latitudes or industrial pollution) or social customs preclude significant exposure of the skin to sunlight, vitamin D must be derived from dietary sources.

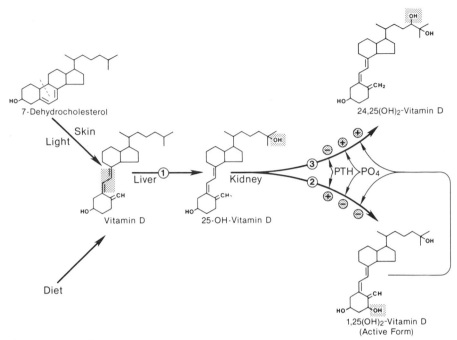

FIGURE 16–5. Synthesis and metabolism of vitamin D. The position of hydroxylation of 25-OH-vitamin D in the kidney is controlled by PTH, phosphate (PO₄), and 1,25-(OH)₂-vitamin D. Shading indicates structural change at each step; the dashed line indicates position of cleavage of 7-dehydrocholesterol to produce vitamin D. Enzymes: (1) 25-hydroxylase; (2) 1α-hydroxylase; (3) 24-hydroxylase.

Regardless of its source, vitamin D is biologically inert and must be activated by two sequential hydroxylations. The first of these reactions occurs in the **liver** and introduces a hydroxyl group at the C-25 position (Fig. 16–5). The product formed, **25-OH-vitamin D**, is the most abundant circulating form of vitamin D and serves as a substrate for the crucial second step in the activation of vitamin D. This step is hydroxylation at the C-1 position to produce **1,25-(OH)₂-vitamin D**, the active form of vitamin D. This reaction occurs only in the **kidney** and is under hormonal control. The kidney can also hydroxylate 25-OH-vitamin D at the C-24 position, but 24,25-(OH)₂-vitamin D has little or no biological activity.

Of the three tissues involved in the synthesis and metabolism of vitamin D, the kidney is the primary site of regulation. The activities of the two renal enzymes, 1-hydroxylase and 24-hydroxylase, are controlled by the same factors; however, they change in opposite directions (Fig. 16–5). The principal regulator of these enzymes is **PTH**, which stimulates 1-hydroxylase and inhibits 24-hydroxylase activities. When PTH levels increase, synthesis of the biologically active 1,25-(OH)₂-vitamin D is favored. Phosphate produces the opposite effect, increasing 24-hydroxylase activity and decreasing that of

1-hydroxylase. Thus, a decline in serum phosphate concentrations produces the same effect as an increase in PTH, although the magnitude of the phosphate-induced change is not as great. A third modulator of vitamin D metabolism is **1,25-(OH)$_2$-vitamin D** itself, which decreases 1-hydroxylase and increases 24-hydroxylase activity. These actions of 1,25-(OH)$_2$-vitamin D appear to result from changes in enzyme biosynthesis rather than allosteric end-product inhibition.

Transport of 1,25-(OH)$_2$-Vitamin D in Blood

As already mentioned, 1,25-(OH)$_2$-vitamin D can be considered a steroid-like hormone, and as are the steroids, it is transported in the circulation largely bound to plasma proteins. Most of this binding occurs to a specific α-globulin, known as **transcalciferin**. This protein also binds vitamin D and 25-OH-vitamin D; in fact, its highest affinity is for 25-OH-vitamin D. However, there is no competition among the various forms of vitamin D for binding, since normally less than 5 per cent of the available binding sites are occupied. Transcalciferin is synthesized in the liver, and its concentration increases moderately during pregnancy. As with other lipophilic hormones, only the free 1,25-(OH)$_2$-vitamin D is biologically active.

Actions of 1,25-(OH)$_2$-Vitamin D

Actions in the Gastrointestinal Tract. The most dramatic, and biologically important, effect of 1,25-(OH)$_2$-vitamin D is to **increase calcium absorption** in the intestine. A deficiency in vitamin D will substantially reduce calcium absorption, so that calcium must be mobilized from bone to maintain plasma calcium concentrations. Both passive diffusion and active transport of calcium are increased by 1,25-(OH)$_2$-vitamin D, although stimulation of the latter is probably more important. The active form of vitamin D also increases sodium-dependent **phosphate absorption** in the intestine, and this action appears to occur independently of the effects on calcium transport.

Studies of the mechanism of action of 1,25-(OH)$_2$-vitamin D have focused on the stimulation of calcium absorption in the intestine. In this tissue, 1,25-(OH)$_2$-vitamin D appears to act like other steroid hormones (Fig. 16–6). It diffuses into the cell and binds to a cytosolic receptor and the hormone-receptor complex then moves into the nucleus, where it activates specific genes leading to the synthesis of new proteins. These new proteins then increase calcium absorption by stimulating the rate-limiting step in this process, the influx of calcium from the intestinal lumen into the cell. The necessity for protein synthesis accounts for the long lag time (over two hours) required for the actions of 1,25-(OH)$_2$-vitamin D in the intestine as well as in other tissues. The nature of the vitamin D-induced proteins and how they stimulate calcium influx are unclear. A calcium-binding protein inducible by 1,25-(OH)$_2$-vitamin D has

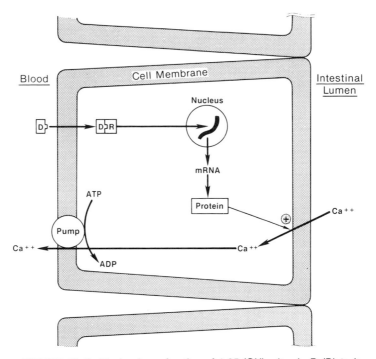

FIGURE 16–6. Mechanism of action of 1,25-(OH)₂-vitamin D (D) to increase calcium absorption in the intestine.

been identified and extensively studied. The amounts of this protein in the intestine correlate well with the rate of calcium absorption, but the exact function of this protein in calcium transport has not yet been determined.

Actions on Bone. The effects of 1,25-(OH)₂-vitamin D on bone are quite similar to those of PTH; it mobilizes bone calcium by stimulating **calcium efflux** from the labile calcium pool and by promoting **bone resorption**. Activated vitamin D also increases the **responsiveness of bone to PTH**. The latter action could account for the effects of 1,25-(OH)₂-vitamin D on calcium efflux from bone, since most *in vivo* studies indicate that PTH must be present for 1,25-(OH)₂-vitamin D to exert an effect on bone.

Other Actions of 1,25-(OH)₂-Vitamin D. Under some circumstances 1,25-(OH)₂-vitamin D will increase the reabsorption of phosphate and calcium by the kidney; the physiological significance of these effects is unclear. Both 1,25-(OH)₂-vitamin D and 24,25-(OH)₂-vitamin D can inhibit PTH secretion, but neither appears to be an important regulator of PTH. Activated vitamin D does have significant effects on muscle. Vitamin D deficiency produces myopathy, and administration of vitamin D restores muscle strength, independently of any effects on plasma calcium and phosphate levels.

Metabolism of 1,25-(OH)$_2$-Vitamin D

The half-life of 1,25-(OH)$_2$-vitamin D is approximately five hours; the pathways involved in its metabolism are unclear. Hydroxylation at the 24-carbon to form 1,24,25-(OH)$_3$-vitamin D appears to be one route of metabolism. Cleavage of the side chain between the C-24 and C-25 positions may be another. Metabolites of 1,25-(OH)$_2$-vitamin D are conjugated as glucuronides and excreted primarily in the bile, so that they appear in the feces.

Control of 1,25-(OH)$_2$-Vitamin D Production

Circulating levels of 1,25-(OH)$_2$-vitamin D vary with calcium and phosphate status. For example, if dietary calcium intake decreases, circulating 1,25-(OH)$_2$-vitamin D levels increase. As with the steroid hormones, the changes in plasma 1,25-(OH)$_2$-vitamin D concentrations result from changes in the rate of synthesis of this hormone. In the case of vitamin D, however, it is the last step in the pathway, the 1-hydroxylation of 25-OH-vitamin D, that is the important control point.

The control of 1,25-(OH)$_2$-vitamin D levels can be largely accounted for by the actions of PTH and phosphate on 1-hydroxylase activity described previously. Changes in calcium status alter 1,25-(OH)$_2$-vitamin D levels via PTH; hypocalcemia increases PTH concentrations, which in turn stimulates 1-hydroxylase activity. This is an appropriate response to hypocalcemia since the increase in 1,25-(OH)$_2$-vitamin D concentrations facilitates calcium absorption in the intestine and promotes calcium efflux from bone. Similarly, a fall in plasma phosphate levels stimulates synthesis of 1,25-(OH)$_2$-vitamin D, which in turn increases phosphate absorption from the intestine.

While PTH and phosphate are the primary regulators of 1,25-(OH)$_2$-vitamin D concentrations in normal adults, other hormones may be important under some circumstances. Plasma concentrations of 1,25-(OH)$_2$-vitamin D are elevated at times of increased calcium need, including periods of rapid growth, late pregnancy, and throughout lactation. These increases in activated vitamin D might be caused by transitory falls in plasma calcium concentrations. Alternatively, there is evidence that growth hormone and prolactin can increase 1-hydroxylase activity. It follows that these hormones could be responsible for the increases in plasma 1,25-(OH)$_2$-vitamin D levels associated with growth and lactation (or pregnancy), respectively.

OVERVIEW OF HORMONAL REGULATION OF CALCIUM AND PHOSPHATE METABOLISM

Although three hormones can affect calcium and phosphate metabolism, they are not of equal physiological importance. Most evidence suggests that

CT plays little or no role in the normal control of calcium and phosphate metabolism. Although CT will protect against hypercalcemia, this condition rarely occurs under normal circumstances. Moreover, neither thyroidectomy nor CT-secreting tumors alter circulating levels of calcium or phosphate. CT may, however, be important in protecting skeletal integrity when there is a large calcium demand on an individual, such as during pregnancy or lactation. PTH and vitamin D do play critical roles in calcium and phosphate metabolism. However, the relative importance of each depends on the nature of the control system: homeostasis or balance.

Control of Calcium Homeostasis

PTH is the principal hormone responsible for calcium homeostasis, the minute-to-minute regulation of plasma calcium concentration. Vitamin D may play a secondary role, but in general, the actions of vitamin D are too sluggish for it to contribute significantly to calcium homeostasis. Perturbations in plasma calcium concentrations are usually corrected within one to two hours and are thus alleviated before an increase in 1,25-$(OH)_2$-vitamin D can stimulate calcium movement into the ECF.

The basic mechanisms controlling calcium homeostasis are illustrated in Figure 16–7 using the response to hypocalcemia as an example. The drop in free plasma calcium concentrations stimulates release of PTH, which then acts on kidney and bone to increase calcium reabsorption and efflux, respectively. Both of these effects increase calcium movement into the ECF within minutes, thus correcting the original deficit. Although the relative importance of kidney and bone in the control of calcium homeostasis remains controversial, bone appears to play the major role. The increase in PTH also stimulates synthesis of 1,25-$(OH)_2$-vitamin D, which promotes both calcium absorption in the intestine and further calcium efflux from bone (Fig. 16–7). However, as already noted, changes in 1,25-$(OH)_2$-vitamin D production normally play only a minor role in calcium homeostasis, because of the time required for any effects to be manifested.

Control of Calcium Balance

Both PTH and 1,25-$(OH)_2$-vitamin D are essential to calcium balance, the process that ensures that calcium intake is equivalent to calcium excretion. Since this process functions over long periods of time (weeks and months), the relative sluggishness of the vitamin D system does not prevent it from contributing to the maintenance of calcium balance. The roles of PTH and vitamin D in calcium balance are illustrated in Figure 16–7. If, for example, there is a decrease in dietary calcium intake, a transient fall in plasma calcium occurs, which stimulates PTH secretion. The rise in PTH concentrations has two effects important for maintenance of calcium balance: it stimulates calcium reab-

CALCIUM HOMEOSTASIS:

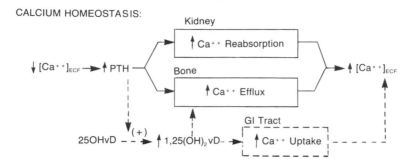

CALCIUM BALANCE:

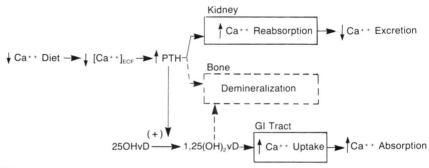

FIGURE 16–7. Mechanisms controlling calcium homeostasis and calcium balance. Processes indicated by dashed lines are not important under physiological conditions but can occur during pathological situations. (vD = vitamin D.)

sorption by the kidney and it increases circulating 1,25-$(OH)_2$-vitamin D levels, which in turn promote calcium absorption by the intestine. These two effects act to correct the deficit in calcium intake by decreasing calcium excretion and increasing the efficiency of calcium absorption, respectively. Note that the increase in PTH levels also promotes bone resorption. Consequently, although bone is not directly involved in regulating calcium balance, this tissue is markedly affected by abnormalities in this process. If calcium excretion exceeds calcium intake for a prolonged period, there is sufficient loss of bone calcium and phosphate to produce pathologic changes in the skeleton.

Control of Phosphate Metabolism

Plasma phosphate concentrations are not as tightly controlled as plasma calcium. For example, the compensatory response to a change in circulating phosphate usually occurs over a number of days. Consequently, the temporal distinctions between phosphate homeostasis and phosphate balance are relatively minor; in fact, the same hormonal mechanisms are responsible for both. A key element in the control of phosphate metabolism is the inverse relationship between the concentrations of calcium and phosphate in the ECF. This inverse relationship occurs because the ions in ECF are in equilibrium with hydroxyapatite crystals in bone. For example, an increase in ECF phosphate promotes hydroxyapatite formation and thus lowers ECF calcium concentrations; conversely, a fall in ECF phosphate increases ECF calcium concentrations.

The overall control of phosphate metabolism is illustrated in Figure 16–8, using the response to a fall in phosphate as an example. Hypophosphatemia has two effects that help to return circulating phosphate concentrations to normal. As just described, it causes an increase in plasma calcium concentrations, which suppresses PTH secretion. The fall in PTH in turn stimulates phosphate reabsorption in the kidney. In addition, since phosphate inhibits 1-hydroxylation of 25-(OH)-vitamin D, hypophosphatemia stimulates the production of 1,25-(OH)$_2$-vitamin D, which then increases phosphate absorption in the intestine. These changes in renal and intestinal function increase ECF phosphate levels, thus alleviating the initial condition. Note that since phosphate intake and excretion are being altered, the same processes (when they are initiated in response to a dietary phosphate deficiency) will produce phosphate balance. It is important to realize that calcium balance is not compromised by these changes. The increase in 1,25-(OH)$_2$-vitamin D stimulates calcium absorption, but the fall in PTH produces a compensatory increase in calcium excretion.

DISORDERS OF CALCIUM AND PHOSPHATE METABOLISM

Abnormalities in all three endocrine systems involved in calcium and phosphate metabolism may occur. However, disorders of calcitonin secretion are extremely rare and cause no obvious abnormalities in the handling of calcium and phosphate.

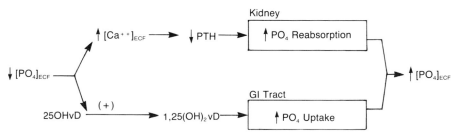

FIGURE 16–8. Mechanisms controlling phosphate metabolism. Note that because PO$_4$ inhibits 1-hydroxylase, a decrease in PO$_4$ stimulates this enzyme. (vD = vitamin D)

Hyperparathyroidism

Excess secretion of PTH is classified as **primary** or **secondary** hyperparathyroidism. The former is caused by a primary defect in the parathyroid glands, which causes excess PTH release. In the latter, the excess PTH secretion is secondary to a defect in calcium metabolism that lowers plasma calcium concentrations.

Primary Hyperparathyroidism. Excess secretion of PTH occurs in about 0.1 per cent of the population. It can be produced by chief cell hyperplasia (affecting all parathyroid glands), by adenomas (limited to one parathyroid gland), or rarely (3 to 4 per cent of the time) by carcinomas. The abnormalities in calcium metabolism produced by primary hyperparathyroidism depend to some extent on the duration of the disease. Acutely, the excess PTH decreases urinary calcium levels by increasing calcium reabsorption and produces hypercalcemia as a result of actions on bone and kidney (Table 16–2). With chronic hyperparathyroidism, both urinary and serum calcium levels are elevated. Under these circumstances, the increase in urinary calcium excretion is secondary to the hypercalcemia; the amount of calcium filtered by the kidney is sufficient to saturate the reabsorption of this ion so that excess calcium appears in the urine.

The symptoms of primary hyperparathyroidism are largely due to the increased calcium levels in plasma and urine and can vary from asymptomatic to severe. The excess urinary calcium often causes polyuria and nephrolithiasis (kidney stones). The hypercalcemia can cause gastrointestinal disorders (peptic ulcers, nausea, and constipation), muscle weakness, and neurological disorders including decreased mentation, poor memory, and depression. Severe bone demineralization can usually be avoided by early detection and treatment, although some evidence of skeletal abnormalities, such as bone pain and frequent fractures, is not uncommon. Surgical removal of the tissue producing the excess PTH will alleviate these symptoms.

Secondary Hyperparathyroidism. In this condition, the excess PTH represents a normal response to hypocalcemia. Thus, secondary hyperparathyroidism can readily be distinguished from primary hyperparathyroidism by

TABLE 16–2. Changes in Serum and Urinary Calcium Concentrations and Serum PTH Levels in Hyperparathyroidism

Condition	Calcium		PTH
	Serum	Urine	
Primary hyperparathyroidism			
Acute	I	D	I
Chronic	I	I	I
Secondary hyperparathyroidism	D	D	I

I = Increased; D = Decreased.

measurement of serum calcium concentrations (Table 16–2). The hypocalcemia responsible for this disease can result from any of a number of conditions. Abnormalities in vitamin D intake or metabolism are a common cause of hypocalcemia and will be considered later. **Renal failure** also causes hypocalcemia and secondary hyperparathyroidism due to renal retention of phosphate. The hyperphosphatemia produces a chronic reduction in ECF calcium. **Insensitivity of target tissues** to PTH can also cause hypocalcemia and hyperparathyroidism; this condition is known as pseudohypoparathyroidism because the clinical manifestations are similar to hypoparathyroidism, even though PTH levels are elevated.

Regardless of the cause, the hypocalcemia of secondary hyperparathyroidism increases neuromuscular excitability and can produce muscle cramps or seizures. Mental changes can include irritability, paranoia, and depression. Abnormal calcification in neural tissues and in the lens of the eye (causing cataracts) can occur with prolonged hypocalcemia. Bone demineralization occurs in some types of secondary hypoparathyroidism (e.g., vitamin D deficiencies) but not in others (e.g., pseudohypoparathyroidism).

Hypoparathyroidism

Hypoparathyroidism can have primary and secondary causes. Hypercalcemia caused by excess bone resorption will result in secondary hypoparathyroidism, but the low PTH is unimportant relative to the other effects of hypercalcemia. Consequently, secondary hypoparathyroidism is not considered to be a significant clinical syndrome.

Primary hypoparathyroidism can be either idiopathic or iatrogenic in origin. In the latter, parathyroid tissue may be removed as a treatment for hyperparathyroidism or inadvertently removed during thyroidectomy. The resulting decrease in PTH secretion causes hypocalcemia, which is responsible for the clinical manifestations of this disease. Most of these symptoms are the same as those in secondary hyperparathyroidism because the basic deficit (hypocalcemia) is the same in both cases. The bone demineralization seen with some forms of secondary hyperparathyroidism is not found in hypoparathyroidism. Hypoparathyroidism is usually treated with dietary calcium supplements and vitamin D (or $1,25\text{-}(OH)_2$-vitamin D). Both treatments promote calcium absorption, and the $1,25\text{-}(OH)_2$-vitamin D also increases the ability of whatever PTH is secreted to promote calcium efflux from bone.

Vitamin D Deficiencies

Any condition that produces a prolonged deficit in $1,25\text{-}(OH)_2$-vitamin D production will compromise absorption of calcium by the intestines and thus disrupt calcium balance. The major clinical manifestations of this dysfunction occur in the bone and are the result of demineralization. These symptoms include bone pain, skeletal deformities, and pathological fractures. Serum calcium levels are slightly below normal but do not decline greatly unless extensive depletion of bone calcium occurs. The mild hypocalcemia produces prolonged secondary hyperparathyroidism, which lowers plasma phosphate by increasing phosphate excretion. If this condition occurs in growing children it is called **rickets**; if in adults, it is usually called **osteomalacia**. In osteomalacia, demineralization is limited to mature bone. In rickets it also occurs at the growing epiphyseal plates, so that the skeletal abnormalities produced by vitamin D deficiency are more severe in children.

A decrease in $1,25$-$(OH)_2$-vitamin D levels can result from a defect at any step in the synthesis of this hormone, but the most common cause is inadequate amounts of vitamin D. This deficiency results from the combination of inadequate exposure to sunlight and insufficient dietary vitamin D and can be remedied by alleviating either of these deficiencies. Because of dietary supplements, vitamin D deficiency is now rare in the United States but is still a significant worldwide health problem. **Liver diseases** (e.g., cirrhosis) can produce a $1,25$-$(OH)_2$-vitamin D deficiency by decreasing formation of 25-OH-vitamin D. A similar problem is sometimes caused by the use of anticonvulsant drugs (e.g., diphenylhydantoin), which increase the activities of liver enzymes that convert vitamin D and 25-OH-vitamin D to inactive metabolites. Finally, decreased 1-hydroxylase activity is sometimes associated with **renal dysfunction**. The resulting low concentrations of $1,25$-$(OH)_2$-vitamin D contribute to the development of calcium abnormalities in such patients.

Vitamin D Excess

The only known cause of abnormally elevated concentrations of $1,25$-$(OH)_2$-vitamin D is ingestion of extremely large doses of vitamin D. This may cause acute vitamin D toxicity, which produces hypercalcemia. The signs and symptoms are similar to those associated with primary hyperparathyroidism, except that bone demineralization does not occur. However, soft tissue calcification can lead to serious complications if vital organs are affected.

REFERENCES

Aurbach, G.D., Marx, S.J., and Spiegel, A.M.: Parathyroid hormones, calcitonin, and the calciferols. In Williams' Textbook of Endocrinology, 7th ed. J.D. Wilson and D.W. Foster, editors. W.B. Saunders Company, Philadelphia, p. 1137, 1985.

Bonner, F. and Coburn, J.W.: Disorders of Mineral Metabolism, Vol II: Calcium Physiology. Academic Press, New York, 1982.

DeLuca, H.F.: The vitamin D hormonal system: Implications for bone diseases. Hospital Practice 15(4):57, 1980.

Parson, J.A.: Endocrinology of Calcium Metabolism. Raven Press, New York, 1982.

Potts, J.T., Jr.: Disorders of bone and bone mineral metabolism: Relation to parathyroid hormone, calcitonin, and vitamin D. In Endocrinology, Vol. 2. L.J. DeGroot, editor. Grune and Stratton, New York, p. 551, 1979.

INDEX

Page numbers in *italics* indicate illustrations. Page numbers followed by t indicate tables.